Workbook for Textbook of Diagnostic Ultrasonography

sixth edition

Sandra L. Hagen-Ansert, MS, RDMS, RDCS
Cardiology Department
Scripps Clinic—Torrey Pines
San Diego, California
Former Office Manager and Clinical Cardiac Sonographer
University Cardiology Associates, Medical University of South Carolina

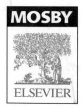
MOSBY

ELSEVIER

MOSBY
ELSEVIER

11830 Westline Industrial Drive
St. Louis, Missouri 63146

WORKBOOK FOR TEXTBOOK OF DIAGNOSTIC
ULTRASONOGRAPHY, SIXTH EDITION

ISBN 13: 978-0-323-04202-4
ISBN 10: 0-323-04202-3

Notice

Knowledge and best practice in this field are constantly changing. As new research and experience broaden our knowledge, changes in practice, treatment, and drug therapy may become necessary or appropriate. Readers are advised to check the most current information provided (i) on procedures featured or (ii) by the manufacturer of each product to be administered, to verify the recommended dose or formula, the method and duration of administration, and contraindications. It is the responsibility of the practitioner, relying on their own experience and knowledge of the patient, to make diagnoses, to determine dosages and the best treatment for each individual patient, and to take all appropriate safety precautions. To the fullest extent of the law, neither the Publisher nor the Author assumes any liability for any injury and/or damage to persons or property arising out of or related to any use of the material contained in this book.

The Publisher

ISBN 13: 978-0-323-04202-4
ISBN 10: 0-323-04202-3

Executive Editor: Jeanne Wilke
Senior Developmental Editor: Linda Woodard
Associate Developmental Editor: Christina Pryor
Publishing Services Manager: Pat Joiner
Project Manager: Gena Magouirk
Design Direction: Andrea Lutes

Printed in USA.

Last digit is the print number: 9 8 7 6 5 4 3 2

Working together to grow
libraries in developing countries

www.elsevier.com | www.bookaid.org | www.sabre.org

ELSEVIER   BOOK AID International   Sabre Foundation

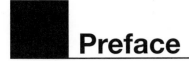

Preface

This workbook was developed to accompany Mosby's *Textbook of Diagnostic Ultrasonography, Sixth Edition.* The chapters in this workbook correlate with those of the primary textbook. The material may serve as a useful review of the respective chapters or for preparation for the national board examinations in diagnostic sonography.

The exercises found in this workbook are designed to provide the reader with a thorough review of terminology, anatomy, physiology, laboratory values, sonographic anatomy and technique, and pathology.

To use this workbook most effectively, the reader should first study the appropriate chapters from *Textbook of Diagnostic Ultrasonography, Sixth Edition.* Each chapter is organized into key term recognition, short answers, and fill-in-the-blank statements. A comprehensive review examination is found at the end of the workbook. Case analysis is provided to give the student an opportunity to analyze clinical symptoms by providing a sonographic interpretation of representative images. All of the answers are found at the back of the workbook.

Sandra L. Hagen-Ansert
MS, RDMS, RDCS

Contents

1 Foundations of Sonography

KEY TERMS

Exercise 1
Match the following basic ultrasound terms with their definitions.

1. _____ acoustic impedance

2. _____ angle of incidence

3. _____ attenuation

4. _____ axial resolution

5. _____ compression

6. _____ crystal

7. _____ decibel (dB)

8. _____ focal zone

9. _____ Fresnel zone

10. _____ frequency

11. _____ intensity

12. _____ interface

13. _____ lateral resolution

14. _____ megahertz (MHz)

15. _____ piezoelectric effect

16. _____ power

17. _____ refraction

18. _____ resolution

19. _____ spatial pulse length

20. _____ transducer

21. _____ wave

A. Change in the direction of propagation of a sound wave transmitted across an interface where the speed of sound varies

B. Angle at which the sound beam strikes the interface

C. Power per unit area

D. Special material in the transducer that has the ability to convert electric impulses into sound waves

E. Propagation of energy that moves back and forth or vibrates at a steady rate

F. The minimum distance between two objects where they still can be displayed as separate objects

G. Any device that converts energy from one form to another

H. Number of cycles per second that a periodic event or function undergoes

I. Measure of a material's resistance to the propagation of sound; expressed as the product of acoustic velocity of the medium and the density of the medium

J. Generation of electric signals as a result of an incident sound beam on a material that has piezoelectric properties

K. The region over which the effective width of the sound beam is within some measure of its width at the focal distance

L. Reduction in the amplitude and intensity of a sound wave as it propagates through a medium

M. Passive force in opposition to another active force; occurs when tissue exerts pressure against the flow

N. Surface forming the boundary between media having different properties

O. Region of increased particle density

P. The product of a number of cycles in the pulse and wavelength of the pulse

Q. Refers to the minimum distance between two structures positioned along the axis of the beam where both structures can be visualized as separate objects

R. Distance over which a wave repeats itself during one period of oscillation

S. Ability of the transducer to distinguish between two structures adjacent to one another

T. Rate of energy flow over the entire beam of sound

22. _____ wavelength

23. _____ resistance

U. Unit used to quantitatively express the ratio of two amplitudes or intensities

V. 1,000,000 Hz

W. The field closest to the transducer during the formation of the sound beam

Exercise 2

Match the following ultrasound terms with their definitions.

1. _____ angle of reflection

2. _____ bulk modulus

3. _____ cycle

4. _____ Fraunhofer zone

5. _____ hertz (Hz)

6. _____ kilohertz (kHz)

7. _____ period

8. _____ pulse duration

9. _____ rarefaction

10. _____ slice thickness

11. _____ velocity

A. The time interval required for generating the transmitted pulse

B. A sequence of events occurring at regular intervals

C. Amount of pressure required to compress a small volume of material a small amount

D. In ultrasound the tissue density determines the speed of the ultrasound wave

E. Unit for frequency, equal to 1 cycle per second

F. Region of decreased particle density

G. Angle of incidence at which the sound beam strikes the interface

H. 1000 Hz

I. The field farthest from the transducer during the formation of the sound beam

J. Thickness of the section in the patient that contributes to echo signals on any one image

K. Duration of a single cycle of a periodic wave of event

Exercise 3

Match the following instrumentation terms with their definitions.

1. _____ aliasing

2. _____ amplitude

3. _____ continuous wave (CW) Doppler

4. _____ Doppler angle

5. _____ Doppler shift

6. _____ dynamic range

7. _____ frame rate

8. _____ gain

9. _____ gray scale

10. _____ laminar

A. Sound is transmitted and received intermittently with one transducer

B. Ability to compensate for attenuation of the transmittal beam as the sound wave travels through tissue in the body

C. Change in frequency of a reflected wave; caused by motion between the reflector and the transducer's beam

D. One transducer continuously transmits sound, and one continuously receives sound; used in high-velocity flow patterns

E. Normal pattern of vessel flow; flow in the center of the vessel is faster than it is at the edges

F. Rate at which images are updated on the display; dependent on frequency of the transducer and depth selection

G. Analysis of the entire frequency spectrum

H. Technical artifact occurring when the frequency change is so large that it exceeds the sampling view and pulse repetition frequency

11. _____ Nyquist sampling limit

12. _____ pulse repetition frequency (PRF)

13. _____ pulsed wave (PW) Doppler

14. _____ real time

15. _____ spectral analysis

16. _____ spectral broadening

17. _____ temporal resolution

18. _____ time gain compensation (TGC)

19. _____ gate

I. In pulse-echo instruments, it is the number of pulses launched per second by the transducer

J. Ability of the system to accurately depict motion

K. Ratio of the largest to smallest signals that an instrument or component of an instrument can respond to without distortion

L. In pulsed Doppler, the Doppler signal must be sampled at least twice for each cycle in the wave if the Doppler frequencies are to be detected accurately

M. Strength of the ultrasound wave measured in decibels

N. Measure of the strength of the ultrasound signal

O. Echo fill-in of the spectral window that is proportional to the severity of the stenosis

P. Ultrasound instrumentation that allows the image to be displayed many times per second to achieve a "real-time" image of anatomic structures and their motion patterns

Q. B-mode scanning technique that permits the brightness of the B-mode dots to be displayed in various shades of gray to represent different echo amplitudes

R. The angle that the reflector path makes with the ultrasound beam; the most accurate velocity is recorded when the beam is parallel to flow

S. The sample site from which the signal is obtained with pulsed Doppler

HISTORY OF ACOUSTICS

Exercise 4

Fill in the blank(s) with the word(s) that best completes the statements or provide a short answer about the history of acoustics.

1. Acoustics is the study of science, engineering, and the art of _____, and _____ sound waves.

2. Ultrasound is defined as sound frequencies beyond the upper limits of human hearing, i.e., greater than

   _____.

3. Name three pioneers who made a significant contribution to ultrasound.

   _____

   _____

4. The terms _____, _____, _____, and _____ have been used to describe an imaging technique used to visualize soft tissue structures of the body by recording the returning reflection of ultrasonic waves directed into the body.

5. The term that applies to the ultrasound evaluation of the cardiac structures is _____.

6. One who performs ultrasound studies and gathers diagnostic data under the direct or indirect supervision of a

   physician is a _____.

7. List the qualities of a sonographer.

_____

_____

_____

MEDICAL TERMS FOR THE SONOGRAPHER

Exercise 5

Match the following medical terms with their definitions.

1. _____ anechoic or sonolucent

2. _____ echogenic or hyperechoic

3. _____ enhancement, increased through transmission

4. _____ fluid level

5. _____ heterogeneous

6. _____ homogeneous

7. _____ hypoechoic

8. _____ infiltrating

9. _____ irregular borders

10. _____ isoechoic

11. _____ loculated mass

12. _____ shadowing

A. Not uniform in texture or composition

B. Usually refers to a diffuse disease process or metastatic disease

C. Echo-producing structure; reflects sound with a brighter intensity

D. Interface between two fluids with different acoustic characteristics. This level will change with patient position.

E. Very close to the normal parenchymal echogenicity pattern

F. Sound that travels through an anechoic (fluid-filled) substance and is not attenuated. There is increased brightness directly beyond the posterior border of the anechoic structure as compared with the surrounding area.

G. Completely uniform in texture or composition

H. Borders are not well defined, are ill defined, or are not present.

I. Low-level echoes within a structure

J. The sound beam is attenuated by a solid or calcified object.

K. Well-defined borders with internal echoes; the septa may be thin (likely benign) or thick (likely malignant).

L. Without internal echoes; the structure is fluid filled and transmits sound easily.

Exercise 6

Provide a short answer that best completes the statements about ultrasound evaluation.

1. Regarding the criteria for identifying abnormalities, identify the three textures for the border of a structure.

_____

_____

_____

2. Regarding the criteria for identifying abnormalities, identify the texture of a structure.

_____

_____

_____

3. Regarding the criteria for identifying abnormalities, identify the three terms that describe the transmission of sound.

_____

_____

_____

4. Identify the sonographic and medical terms that describe the characteristics of an organ or mass.

_____

_____

_____

5. Define the characteristics of a cystic mass.

_____

_____

_____

6. Define the characteristics of a solid mass.

_____

_____

_____

7. Define the characteristics of a complex mass.

_____

_____

_____

INSTRUMENTATION

Exercise 7

Fill in the blank(s) with the word(s) that best completes the statements or provide a short answer about ultrasound instrumentation.

1. As the ceramic element vibrates, it periodically presses against and pulls away from the adjacent medium with

   resultant particle _____ and _____ in the medium.

2. A transducer converts _____ energy into _____ energy.

3. A propagation of energy that moves back and forth or vibrates at a steady rate is a _____.

4. The time required to produce each cycle depends on the _____ of the transducer.

5. Ultrasound is a form of nonionizing radiation in which _____ pressure waves of high frequency are transmitted through a medium.

6. The distance between two peaks over a period of time is the _____.

7. The wavelength is inversely related to frequency, which means that the higher the frequency, the

   _____ the wavelength.

8. As frequencies become higher, the pulse duration _____, yielding a decrease in the depth of field.

9. The rate at which energy is transmitted is referred to as the _____.

10. Power per unit area is defined as _____.

11. If you double the power, the intensity also _____.

12. The piezoelectric effect was first described by the _____ brothers in 1880.

13. Lung and bowel have a detrimental effect on the ultrasound beam, causing _____ transmission of sound.

14. Bone conducts sound at a _____ speed than soft tissue.

15. Normal transmission of sound through soft tissue travels at _____ m/sec.

16. The acoustic impedance is the product of the _____ in a medium and the density of that medium.

17. Reflections most frequently received are those that occurred at a(n) _____ incidence. *The angle of*

   reflection is equal to the _____.

18. The sum of acoustic energy losses resulting from absorption, scattering, and reflection is the _____.

19. The minimum reflector separation along the sound path required to produce separate echoes is the

_____ resolution.

20. The _____ resolution is the ability to produce separate echoes perpendicular to the sound path and is

affected by transducer diameter and focusing.

21. Lateral resolution is determined by _____.

22. The _____ resolution of an ultrasound system refers to the minimum distance between two objects
where they can be displayed as separate structures.

23. Identify the criteria that determine the type of transducer selected for a particular examination.

_____

_____

_____

_____

24. The number of pulses launched per second is the _____.

25. If the gain is set too_____, artifactual echo noise will be displayed throughout the image.

26. A one-dimensional image displaying the amplitude strength of the returning echo signals along the vertical axis

and the time (distance) along the horizontal axis is produced by _____.

27. The intensity (amplitude) of an echo by varying the brightness of a dot to correspond to echo strength is displayed

by the _____ method.

28. The condition of assigning each level of amplitude a particular shade of gray is referred to as the _____.

29. The _____displays time along the horizontal axis and depth along the vertical axis to depict movement, especially in cardiac structures.

30. A dynamic presentation of multiple image frames per second over selected areas of the body is provided by

_____ imaging.

31. With pulsed Doppler, for accurate detection of Doppler frequencies to occur, the Doppler signal must be sampled

at least _____ for each cycle in the wave.

32. When the Nyquist limit is exceeded, an artifact called _____ occurs.

EQUIPMENT ARTIFACTS

Exercise 8

Provide a short answer that best completes the statements about equipment artifacts.

1. List the four types of equipment artifacts.

_____

_____

_____

_____

2. List the two types of technique artifacts.

_____

_____

_____

3. List the moving artifact.

_____

_____

_____

_____

4. List the sound-tissue artifacts.

_____

_____

_____

_____

Introduction to Physical Findings, Physiology, and Laboratory Data of the Abdomen

2

KEY TERMS

Exercise 1

Match the following terms related to symptoms and systems with their definitions.

1. _E_ auscultation
2. _I_ dysuria
3. _G_ epigastric
4. _A_ hematochezia
5. _K_ hypertension
6. _F_ hypotension
7. _D_ sphygmomanometer
8. _J_ suprapubic
9. _L_ tachycardia
10. _B_ tympany
11. _H_ umbilical
12. _C_ urinary incontinence

A. Passage of bloody stools
B. Preponderant sound heard over hollow organs
C. The uncontrollable passage of urine
D. Device used to measure blood pressure
E. Procedure of listening to the heart sounds with a stethoscope
F. Low blood pressure
G. Above the umbilicus and between the costal margins
H. Around the navel
I. Painful or difficult urination
J. Above the symphysis pubis
K. Blood pressure greater than 130/70 mm Hg
L. Heart rate more than 100 beats/min

Exercise 2

Match the following physiology terms with their definitions.

1. _F_ acidic
2. _U_ alkaline
3. _D_ anemia
4. _L_ bile
5. _H_ buffer
6. _N_ erythrocytes
7. _B_ erythropoiesis
8. _C_ hematocrit

A. Overproduction of red blood cells
B. Production of red blood cells
C. Special hepatic cells that remove bile pigment, old blood cells, and the byproducts of phagocytosis from the blood and deposit them into the bile ducts
D. Abnormal condition where blood lacks either a normal number of red blood cells or normal concentration of hemoglobin
E. Protein in red blood cells that picks up oxygen and releases it in the capillaries of tissue
F. A type of solution that contains more hydrogen ions than hydroxyl ions
G. Platelets in blood

9. __E__ hemoglobin

10. __C__ Kupffer cells

11. __M__ leukopoiesis

12. __I__ leukocytes

13. __A__ polycythemia

14. __G__ thrombocytes

H. Chemical compound that can act as a weak acid or a base to combine with excess hydrogen or hydroxyl ions to neutralize the pH in blood

I. White blood cells

J. A type of solution that contains more hydroxyl ions than hydrogen ions

K. The percent of the total blood volume containing the red blood cells, white blood cells, and the platelets

L. Bile pigment, old blood cells, and the byproducts of phagocytosis together

M. White blood cell formation stimulated by the presence of bacteria

N. Red blood cells

THE HEALTH HISTORY AND SYMPTOMS EXPLORATION

Exercise 3

Fill in the blank(s) with the word(s) that best completes the statements or provide a short answer about the health history and symptoms of the gastrointestinal, genitourinary, and urinary systems.

1. A red swollen leg in a patient experiencing leg pain is a(n) __objective__ finding.

2. List four important steps in the patient interview process.

_____

_____

3. Normal body temperature ranges from __96.7__ to __100.5__ degrees.

4. The patient's __pulse__ reflects the amount of blood ejected with each heartbeat.

5. A normal pulse for an adult is between __60__ and __100__ beats/min.

6. A respiratory rate of __16__ to __20__ breaths/minute is normal for an adult.

7. The __systolic__ reading reflects the maximum pressure exerted on the arterial wall at the peak of the left ventricular contraction.

8. The minimum pressure exerted on the arterial wall during left ventricular relaxation is the __diastolic__ reading.

9. List five factors that should be evaluated when inspecting the abdomen.

__Symm, shape + contour, umb mid + inv, skin smooth + unif in color, dilated veins, surgical scars__

10. The most significant signs and symptoms related to the GI system are:

__abd'l pain, diar, n + v, hematochezia__

11. Kidney dysfunction can cause trouble with _____conc._____, _____mem loss_____, or _____disorientation_____

12. Two common signs and symptoms related to urinary dysfunction are _____dysur_____ and _____urin. incont_____

LABORATORY TESTS

Exercise 4
Match the following laboratory tests with their definitions.

1. __B__ bilirubin

2. __E__ cholesterol

3. __G__ glucose

4. __D__ alkaline phosphatase

5. __A__ aspartate aminotransferase

6. __F__ alanine aminotransferase

7. __I__ prothrombin time

8. __C__ urinary bile and bilirubin

9. __H__ urinary urobilinogen

A. This enzyme is increased in the presence of liver cell necrosis secondary to viral hepatitis, toxic hepatitis, and other acute forms.

B. This is derived from the breakdown of hemoglobin in red blood cells and is excreted by the liver in the bile.

C. There may be spillover into the blood in obstructive liver disease or where there is an excess of red blood cell destruction.

D. This is found in the serum and the value rises in disorders of the liver and biliary tract when excretion is impaired (i.e., obstruction).

E. This is found in the blood and in all cells. Hepatic disease may alter its metabolism.

F. This enzyme rises higher than AST in cases of hepatitis. It falls slowly and reaches normal levels in 2 to 3 months.

G. Chronic liver disease and severe diabetes will cause an increase in this level.

H. This test may be used to differentiate between complete and incomplete obstruction of the biliary tract.

I. This is converted to thrombin in the clotting process and this is made possible by the action of vitamin K that is absorbed in the intestine and stored in the liver.

3 Anatomic and Physiologic Relationships within the Abdominal Cavity

KEY TERMS

Exercise 1

Match the following terms with their definitions.

1. ___F___ homeostasis

2. ___C___ intertubercular plane

3. ___A___ metabolism

4. ___E___ subcostal plane

5. ___D___ transpyloric plane

6. ___B___ vital signs

A. Physical and chemical changes that occur within the body

B. Medical measurements to ascertain how the body is functioning

C. Lowest horizontal line joins the tubercles on the iliac crests

D. Horizontal plane that passes through the pylorus, the duodenal junction, the neck of the pancreas, and the hilum of the kidneys

E. Upper horizontal line joins the lowest point of the costal margin on each side of the body

F. Maintenance of normal body physiology

Exercise 2

Match the following abdominal and pelvic cavity terms with their definitions.

1. ___J___ diaphragm

2. ___D___ inguinal ligament

3. ___K___ lateral arcuate ligament

4. ___A___ left crus of the diaphragm

5. ___G___ linea alba

6. ___C___ linea semilunaris

7. ___B___ medial arcuate ligament

8. ___H___ median arcuate ligament

9. ___N___ pelvic cavity

10. ___E___ rectouterine space

11. ___P___ rectus abdominis muscle

12. ___F___ right crus of the diaphragm

13. ___L___ scrotal cavity

A. Arises from the sides of the bodies of the first two lumbar vertebrae

B. Thickened upper margin of the fascia covering the anterior surface of the psoas muscle

C. Extends from the ninth costal cartilage to the pubic tubercle

D. Ligament between the anterior superior iliac spine and the pubic tubercle

E. Posterior pouch between the uterus and rectum

F. Arises from the sides of the bodies of the first three lumbar vertebrae

G. Fibrous band of tissue that stretches from the xiphoid to the symphysis pubis

H. Connects the medial borders of the two crura as they cross anterior to the aorta

I. Anterior pouch between the uterus and bladder

J. Broad muscle that separates the thoracic and abdominopelvic cavities and forms the floor of the thoracic cavity

K. Thickened upper margin of the fascia covering the anterior surface of the quadratus lumborum muscle

L. In the male, a small outpocket of the pelvic cavity containing the testes

M. Triangular opening in the external oblique aponeurosis

14. __M__ superficial inguinal ring

15. __I__ uterovesical space

16. __O__ viscera

N. Lower portion of the abdominopelvic cavity that contains part of the large intestine, the rectum, urinary bladder, and reproductive organs

O. The internal organs

P. Muscle of the anterior abdominal wall

Exercise 3

Match the following abdominal cavity terms with their definitions.

1. __B__ anterior pararenal space

2. __G__ ascites

3. __L__ epiploic foramen

4. __A__ falciform ligament

5. __E__ gastrosplenic ligament

6. __M__ greater omentum

7. __D__ greater sac

8. __H__ lesser omentum

9. __R__ lesser sac

10. __J__ lienorenal ligament

11. __S__ ligamentum teres

12. __C__ mesothelium

13. __N__ Morison's pouch

14. __I__ parietal peritoneum

15. __F__ perirenal space

16. __P__ peritoneal cavity

17. __O__ peritoneal recess

18. __K__ posterior pararenal space

19. __Q__ visceral peritoneum

A. Attaches the liver to the anterior abdominal wall and undersurface of the diaphragm

B. Located between the anterior surface of the renal fascia and the posterior area of the peritoneum

C. Single layer of cells that forms the peritoneum

D. Primary compartment of the peritoneal cavity; extends across the anterior abdomen from the diaphragm to the pelvis

E. Ligaments between the stomach and the spleen; helps support the stomach and spleen

F. Located directly around the kidney; completely enclosed by renal fascia

G. Accumulation of fluid

H. Attaches to the lesser curvature of the stomach

I. Layer of the peritoneum that lines the abdominal wall

J. Ligament between the spleen and kidney

K. Found between the posterior renal fascia and the muscles of the posterior abdominal wall

L. Opening to the lesser sac

M. Attaches to the greater curvature of the stomach

N. Right posterior subphrenic space lies between the right lobe of the liver, anterior to the kidney

O. Slitlike spaces near the liver; potential space for fluid to accumulate

P. Potential space between the parietal and visceral peritoneal layers

Q. Layer of peritoneum that covers the abdominal organs

R. Peritoneal pouch located behind the lesser omentum and stomach

S. Termination of the falciform ligament seen in the left lobe of the liver

BODY SYSTEMS

Exercise 4

Complete the following table by identifying the body system and its functions.

System	Components	Functions
1.	Skeletal, cardiac, smooth muscle	
2.	Pituitary, adrenal, thyroid, pancreas, parathyroid, ovaries, testes, pineal, and thymus gland	
3.	Heart, blood vessels, blood; lymph and lymph structures	
4.	Mouth, tongue, teeth, salivary glands, pharynx, esophagus, stomach, liver, gallbladder, pancreas, and small and large intestines	
5.	Kidney, bladder, ureters	
6.	Testes, scrotum, spermatic cord, vas deferens, ejaculatory duct, penis, epididymis, prostate, uterus, ovaries, fallopian tubes, vagina, breast	

ANATOMIC DIRECTIONS

Exercise 5

Fill in the blank(s) with the word(s) that best completes the statements about the anatomic directions.

1. The front (belly) surface of the body is _____.

2. When a structure is closer to the body midline or point of attachment to the trunk, it is described

   as _____.

3. The top of the head is the most _____ point of the body.

4. Structures located toward the surface of the body are _____.

5. The back surface of the body is _____.

6. The sphincter of Oddi is _____ to the common bile duct.

7. The bottom of the feet is the _____ point of the body.

8. Structures located farther inward (away from the body surface) are _____.

9. The hepatic artery is _____ to the common duct.

10. Towards the head is _____.

11. The structure is _____ if it is towards the side of the body.

12. Towards the tail, or_____, is sometimes used instead of inferior.

Exercise 6

Match the following anatomic terms with their region.

1. _____ thoracic

2. _____ popliteal

3. _____ perineal

4. _____ pelvic

5. _____ mammary

6. _____ lumbar

7. _____ leg

8. _____ groin and/or inguinal

9. _____ femoral

10. _____ costal

11. _____ cervical

12. _____ celiac

13. _____ brachial

14. _____ axillary

15. _____ abdominal

A. Loin; the region of the lower back and side, between the lowest rib and the pelvis

B. Pelvis; the bony ring that girdles the lower portion of the trunk

C. Thigh; the part of the lower extremity between the hip and the knee

D. Area behind the knee

E. Abdomen

F. Depressed region between the abdomen and the thigh

G. Breasts

H. Neck region

I. Lower extremity, especially from the knee to the foot

J. Ribs

K. Area of armpit

L. Region between the anus and the pubic arch; includes the region of the external reproductive structures

M. Arm

N. Portion of trunk below the diaphragm

O. Chest; the part of the trunk below the neck and above the diaphragm

Exercise 7

Fill in the blank(s) with the word(s) that best completes the statements about the body cavity or anatomic structure.

1. The two principal body cavities are the _____ and the_____.

2. The bony dorsal cavity may be subdivided into the_____, which holds the brain, and the *vertebral* or *spinal canal,* which contains the spinal cord.

3. The _____ is located near the anterior body surface and is subdivided into the _____ and

   the_____.

4. The thoracic and abdominopelvic cavities are separated by a broad muscle, the _____, which forms the floor of the thoracic cavity.

5. Divisions of the thoracic cavity are the_____, each containing a lung, with the mediastinum between them.

6. The heart is surrounded by another cavity called the_____.

Exercise 8

Fill in the blank(s) with the word(s) that best completes the statements about the abdominal cavity.

1. The abdominal cavity is bounded superiorly by the _____; anteriorly by the _____ muscles; posteriorly by the vertebral column, ribs, and iliac fossa; and inferiorly by the _____.

2. The liver lies posterior to the lower ribs with the majority of the right lobe in the right _____ and_____; the left lobe lies in the _____ and _____.

3. The _____kidney lies slightly lower than the left.

4. The aorta lies _____to the spine, slightly to the _____of the midline in the abdomen.

5. The inferior vena cava lies to the _____of the spine.

6. The dome-shaped muscle that separates the thorax from the abdominal cavity is the _____.

7. The _____ crus of the diaphragm arises from the sides of the bodies of the first three lumbar vertebrae.

8. The medial borders of the two crura as they cross anterior to the aorta are connected by the _____.

9. The fibrous band that stretches from the xiphoid to the symphysis pubis is the _____.

10. A sheath formed by the aponeuroses of the muscles of the lateral group is the _____ muscle.

11. Part of the abdominal cavity proper and lying between the iliac fossae, superior to the pelvic brim, is the

    _____.

12. The _____ contains the pelvic cavity and is found inferior to the brim of the pelvis.

13. Identify the organs contained within the pelvic cavity.

    _____

    _____

    _____

14. The peritoneum passes from the bladder to the uterus to form the _____ pouch.

15. Between the uterus and the rectum the peritoneum forms the deep _____ pouch.

16. The _____ tubes extend laterally from the fundus of the uterus and are enveloped by a fold of peritoneum known as the broad ligament.

17. A muscular "sling" composed of the _____ and _____ muscles forms the inferior boundary of the true pelvis and separates it from the perineum.

18. The muscles that lie along the posterior and lateral margins of the pelvis major are the _____ and

    _____.

19. The _____ muscles form the posterior pelvic wall.

20. The _____ peritoneum is the portion that lines the abdominal wall, but does not cover a viscus; the

    _____ peritoneum is the portion that covers an organ.

21. The _____ omentum is attached to the greater curvature of the stomach and hangs down like an apron
    in the space between the small intestine and anterior abdominal wall.

22. An extensive peritoneal pouch located behind the lesser omentum and stomach is the _____ sac.

23. The opening to the lesser sac in the abdomen is the _____ .

24. The peritoneal ligaments are two-layered folds of _____ that attach the lesser mobile solid viscera to the
    abdominal walls.

25. The liver is attached by the _____ ligament to the anterior abdominal wall and to the undersurface
    of the diaphragm.

26. The _____ lies in the free borders of this ligament.

27. The visceral peritoneum covers the spleen and is reflected onto the greater curvature of the stomach as the anterior

    layer of the _____ ligament.

Exercise 9
Fill in the blank(s) with the word(s) that best completes the statements about the potential spaces in the body.

1. The right and left anterior _____ spaces lie between the diaphragm and the liver, one on each side of
   the falciform ligament.

2. The right posterior subphrenic space that lies between the right lobe of the liver, the right kidney, and the right colic

   flexure is also called _____ .

3. The omental bursa normally has some empty places known as _____ .

4. The _____ lateral paracolic gutter communicates with the right posterior subphrenic space.

5. The protrusion of part of the abdominal contents beyond the normal confines of the abdominal wall is a

   _____ .

Exercise 10
Fill in the blank(s) with the word(s) that best completes the statements or provide a short answer about the
retroperitoneum.

1. The retroperitoneal cavity contains these anatomic structures:

   _____

   _____

   _____

2. The _____ is located between the anterior surface of the renal fascia (Gerota's fascia) and the posterior area of the peritoneum.

3. The _____ is found between the posterior renal fascia and the muscles of the posterior abdominal wall.

4. The _____ space is located directly around the kidney and is completely enclosed by renal fascia.

Exercise 11

Fill in the blank(s) with the word(s) that best completes the statements or provide a short answer.

1. There are many forms of anatomy and physiology: _____ studies the body by dissection of tissue,

   _____ studies parts of the tissue under the microscope, _____ studies the development

   before birth, and _____ is the study of the disease process.

2. Within the human body, the next most complex basic unit of structure and function is a microscopic part

   called a _____ .

3. Cells are organized into layers or masses that have common functions known as a _____ .

4. The four primary types of tissues in the body are _____ , _____ , _____ , and

   _____ tissues.

5. Groups of different tissues combine together to form _____ -complex structures with specialized functions, such as the liver, pancreas, or uterus.

6. A coordinated group of organs are arranged into organ or _____ .

7. All of the physical and chemical changes that occur within the body are referred to as _____ .

8. These vital signs include measuring _____ and _____ and observing rates and types

   of _____ and _____ movements.

Exercise 12

Label the following illustrations.

1.   Anterior and lateral view of the body.

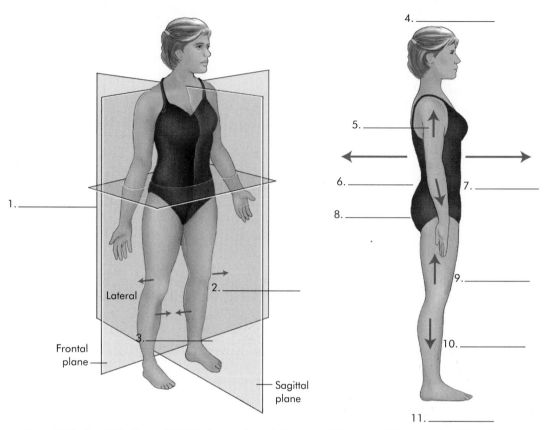

1. _____

Lateral

Frontal
plane

Sagittal
plane

2. _____

3. _____

4. _____

5. _____

6. _____

7. _____

8. _____

9. _____

10. _____

11. _____

From Thibodeau GA, Patton KT: *The human body in health and disease,* ed 5, St. Louis, 2005, Mosby.

2.   Surface landmarks of the anterior abdominal wall.

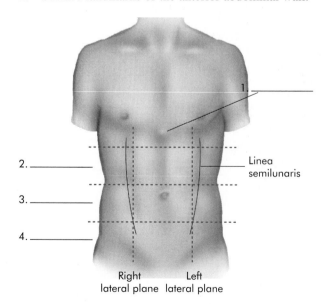

1. _____

2. _____

3. _____

4. _____

Linea
semilunaris

Right
lateral plane

Left
lateral plane

3.   Regions of the abdominal wall.

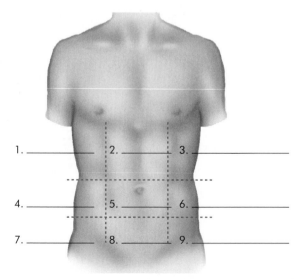

1. _____   2. _____   3. _____

4. _____   5. _____   6. _____

7. _____   8. _____   9. _____

4. Body cavities.

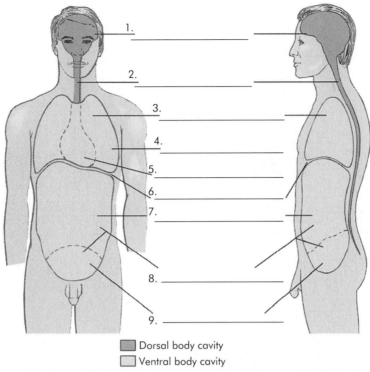

1. _____

2. _____

3. _____

4. _____

5. _____

6. _____

7. _____

8. _____

9. _____

■ Dorsal body cavity
□ Ventral body cavity

From Thibodeau GA, Patton KT: *The human body in health and disease,* ed 5, St. Louis, 2005, Mosby.

5. Inferior view of the diaphragm.

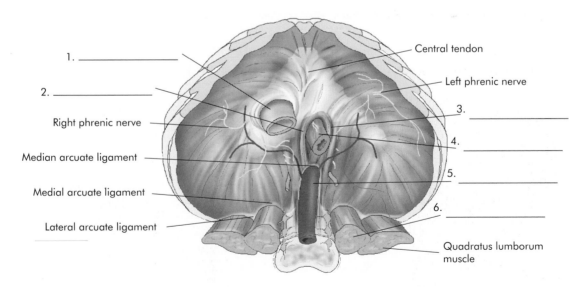

1. _____

2. _____

Right phrenic nerve

Median arcuate ligament

Medial arcuate ligament

Lateral arcuate ligament

Central tendon

Left phrenic nerve

3. _____

4. _____

5. _____

6. _____

Quadratus lumborum muscle

6. Lateral midsagittal view of the female pelvis.

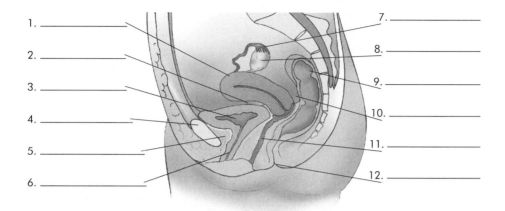

1. _____
2. _____
3. _____
4. _____
5. _____
6. _____

7. _____
8. _____
9. _____
10. _____
11. _____
12. _____

7. Lateral and inferior views of the pelvis.

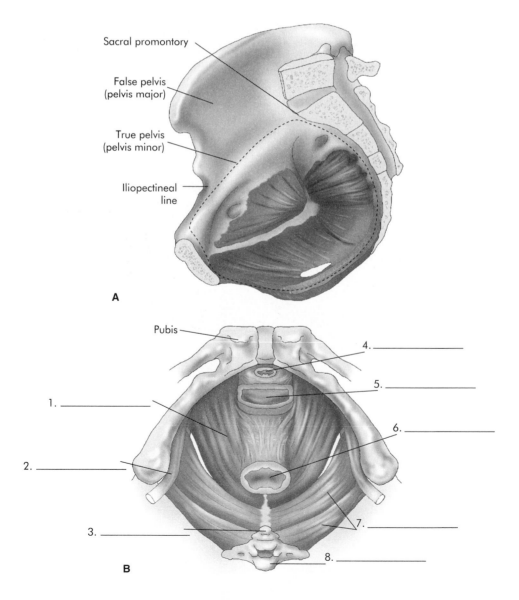

Sacral promontory

False pelvis
(pelvis major)

True pelvis
(pelvis minor)

Iliopectineal
line

A

Pubis

4. _____
5. _____
6. _____

1. _____

2. _____

7. _____

3. _____

8. _____

B

8. Lateral view of the peritoneum.

1. _____
21. _____
20. _____
19. _____
18. _____
17. _____
16. _____
15. _____
14. _____
13. _____
12. _____
11. _____
10. _____

2. _____
3. _____
4. _____
5. _____
6. _____
7. _____
8. _____
9. _____

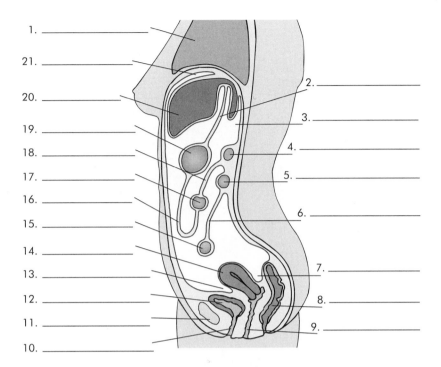

9. Axial view of the peritoneum.

8. _____
7. _____
6. _____
5. _____

1. _____
2. _____
3. _____
4. _____

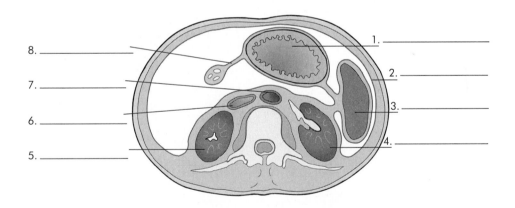

10. Upper abdominal dissection.

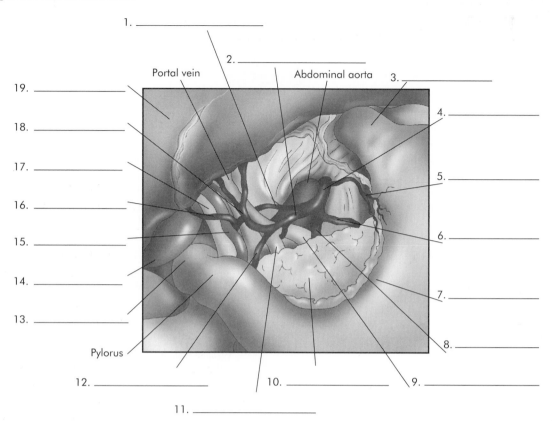

1. _____

2. _____

Portal vein   Abdominal aorta   3. _____

19. _____   4. _____

18. _____

17. _____   5. _____

16. _____

15. _____   6. _____

14. _____   7. _____

13. _____   8. _____

Pylorus

12. _____   10. _____   9. _____

11. _____

11. Transverse view of the falciform ligament.

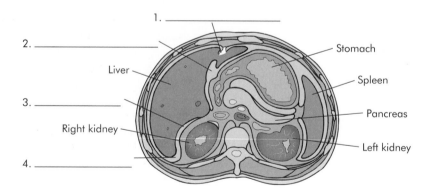

1. _____

2. _____   Stomach

Liver   Spleen

3. _____   Pancreas

Right kidney   Left kidney

4. _____

KEY TERMS

Exercise 1

Match the following arterial terms with their definitions.

1. _____ aorta

2. _____ celiac axis

3. _____ common femoral arteries

4. _____ gastroduodenal artery

5. _____ hepatic artery

6. _____ iliac arteries

7. _____ inferior mesenteric artery

8. _____ left gastric artery

9. _____ left renal artery

10. _____ right renal artery

11. _____ splenic artery

12. _____ superior mesenteric artery

A. Common hepatic artery arises from the celiac trunk and courses to the right of the abdomen and branches into the GDA and proper HA

B. Arises from the posterolateral wall of the aorta directly into the hilus of the kidney

C. Vessels originating from the iliac arteries and seen in the inguinal region into the upper thigh

D. Leaves the posterolateral wall of the aorta; travels posterior to the inferior vena cava to enter the hilum of the kidney

E. First major anterior artery to arise from the abdominal aorta inferior to the diaphragm; it branches into the hepatic, splenic, and left gastric arteries

F. Arises from the anterior aortic wall at the level of the third or fourth lumbar vertebra to supply the left transverse colon, descending colon, sigmoid colon, and rectum

G. Arises from the celiac trunk to supply the spleen

H. Branch of the common hepatic artery to supply the stomach and duodenum

I. Largest arterial structure in the body; arises from the extremities, and abdominopelvic cavity

J. Originate from the bifurcation of the aorta at the level of the umbilicus

K. Arises inferior to the celiac axis from the anterior wall of the abdominal aorta; travels parallel to the aorta to supply the small bowel, cecum, ascending colon, and transverse colon; lies posterior to the body of the pancreas

L. Small branch of the celiac axis that feeds the stomach

Exercise 2

Match the following venous terms with their definitions.

1. _____ confluence of the splenic and portal veins

2. _____ femoral veins

3. _____ hepatic veins

4. _____ iliac veins

5. _____ inferior vena cava

6. _____ left portal vein

7. _____ left renal vein

8. _____ portal venous system

9. _____ right renal vein

10. _____ splenic vein

11. _____ superior mesenteric vein

A. Upper part of the venous drainage system of the lower extremity found in the upper thigh and groin

B. Principal venous vessel that returns blood from the lower half of the body from the confluence of the right and left common iliac veins; flows posterior to the liver to enter the right atrium of the heart

C. Drains the small bowel and cecum and transverse and sigmoid colon; travels vertically to join the splenic and portal veins; serves as a posterior landmark to the body of the pancreas and anterior border to the uncinate process of the head

D. Leaves the renal hilum and travels anterior to the aorta, posterior to the superior mesenteric artery to empty into the lateral wall of the inferior vena cava

E. Junction of the splenic and portal veins that occurs in the midabdomen and serves as a posterior border of the pancreas

F. Supplies the left lobe of the liver

G. Leaves the renal hilum to flow directly into the IVC

H. Largest tributaries that drain the liver and empty into the inferior vena cava at the level of the diaphragm

I. Comprises the splenic, inferior mesenteric, superior mesenteric, and portal veins

J. Receive tributaries from the lower extremities and drain into the inferior vena cava

K. Drains blood from the spleen and part of the stomach; forms the posteromedial border of the pancreas as it travels horizontally across the abdomen; joins the superior mesenteric vein to form the main portal vein

Exercise 3

Match the following ligaments and other structures with their definitions.

1. _____ caudate lobe

2. _____ collateral vessels

3. _____ crus of the diaphragm

4. _____ dome of liver

5. _____ falciform ligament

6. _____ ligamentum teres

7. _____ ligamentum venosum

8. _____ main portal vein

9. _____ Morison's pouch

A. Termination of the falciform ligament, seen in the left lobe of the liver

B. Where the triad of the portal vein, common bile duct, and hepatic artery enter the liver

C. Muscular structures seen in the upper abdomen at the level of the celiac axis; aligns the vertebral column before crossing the midline posterior to the inferior vena cava and anterior to the aorta

D. Attaches the liver to the anterior abdominal wall and undersurface of the diaphragm

E. Group of muscles that originate at the hilum of the kidneys and lie lateral to the spine

F. Echogenic linear structure found anterior to the caudate lobe and posterior to the left lobe of the liver

G. Central area of the spleen that allows the vascular and lymph structure to emerge or enter

10. _____ porta hepatis

11. _____ psoas major muscle

12. _____ right portal vein

13. _____ splenic hilum

H. Smallest lobe of the liver; lies posterior to the left lobe and anterior to the inferior vena cava; superior border is the ligamentum venosum

I. Formed by the union of the splenic vein and superior mesenteric vein; serves as the posterior border of the pancreas

J. Supplies the right lobe of the liver

K. Most superior aspect of the liver at the level of the diaphragm

L. Small peritoneal recess located anterior to the right kidney and inferior to the liver

M. Ancillary vessels that develop when portal hypertension occurs

Exercise 4

Fill in the blank(s) with the word(s) that best completes the statements about abdominal scanning.

1. All transverse supine scans are oriented with the liver on the _____ of the screen.

2. Longitudinal scans present the patient's head to the _____ and feet to the _____ of the screen and use the xiphoid, umbilicus, or symphysis to denote the midline of the scan plane.

3. The position of the patient should be described in relation to the _____.

4. Variations in the patient's respiration may also help eliminate _____ interference and improve image quality.

5. Patients should be instructed not to eat or drink anything for _____ hours before the abdominal ultrasound procedure.

6. Identify the structures that are included in a survey of the baseline upper abdominal ultrasound examination.

   _____

   _____

   _____

7. In Doppler imaging, flow towards the transducer is positive, or _____, whereas flow away from the transducer is negative, or _____.

8. Arterial flow pulsates with the cardiac cycle and shows its maximal peak during the _____ part of the cycle.

9. A phasic pattern may be seen in the _____ (near the heart) that is associated with overload of the right ventricle.

EXERCISE 5

Label the following illustrations.
1. Various standard patient positions for the ultrasound examination.

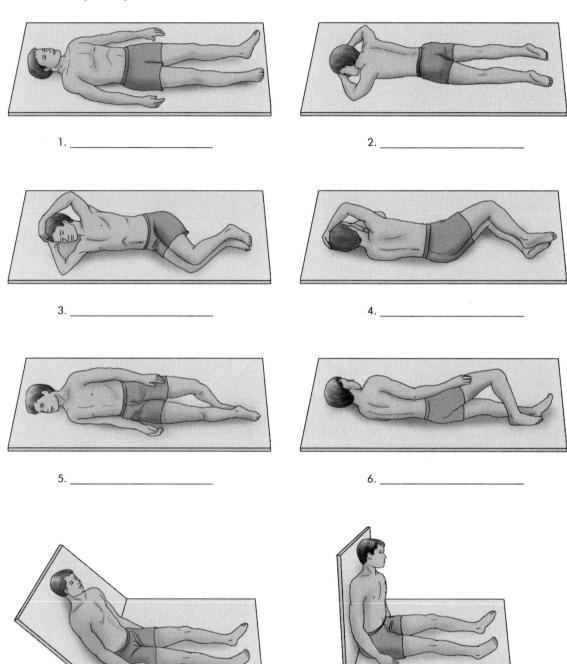

1. _____

2. _____

3. _____

4. _____

5. _____

6. _____

7. _____

8. _____

2. Cross section of the abdomen at the level of the tenth intervertebral disk.

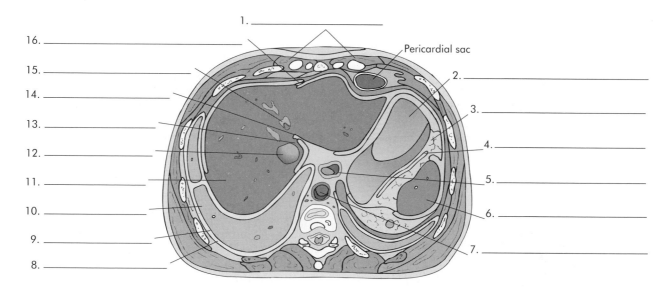

1. _____

16. _____

Pericardial sac

15. _____

2. _____

14. _____

3. _____

13. _____

4. _____

12. _____

5. _____

11. _____

6. _____

10. _____

7. _____

9. _____

8. _____

3. Cross section of the abdomen at the level of the eleventh thoracic disk.

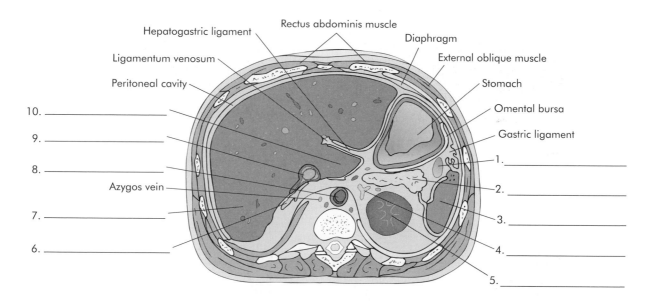

Hepatogastric ligament   Rectus abdominis muscle

Ligamentum venosum   Diaphragm

Peritoneal cavity   External oblique muscle

10. _____   Stomach

9. _____   Omental bursa

8. _____   Gastric ligament

Azygos vein   1. _____

7. _____   2. _____

6. _____   3. _____

4. _____

5. _____

4. Cross section of the abdomen at the level of the twelfth thoracic vertebra.

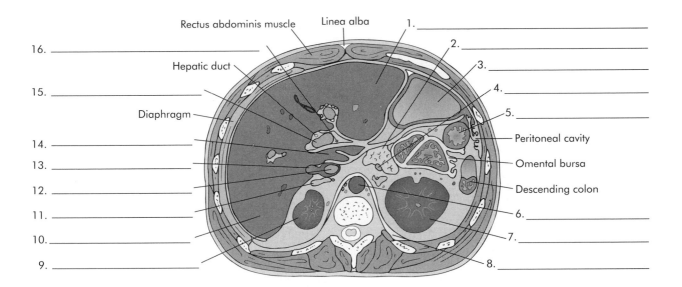

Rectus abdominis muscle   Linea alba   1. _____

16. _____   2. _____

Hepatic duct   3. _____

15. _____   4. _____

Diaphragm   5. _____

14. _____   — Peritoneal cavity

13. _____   — Omental bursa

12. _____   — Descending colon

11. _____   6. _____

10. _____   7. _____

9. _____   8. _____

5. Cross section of the abdomen at the first lumbar vertebra.

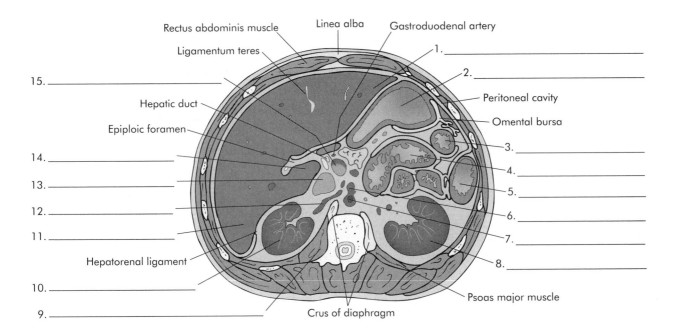

Rectus abdominis muscle   Linea alba   Gastroduodenal artery

Ligamentum teres   1. _____

15. _____   2. _____

Hepatic duct   — Peritoneal cavity

Epiploic foramen   — Omental bursa

14. _____   3. _____

13. _____   4. _____

12. _____   5. _____

11. _____   6. _____

Hepatorenal ligament   7. _____

10. _____   8. _____

9. _____   Psoas major muscle

Crus of diaphragm

6. Cross section of the abdomen at the level of the second lumbar vertebra.

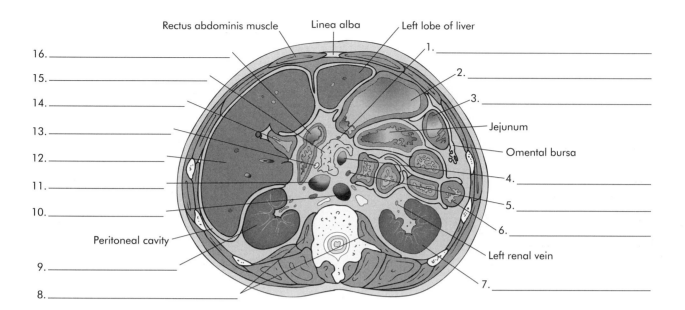

Rectus abdominis muscle   Linea alba   Left lobe of liver

16. _____

15. _____

14. _____

13. _____

12. _____

11. _____

10. _____

Peritoneal cavity

9. _____

8. _____

1. _____

2. _____

3. _____

Jejunum

Omental bursa

4. _____

5. _____

6. _____

Left renal vein

7. _____

7. Cross section of the abdomen at the level of the third lumbar vertebra.

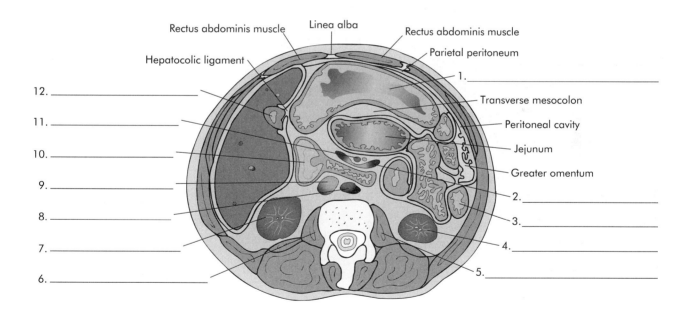

Rectus abdominis muscle   Linea alba   Rectus abdominis muscle

Hepatocolic ligament   Parietal peritoneum

12. _____

11. _____

10. _____

9. _____

8. _____

7. _____

6. _____

1. _____

Transverse mesocolon

Peritoneal cavity

Jejunum

Greater omentum

2. _____

3. _____

4. _____

5. _____

8. Cross section of the abdomen at the level of the third lumbar disk.

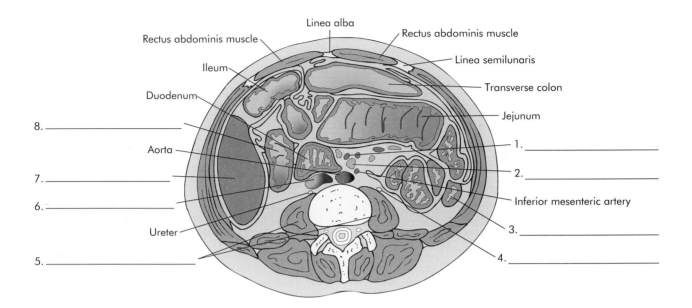

Linea alba

Rectus abdominis muscle

Ileum

Duodenum

8. _____

Aorta

7. _____

6. _____

Ureter

5. _____

Rectus abdominis muscle

Linea semilunaris

Transverse colon

Jejunum

1. _____

2. _____

Inferior mesenteric artery

3. _____

4. _____

9. Cross section of the pelvis taken at the lower margin of the fifth lumbar vertebra and disk.

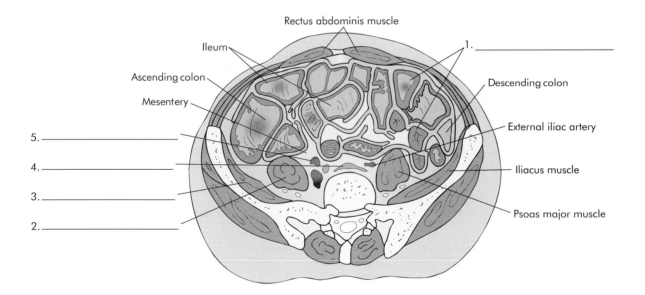

Rectus abdominis muscle

Ileum

Ascending colon

Mesentery

5. _____

4. _____

3. _____

2. _____

1. _____

Descending colon

External iliac artery

Iliacus muscle

Psoas major muscle

10. Cross section of the female pelvis just below the junction of the sacrum and coccyx.

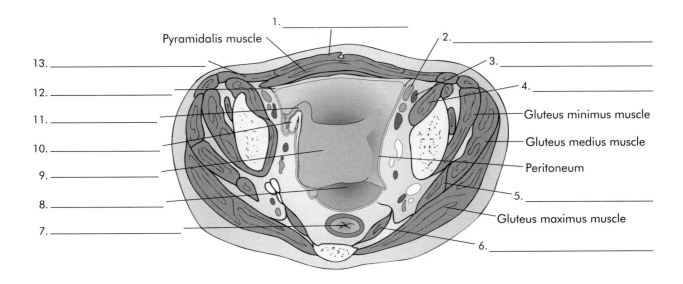

Pyramidalis muscle
1. _____
2. _____
3. _____
4. _____
13. _____
12. _____
11. _____
Gluteus minimus muscle
Gluteus medius muscle
10. _____
Peritoneum
9. _____
5. _____
8. _____
Gluteus maximus muscle
7. _____
6. _____

11. Cross section of the female pelvis taken through the lower part of the coccyx and the spine of the ischium.

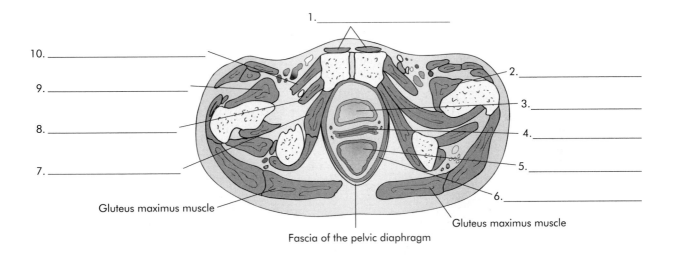

1. _____
10. _____
2. _____
9. _____
3. _____
8. _____
4. _____
5. _____
7. _____
6. _____
Gluteus maximus muscle
Gluteus maximus muscle
Fascia of the pelvic diaphragm

12. Sagittal section of the abdomen taken along the right abdominal border.

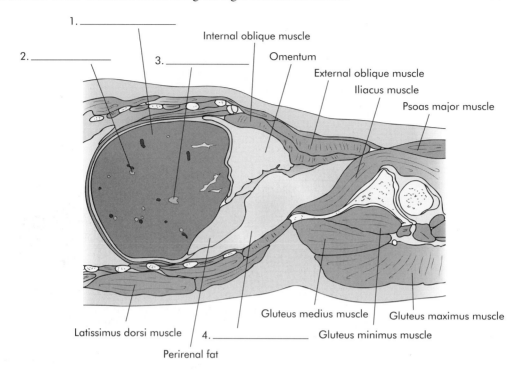

1. _____

2. _____

3. _____

Internal oblique muscle

Omentum

External oblique muscle

Iliacus muscle

Psoas major muscle

Latissimus dorsi muscle

4. _____

Perirenal fat

Gluteus medius muscle

Gluteus minimus muscle

Gluteus maximus muscle

13. Sagittal section of the abdomen 8 cm from the midline.

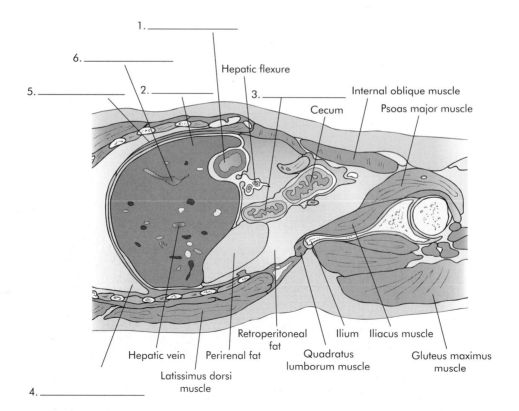

1. _____

6. _____

5. _____

2. _____

Hepatic flexure

3. _____

Cecum

Internal oblique muscle

Psoas major muscle

Hepatic vein

Perirenal fat

Retroperitoneal fat

Quadratus lumborum muscle

Ilium

Iliacus muscle

Gluteus maximus muscle

Latissimus dorsi muscle

4. _____

14. Sagittal section of the abdomen 7 cm from the midline.

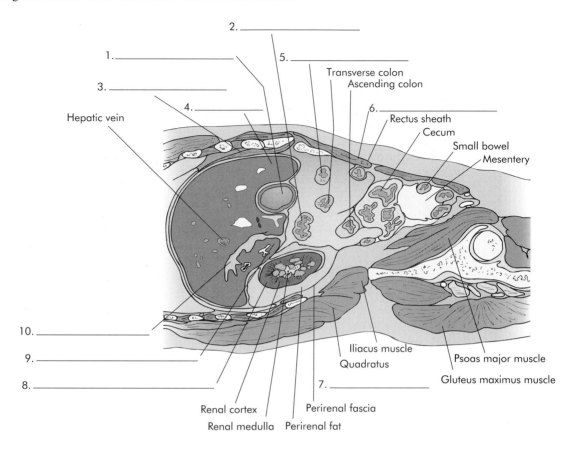

2. _____
1. _____
5. _____
3. _____
Transverse colon
Ascending colon
4. _____
6. _____
Rectus sheath
Cecum
Hepatic vein
Small bowel
Mesentery
10. _____
9. _____
Iliacus muscle
Psoas major muscle
Quadratus
Gluteus maximus muscle
8. _____
7. _____
Renal cortex
Perirenal fascia
Renal medulla   Perirenal fat

15. Sagittal section of the abdomen 6 cm from the midline.

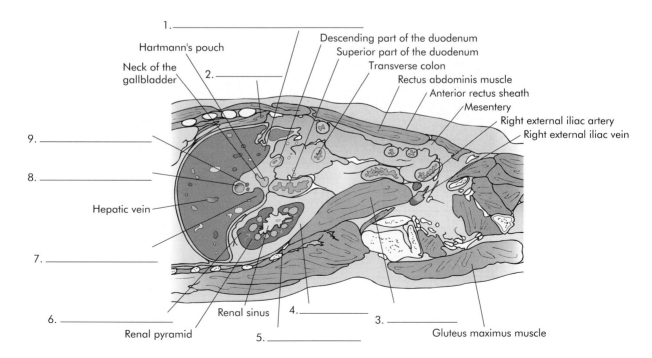

1. _____
Hartmann's pouch
Descending part of the duodenum
Superior part of the duodenum
Neck of the
gallbladder
2. _____
Transverse colon
Rectus abdominis muscle
Anterior rectus sheath
Mesentery
Right external iliac artery
Right external iliac vein
9. _____
8. _____
Hepatic vein
7. _____
6. _____
Renal sinus
4. _____
3. _____
Renal pyramid
5. _____
Gluteus maximus muscle

16. Sagittal section of the abdomen 3 cm from the midline.

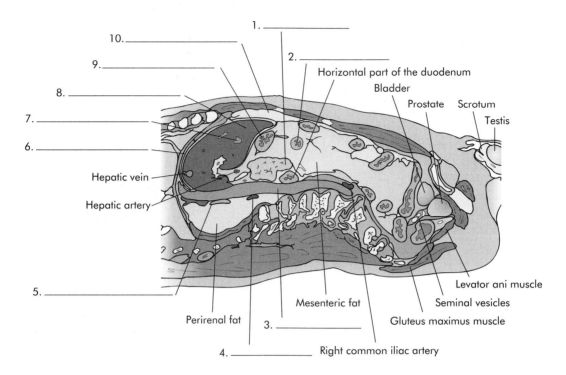

1. _____
10. _____
9. _____
8. _____
7. _____
6. _____
Hepatic vein
Hepatic artery
5. _____

2. _____
Horizontal part of the duodenum
Bladder
Prostate   Scrotum
Testis

Perirenal fat
3. _____
4. _____ Right common iliac artery
Mesenteric fat
Gluteus maximus muscle
Seminal vesicles
Levator ani muscle

17. Sagittal section of the abdomen 1 cm from the midline.

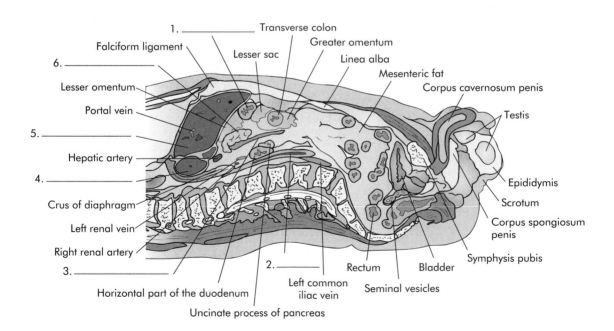

1. _____ Transverse colon
Falciform ligament
Lesser sac
Greater omentum
Linea alba
Mesenteric fat
Corpus cavernosum penis
6. _____
Lesser omentum
Portal vein
5. _____
Hepatic artery
4. _____
Crus of diaphragm
Left renal vein
Right renal artery
3. _____
Horizontal part of the duodenum
Uncinate process of pancreas
2. _____
Left common iliac vein
Rectum
Seminal vesicles
Bladder
Testis
Epididymis
Scrotum
Corpus spongiosum penis
Symphysis pubis

18. Midline sagittal section of the abdomen.

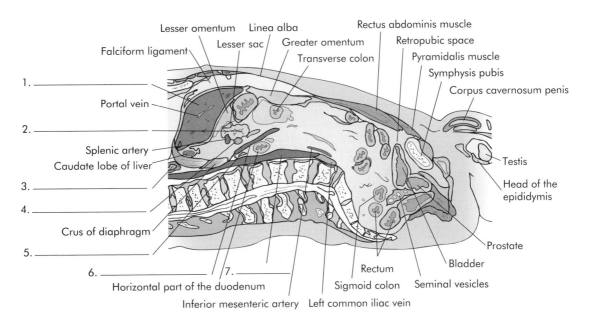

Lesser omentum   Linea alba   Rectus abdominis muscle

Falciform ligament   Lesser sac   Greater omentum   Retropubic space

Pyramidalis muscle

Transverse colon   Symphysis pubis

Corpus cavernosum penis

1. _____

Portal vein

2. _____

Splenic artery   Testis

Caudate lobe of liver   Head of the
epididymis

3. _____

4. _____

Crus of diaphragm

Prostate

5. _____   Bladder

6. _____   7. _____

Horizontal part of the duodenum   Rectum

Sigmoid colon   Seminal vesicles

Inferior mesenteric artery   Left common iliac vein

19. Sagittal section of the abdomen along the left abdominal border.

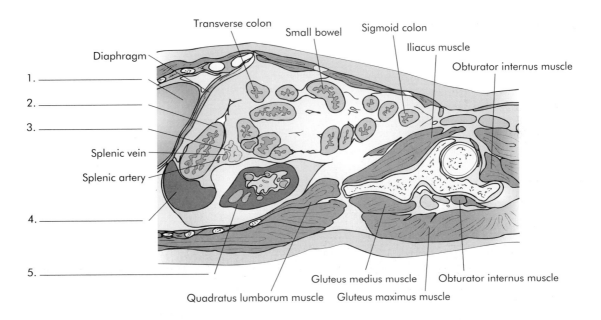

Transverse colon   Sigmoid colon

Small bowel   Iliacus muscle

Diaphragm   Obturator internus muscle

1. _____

2. _____

3. _____

Splenic vein

Splenic artery

4. _____

5. _____   Obturator internus muscle

Gluteus medius muscle

Quadratus lumborum muscle   Gluteus maximus muscle

5 The Vascular System

KEY TERMS

Exercise 1

Match the following structural terms with their definitions.

1. __A__ vasa vasorum

2. __F__ tunica media

3. __E__ tunica adventitia

4. __B__ tunica intima

5. __D__ anastomosis

6. __C__ capillaries

A. The tiny arteries and veins that supply the walls of blood vessels

B. Inner layer of the vascular system

C. Minute vessels that connect the arterial and venous systems

D. A communication between two blood vessels without any intervening capillary network

E. Outer layer of the vascular system, contains the vasa vasorum

F. Middle layer of the vascular system; veins have thinner tunica media than arteries

Exercise 2

Match the following arterial terms with their definitions.

1. __H__ superior mesenteric artery

2. __D__ arteries

3. __M__ left hepatic artery

4. __I__ common iliac arteries

5. __A__ right renal artery

6. __G__ gastroduodenal artery

7. __L__ aorta

8. __J__ inferior mesenteric artery

9. __B__ left gastric artery

10. __N__ splenic artery

11. __E__ common hepatic artery

12. __C__ right hepatic artery

13. __K__ left renal artery

14. __F__ right gastric artery

A. Arises from the lateral wall of the aorta, travels posterior to the inferior vena cava to supply the kidney

B. Arises from the celiac axis to supply the stomach and lower third of the esophagus

C. Supplies the gallbladder via the cystic artery

D. Vascular structures that carry blood away from the heart

E. Arises from the celiac trunk to supply the liver

F. Supplies the stomach

G. Branch of the common hepatic artery that supplies the stomach and duodenum

H. Arises inferior to the celiac axis to supply the proximal half of the colon and the small intestine

I. The abdominal aorta bifurcates at the level of the umbilicus into common iliac arteries to supply blood to the lower extremities

J. Arises from the anterior aortic wall at the level of the third or fourth lumbar vertebra to supply the left transverse colon, descending colon, sigmoid colon, and rectum

K. Arises from the posterolateral wall of the aorta directly into the hilus of the kidney

L. Largest arterial structure in the body; arises from the left ventricle to supply blood to the head, upper and lower extremities, and abdominopelvic cavity

M. Small branch supplying the caudate and left lobes of the liver

N. Arises from the celiac trunk to supply the spleen

Exercise 3

Match the following venous terms with their definitions.

1. _____ splenic vein

2. _____ hepatic veins

3. _____ portal vein

4. _____ right renal vein

5. _____ veins

6. _____ inferior mesenteric vein

7. _____ left renal vein

8. _____ superior mesenteric vein

9. _____ inferior vena cava

A. Drains the spleen; travels horizontally across abdomen (posterior to the pancreas) to join the superior mesenteric vein to form the portal vein

B. Collapsible vascular structures that carry blood back to the heart

C. Formed by the union of the superior mesenteric vein and splenic vein near the porta hepatis of the liver

D. Drains the left third of the colon and upper colon and joins the splenic vein

E. Drains the proximal half of the colon and small intestine, travels vertically (anterior to the inferior vena cava) to join the splenic vein to form the portal veins

F. Three large veins that drain the liver and empty into the inferior vena cava at the level of the diaphragm

G. Leaves the renal hilum, travels anterior to the aorta and posterior to the superior mesenteric artery to enter the lateral wall of the inferior vena cava

H. Largest venous abdominal vessel that conveys blood from the body below the diaphragm to the right atrium of the heart

I. Leaves the renal hilum to enter the lateral wall of the inferior vena cava

Exercise 4

Match the following pathology terms with their definitions.

1. _____ cystic medial necrosis

2. _____ abdominal aortic aneurysm

3. _____ Budd-Chiari syndrome

4. _____ arteriosclerosis

5. _____ fusiform aneurysm

6. _____ TIPS

7. _____ saccular aneurysm

8. _____ atherosclerosis

9. _____ cavernous transformation of the portal vein

10. _____ dissecting aneurysm

11. _____ arteriovenous fistula

12. _____ portal venous hypertension

A. A disease of the arterial vessels marked by thickening, hardening, and loss of elasticity in the arterial walls

B. Condition in which the aortic wall becomes irregular from plaque formation

C. Tear in the intima and/or media of the abdominal aorta

D. Permanent localized dilatation of an artery, with an increase of 1.5 times its normal diameter

E. Periportal collateral channels in patients with chronic portal vein obstruction

F. Circumferential enlargement of a vessel with tapering at both ends

G. Weakening of the arterial wall

H. Pulsatile hematoma that results from leakage of blood into soft tissue abutting the punctured artery with fibrous encapsulation and failure of the vessel wall to heal.

I. Transjugular intrahepatic portosystemic shunt

J. Most commonly results from intrinsic liver disease; however, also results from obstruction of the portal vein, hepatic veins, inferior vena cava, or prolonged congestive heart failure; may cause flow reversal to the liver, thrombosis of the portal system, or cavernous transformation of the portal vein

13. _____ pseudoaneurysm

14. _____ Marfan syndrome

K. Communication between an artery and a vein

L. Localized dilatation of the vessel

M. Thrombosis of the hepatic veins

N. Hereditary disorder of connective tissue, bones, muscles, ligaments, and skeletal structures

Exercise 5

Match the following abdominal Doppler terms with their definitions.

1. _____ resistive

2. _____ hepatopetal

3. _____ nonresistive

4. _____ resistive index

5. _____ spectral broadening

6. _____ hepatofugal

7. _____ Doppler sample volume

A. Vessels that have high diastolic component and supply organs that need constant perfusion (i.e., internal carotid artery, hepatic artery, and renal artery)

B. Flow toward the liver

C. Peak systole minus peak diastole divided by peak systole ([S − D] ÷ S = RI); an RI of 0.7 or less indicates good perfusion; an RI of 0.7 or higher indicates decreased perfusion

D. Flow away from the liver

E. Vessels that have little or reversed flow in diastole and supply organs that do not need a constant blood supply (i.e., external carotid artery and brachial arteries)

F. Increased turbulence is seen within the spectral tracing that indicates flow disturbance

G. The sonographer selects the exact site to record Doppler signals and sets the sample volume (gate) at this site.

Exercise 6

Label the following illustrations.

1. The abdominal arterial vascular system and its tributaries.

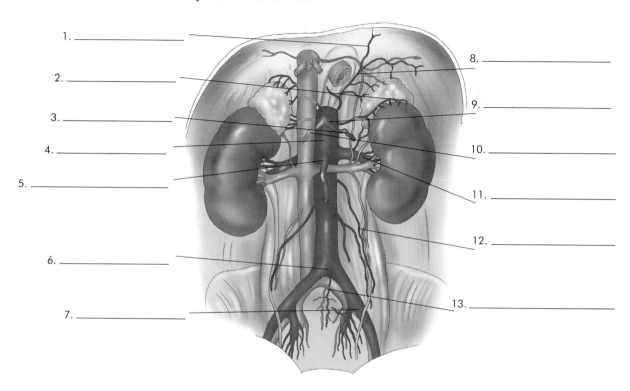

1. _____
2. _____
3. _____
4. _____
5. _____
6. _____
7. _____
8. _____
9. _____
10. _____
11. _____
12. _____
13. _____

2. The celiac artery and its branches.

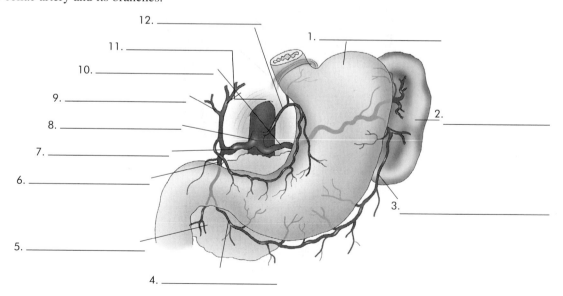

12. _____
11. _____
10. _____
9. _____
8. _____
7. _____
6. _____
5. _____
4. _____
1. _____
2. _____
3. _____

3. The superior mesenteric artery.

17. _____

16. _____

15. _____

14. _____

13. _____

12. _____

11. _____

10. _____

9. _____

8. _____

7. _____

6. _____

5. _____

4. _____

3. _____

2. _____

1. _____

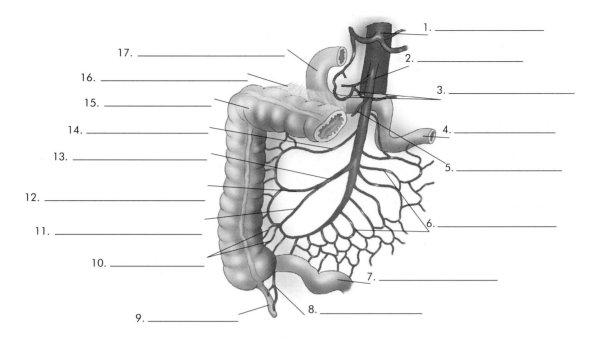

4. The abdominal venous system and its tributaries.

10. _____

9. _____

8. _____

7. _____

6. _____

1. _____

2. _____

3. _____

4. _____

5. _____

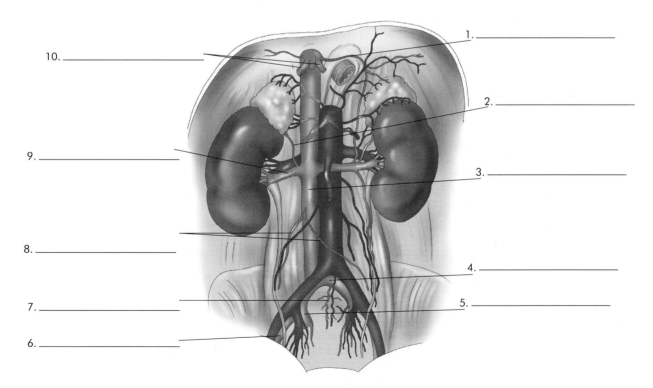

5. The portal vein.

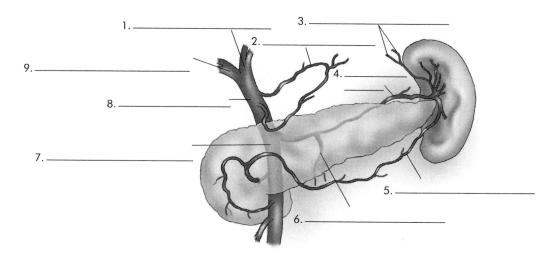

1. _____
2. _____
3. _____
4. _____
5. _____
6. _____
7. _____
8. _____
9. _____

Exercise 7

Fill in the blank(s) with the word(s) that best completes the statements about the arterial and venous structures.

1. The root of the aorta arises from the _____ outflow tract in the heart.

2. The _____ passes anterior to the third part of the duodenum and posterior to the neck of the pancreas, where it joins the splenic vein to form the main portal vein.

3. The _____ supplies the gallbladder via the cystic artery and the liver.

4. The aorta continues to flow in the _____ cavity anterior and slightly _____ of the vertebral column.

5. The _____ trunk is the first anterior branch of the aorta, arising 1 to 2 cm inferior to the diaphragm.

6. The _____ flows from the kidney posterior to the superior mesenteric artery and anterior to the aorta to enter the lateral wall of the inferior vena cava.

7. The diameter of the abdominal aorta measures approximately _____ with tapering to

   _____ after it proceeds inferiorly to the bifurcation into the iliac arteries.

8. The _____ is the second anterior branch, arising approximately 2 cm from the celiac trunk.

9. Portal veins become _____ as they progress into the liver from the porta hepatis.

10. The _____ courses from the aorta posterior to the inferior vena cava and anterior to the vertebral column in a posterior and slightly caudal direction to enter the hilus of the kidney.

11. The _____ courses along the upper border of the head of the pancreas, behind the posterior layer of the peritoneal bursa, to the upper margin of the superior part of the duodenum, which forms the lower boundary of the epiploic foramen.

12. Three arterial branches arise from the superior border of the aortic arch to supply the head, neck, and upper

    extremities: the _____, _____, and _____.

13. The _____ is formed posterior to the pancreas by the union of the superior mesenteric vein and splenic veins at the level of L2.

14. The _____ artery takes a somewhat tortuous course horizontally to the left as it forms the superior border of the pancreas.

15. The portion of the femoral artery posterior to the knee is the _____ .

16. The _____ originate in the liver and drain into the inferior vena cava at the level of the diaphragm.

Exercise 8

Provide a short answer for each anatomy and physiology question.

1. List the five sections into which the aorta is divided.

_____

_____

_____

_____

2. Describe the specific differences between the arteries and the veins.

_____

_____

_____

_____

3. List the four branches of the aorta that supply other visceral organs and the mesentery.

_____

_____

_____

_____

4. Describe the function of the circulatory system.

_____

_____

_____

_____

5. List the characteristics of a vein.

_____

_____

_____

_____

6. Describe the effect of gain settings when performing an abdominal aortic ultrasound.

_____

_____

_____

_____

7. Describe how blood is transported from the artery and returned by the veins.

_____

_____

_____

_____

8. Describe the function of the capillaries.

_____

_____

_____

_____

SONOGRAPHIC TECHNIQUE

Exercise 9

Fill in the blank(s) with the word(s) that best completes the statements or provide a short answer about the vascular and abdominal sonographic evaluations.

1. Describe how Doppler is used to distinguish the presence or absence of flow in a vessel from nonvascular structures.

_____

_____

_____

2. A flow disturbance (increased velocity or obstruction of flow) may result from the formation of an atheroma, AV fistula, _____, or aneurysmal dilation.

3. Describe the technique that should be used to image the inferior vena cava.

_____

_____

_____

_____

4. Nonresistive vessels have a high _____ component and supply organs that need constant perfusion, such as the internal carotid artery, the hepatic artery, and the renal artery.

5. Resistive vessels have very little or even reversed flow in diastole and supply organs that do not need a constant blood supply, such as the _____ carotid and the iliac and brachial arteries.

6. Explain how one can differentiate the inferior vena cava from the aorta.

_____

_____

_____

_____

7. _____ is a pattern of blood flow, typically seen in large arteries, in which most cells are moving at the same velocity across the entire diameter of the vessel. In other vessels the different velocities are the result of friction between the cells and arterial walls.

8. Doppler only records accurate velocity patterns when the beam is _____ to the flow.

9. The flow pattern of the proximal abdominal aorta above the renal arteries shows a high _____ peak and a relatively low _____ component.

10. The main renal artery has a _____ impedance (nonresistive) pattern with significant diastolic flow—usually 30% to 50% of peak systole.

11. During rejection, the vascular impedance _____, resulting in a decrease or even reversal of the diastolic flow.

12. The portal vein shows a relatively _____ flow at low velocities, which may vary slightly with respirations.

13. Cavernous transformation of the portal vein demonstrates _____ collateral channels in patients with chronic portal vein obstruction.

14. With a recanalized _____ vein, the main portal vein and the left portal vein show normal flow, but the flow in the right portal vein is reversed.

Exercise 10

Fill in the blank(s) with the word(s) that best completes the statements or provide a short answer about vascular pathology.

1. The most common causes of aneurysms are _____ and _____.

2. The large aneurysm may rupture into the peritoneal cavity or retroperitoneum, causing _____ and a

   drop in _____.

3. The normal measurement for an adult abdominal aorta is less than 3 cm, measuring from _____ to

   _____ walls.

4. Thrombus usually occurs along the _____ or _____ wall.

5. A _____ is a pulsatile hematoma that results from the leakage of blood into the soft tissue abutting the punctured artery, with subsequent fibrous encapsulation and failure of the vessel wall defect to heal.

6. What are the clinical findings in a patient with a dissecting aneurysm?

7. Describe the three locations where a dissection of the aorta may occur.

   _____

   _____

   _____

   _____

8. Describe other pseudopulsatile abdominal masses that may simulate an aortic aneurysm.

   _____

   _____

   _____

9. In patients with right ventricular failure, the inferior vena cava does not _____ with collapse.

10. Describe the complications of inferior vena caval thrombosis.

    _____

    _____

    _____

    _____

11. The most common origin of pulmonary emboli is venous thrombosis from the _____ extremities.

Exercise 11

Provide a short answer for each question after evaluating the images.

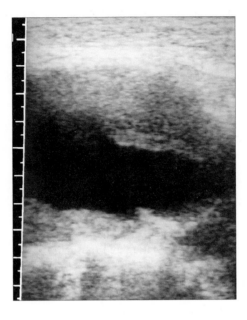

1. A 63-year-old man presents with a pulsatile abdominal mass. What does this longitudinal image of the abdomen demonstrate?

_____

_____

_____

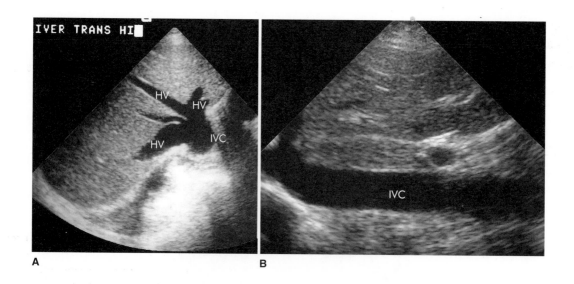

A   B

2. How can the sonographer know if this inferior vena cava is dilated?

_____

_____

_____

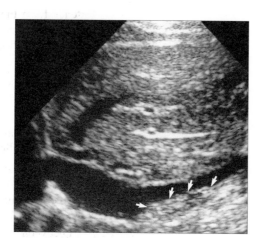

3. What are the arrows pointing to?

_____

_____

_____

6 The Liver

Exercise 1

Match the following anatomic terms with their definitions.

1. __C__ bare area

2. __A__ caudate lobe

3. __N__ epigastrium

4. __G__ falciform ligament

5. __M__ left hypochondrium

6. __D__ left lobe of the liver

7. __H__ left portal vein

8. __I__ ligamentum teres

9. __B__ ligamentum venosum

10. __F__ main lobar fissure

11. __J__ main portal vein

12. __K__ right hypochondrium

13. __E__ right lobe of the liver

14. __L__ right portal vein

A. Small lobe of the liver situated on the posterosuperior surface of the left lobe; the ligamentum venosum is the anterior border

B. Separates left lobe from caudate lobe; shown as echogenic line on the transverse and sagittal images

C. Area superior to the liver that is not covered by peritoneum so inferior vena cava may enter the chest

D. Lies in the epigastrium and left hypochondrium

E. Largest of the lobes of the liver

F. Boundary between the right and left lobes of the liver; seen as hyperechoic line on the sagittal image extending from the portal vein to the neck of the gallbladder

G. Extends from the umbilicus to the diaphragm in a sagittal plane and contains the ligamentum teres

H. Supplies the left lobe of the liver

I. Appears as bright echogenic foci on transverse image; along with falciform ligament divides medial and lateral segments of left lobe of liver

J. Enters the liver at the porta hepatis

K. Right upper quadrant of the abdomen that contains the liver and gallbladder

L. Supplies the right lobe of the liver; branches into anterior and posterior segments

M. Left upper quadrant of the abdomen that contains the left lobe of the liver, spleen, and stomach

N. Area between the right and left hypochondrium

Exercise 2

Match the following physiology and laboratory terms with their definitions.

1. ___H___ alkaline phosphatase

2. ___B___ ALT

3. ___D___ AST

4. ___A___ bilirubin

5. ___J___ BUN

6. ___I___ hepatocellular disease

7. ___F___ hepatocyte

8. ___E___ hepatofugal

9. _____ hepatopetal

10. ___G___ hyperglycemia

11. ___M___ hypoglycemia

12. ___C___ liver function tests

13. ___K___ obstructive disease

A. Broken down product of hemoglobin; excreted by liver and stored in the gallbladder

B. Alanine aminotransferase—enzyme of the liver

C. Specific laboratory tests that look at liver function (aspartate or alanine aminotransferase, lactic acid dehydrogenase, alkaline phosphatase, and bilirubin)

D. Aspartate aminotransferase—enzyme of the liver

E. Flow away from the liver

F. A parenchymal liver cell that performs all functions ascribed to the liver

G. Uncontrolled increase in glucose

H. Enzyme of the liver

I. Refers to liver cells or hepatocytes as primary problem

J. Blood urea nitrogen

K. Refers to bile excretion blocked within the liver or biliary system

L. Flow toward the liver

M. Deficiency of glucose

Exercise 3

Match the following pathology terms with their definitions.

1. _____ bull's-eye (target) lesion

2. _____ collateral circulation

3. _____ diffuse hepatocellular disease

4. _____ extrahepatic

5. _____ intrahepatic

6. _____ metastatic disease

7. _____ neoplasm

8. _____ pyogenic abscess

A. Outside the liver

B. Hypoechoic mass with an echogenic central core (abscess, metastases)

C. Refers to any new growth (benign or malignant)

D. Within the liver

E. Most common form of neoplasm of the liver; primary sites are colon, breast, and lung

F. Affects hepatocytes and interferes with liver function

G. Pus-forming collection of fluid

H. Develops when normal venous channels become obstructed

COLOR

Exercise 4

Label the following illustrations.

1.   Anterior view of the liver.

from the front

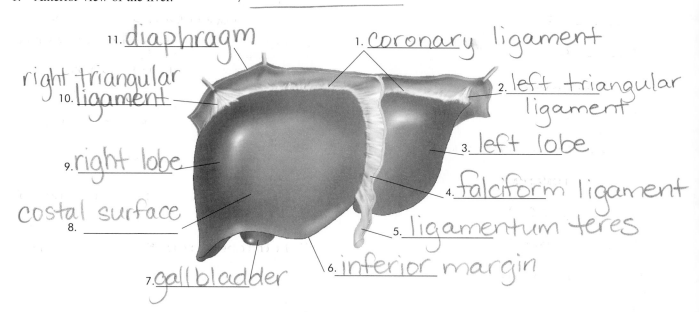

11. diaphragm

right triangular
10. ligament

9. right lobe

costal surface
8.

7. gallbladder

1. coronary ligament

2. left triangular
   ligament

3. left lobe

4. falciform ligament

5. ligamentum teres

6. inferior margin

2.   Superior view of the liver.

belly

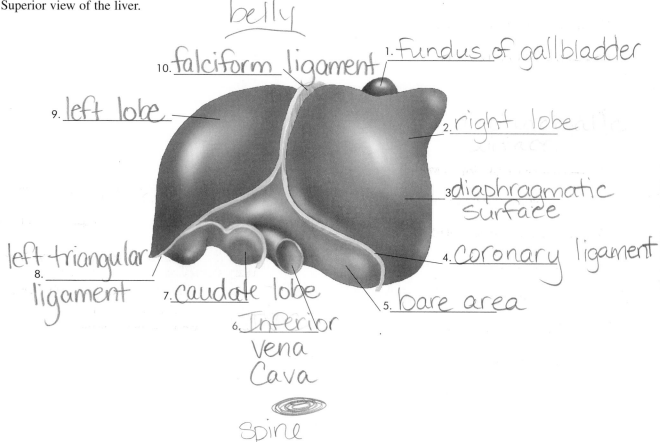

10. falciform ligament

9. left lobe

left triangular
8.
ligament

7. caudate lobe

6. Inferior
   Vena
   Cava

spine

1. fundus of gallbladder

2. right lobe

3. diaphragmatic
   surface

4. coronary ligament

5. bare area

from the back
hepatic duct

3. Interior view of the visceral surface of the liver.

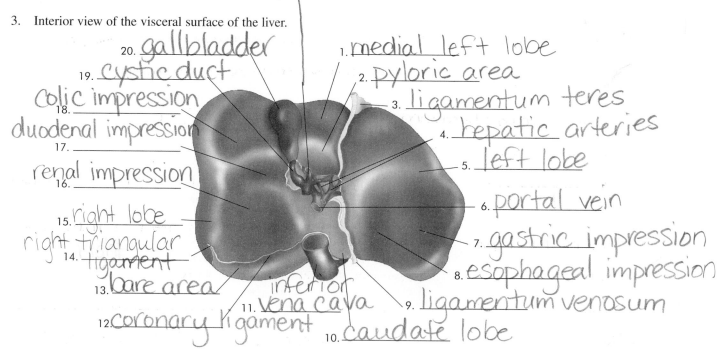

20. gallblladder
19. cystic duct
18. colic impression
17. duodenal impression
16. renal impression
15. right lobe
14. right triangular ligament
13. bare area
12. coronary ligament
11. inferior vena cava
10. caudate lobe

1. medial left lobe
2. pyloric area
3. ligamentum teres
4. hepatic arteries
5. left lobe
6. portal vein
7. gastric impression
8. esophageal impression
9. ligamentum venosum

4. Posterior view of the diaphragmatic surface of the liver.

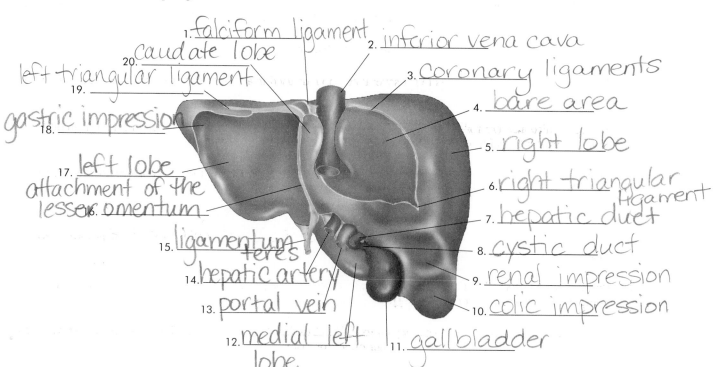

20. caudate lobe
19. left triangular ligament
18. gastric impression
17. left lobe
16. attachment of the lesser omentum
15. ligamentum teres
14. hepatic artery
13. portal vein
12. medial left lobe

1. falciform ligament
2. inferior vena cava
3. coronary ligaments
4. bare area
5. right lobe
6. right triangular ligament
7. hepatic duct
8. cystic duct
9. renal impression
10. colic impression
11. gallbladder

Exercise 5

Fill in the blank(s) with the word(s) that best completes the statements about the anatomy and physiology of the liver.

1. A congenital variant, _____, can sometimes be seen as an anterior projection of the liver and may extend inferiorly as far as the iliac crest.

2. The liver is covered by a thin connective tissue layer called _Glisson's_ capsule.

3. The _main lobar_ fissure is the boundary between the right and left lobes of the liver.

4. The _falciform_ ligament extends from the umbilicus to the diaphragm in a parasagittal plane and contains the ligamentum teres.

5. The _ligamentum teres_ appears as a bright echogenic focus on the sonogram and is seen as the rounded termination of the falciform ligament.

6. The fissure for the _ligamentum venosum_ separates the left lobe from the caudate lobe.

7. The hepatic veins are divided into three components: _right_, _middle_, and _left_.

8. The liver is a major center of _metabolism_, which may be defined as the physical and chemical process whereby foodstuffs are synthesized into complex elements.

9. Through the process of _digestion_, the liver expels these waste products from the body via its excretory product, bile, which also plays an important role in fat absorption.

10. A pigment released when the red blood cells are broken down is _bilirubin_.

11. The liver is a _storage_ site for several compounds used in a variety of physiologic activities throughout the body.

12. The liver is also a center for _detoxification_ of the waste products of metabolism accumulated from other sources in the body and foreign chemicals that enter the body.

13. Diseases affecting the liver may be classified as _hepatocellular_ when the liver cells or hepatocytes are the immediate problem; or _obstructive_ when bile excretion is blocked.

14. Raw materials in the form of _carbohydrates_, _fats_, and _amino acids_ are absorbed from the intestine and transported to the liver via the circulatory system.

15. Sugars may be absorbed from the blood in several forms, but only _glucose_ can be used by cells throughout the body as a source of energy.

16. Dietary fats are converted in the hepatocytes to _lipoproteins_, in which form fats are transported throughout the body to sites where they are used by other organs or stored.

17. The accompanying loss of oncotic pressure in the vascular system allows fluid to migrate into the interstitial space, resulting in _edema_ in dependent areas.

18. Because the liver is a major center of metabolism, large quantities of _enzymes_ are present in hepatocytes, and these leak into the bloodstream when the liver cells are damaged or destroyed by disease.

19. In severe hepatocellular destruction, such as acute viral or toxic hepatitis, striking elevation of _____AST_____ and _____ALT_____ may be seen.

20. Marked elevation of ___alkaline phosphatase___ is typically associated with biliary obstruction or the presence of mass lesions in the liver.

21. Hemoglobin released from the red cells is converted to _bilirubin_ within the reticuloendothelial system and is then released into the bloodstream.

22. Elevation of serum bilirubin results in _jaundice_, which is a yellow coloration of the skin, sclerae, and body secretions.

Exercise 6

Provide a short answer for each anatomy and physiology question.

1. Name the landmarks of the liver.

_____

_____

_____

_____

2. Identify at least three characteristics of the right lobe of the liver.

1) largest lobe (6:1 - right:left size ratio)

2) in rt. hypochondrium

3) post. surface marked by 3 fossae (porta hep, GB & IVC fossae)

4) ant. border is falc. lig

3. Identify at least three characteristics of the left lobe of the liver.

1) always smaller than rt.

2) varies in size & shape

3) larger left = better visualization of pancreas

4) lies in epig. & lt. hyp. regions

4. Name the ligaments and fissures found within the hepatic parenchyma.

_____

_____

_____

_____

5. Explain how one can distinguish hepatic veins from portal veins.

HEP

PORT

HEP	PORT
1) course b/t hep lobes + segments	1) course w/in lobar segments
2) drain toward rt. atrium	2) emanate from porta hepatis
3) ↑ in caliber tow. diaphragm	3) ↑ in caliber at level of porta hep.
4) do not have high-amp reflections	4) have high-amp, reflections
	5) course centrally w/in segments

6. List the seven liver function tests established to analyze how the liver is performing under normal and diseased conditions.

_____

_____

_____

_____

SONOGRAPHIC EVALUATION

Exercise 7

Fill in the blank(s) with the word(s) that best completes the statements or provide a short answer about the sonographic techniques in liver examination.

1. Explain why the evaluation of the hepatic structures is one of the most important procedures in sonography.

_____

_____

_____

2. Within the homogeneous parenchyma lie the thin-walled *hepatic veins*, the brightly reflective *portal veins*, the *hepatic* arteries, and the *hepatic* duct.

3. The portal flow is shown to be _____ (toward the liver), whereas the hepatic venous flow is

_____ (away from the liver).

4. Near the porta hepatis, the hepatic duct can be seen along the *anterior* lateral border of the portal vein, whereas the hepatic artery can be seen along the anterior *medial* border.

5. Describe how time gain compensation should be adjusted to balance the far-gain and the near-gain echo signals?

_____

_____

_____

6. Generally a wider pie sector or curved linear array transducer is the most appropriate to optimally image the

   _____ of the abdomen.

7. To image the far field better, a _____ array transducer with a longer focal zone is used.

PATHOLOGY

Exercise 8

Fill in the blank(s) with the word(s) that best completes the statements or provide a short answer about the pathology of the liver.

1. List the four criteria assessed when evaluating the liver parenchyma.

   _____

   _____

   _____

2. Hepatocellular disease affects the *hepatocytes* and interferes with liver function enzymes.

3. The hepatic enzyme levels are elevated with *cell* _____ necrosis.

4. Fatty infiltration implies increased _____ in the hepatocytes and results from significant injury to the liver or a systemic disorder leading to impaired or excessive metabolism of fat.

5. Describe the sonographic findings of fatty infiltration of the liver.

   _____

   _____

   _____

6. In focal sparing, the most common affected areas are anterior to the _____ or the portal vein and the

   posterior portion of the _____ of the liver.

7. On ultrasound examination, the liver parenchyma in chronic hepatitis is _____ with _____ brightness of the portal triads, but the degree of attenuation is not as great as seen in fatty infiltration.

8. Cirrhosis is a chronic degeneration of the liver in which the lobes are covered with fibrous tissue, the parenchyma

   _____, and the lobules are infiltrated with _____.

9. List the sonographic findings of cirrhosis of the liver.

   _____

   _____

   _____

10. Glycogen storage disease is associated with _____, focal nodular _____, and hepatomegaly.

11. List the differential considerations for focal diseases of the liver.

_____

_____

_____

12. List the criteria that should be used by the sonographer to differentiate whether the mass is extrahepatic or intrahepatic.

_____

_____

_____

13. List the symptoms that are revealed in the clinical findings of a patient who has inflammatory disease of the liver.

_____

_____

_____

14. A _____ is any new growth of new tissue, either benign or malignant.

15. A _____ is a benign, congenital tumor consisting of large, blood-filled cystic spaces.

16. The pathogenesis of hepatocellular carcinoma is related to _____, chronic _____ virus infection, and hepatocarcinogens in food.

17. Describe the pathologic patterns seen in carcinoma of the liver.

_____

_____

_____

18. The liver is the third most common organ injured in the abdomen after the _____ and the

_____.

19. Describe the complications of liver transplantation as seen on an ultrasound.

_____

_____

_____

20. An increase in portal venous pressure or hepatic venous gradient is defined as _____.

21. Portal hypertension may also develop when hepatopetal flow is impeded by _____ or _____ invasion.

22. The umbilical vein may become _____ secondary to portal hypertension.

23. The pulse repetition frequency allows one to record lower velocities as the PRF is _____.

24. The Doppler sample volume should be _____ than the diameter of the lumen.

25. Explain what color Doppler velocity is dependent upon.

_____

_____

_____

26. Acute abdominal pain, massive ascites, and hepatomegaly secondary to thrombosis of the hepatic veins or inferior

vena cava characterizes _____ syndrome, which has a poor prognosis.

Exercise 9

Provide a short answer for each question after evaluating the images.

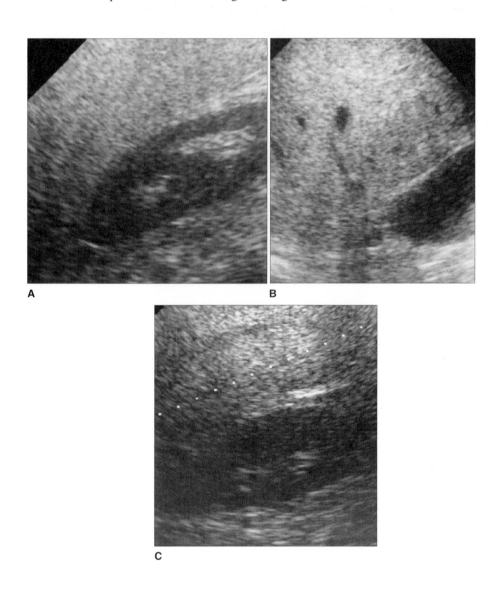

A

B

C

1. What liver disease is present in these images?

_____

_____

_____

_____

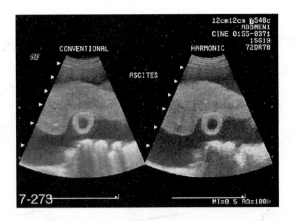

2. Describe the abnormality in this image. Does the patient show signs of acute cholecystitis?

_____

_____

_____

_____

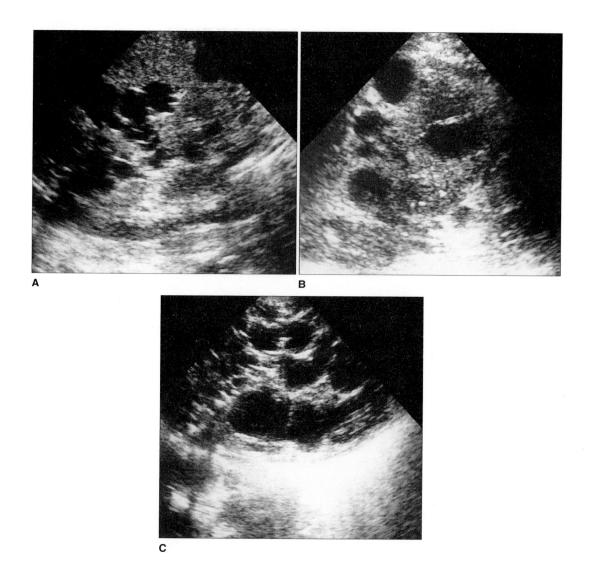

A

B

C

3. Multiple images over the right upper quadrant demonstrate what abnormality of the liver? What other area should the sonographer investigate?

_____

_____

_____

_____

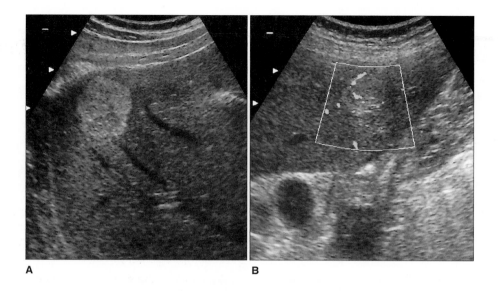

A   B

4. Describe the lesion seen in the right upper quadrant and list the most likely differentials in this asymptomatic patient.

_____

_____

_____

_____

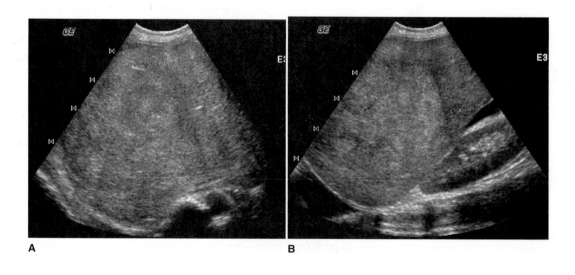

A   B

5. A patient with a history of cirrhosis shows evidence of hepatomegaly. What are the possible sonographic findings?

_____

_____

_____

7 The Gallbladder and the Biliary System

KEY TERMS

Exercise 1
Match the following anatomic and physiologic terms with their definitions.

1. __C__ ampulla of Vater
2. __L__ bilirubin
3. __M__ cholecystectomy
4. __A__ common bile duct
5. __F__ common duct
6. __O__ common hepatic duct
7. __G__ cystic duct
8. __B__ gallbladder
9. __I__ Hartmann's pouch
10. __E__ Heister's valve
11. __D__ hydrops
12. __J__ pancreatic duct
13. __N__ phrygian cap
14. __H__ porta hepatis
15. __K__ sphincter of Oddi

A. Extends from the point where the common hepatic duct meets the cystic duct; drains into the duodenum after it joins with the main pancreatic duct
B. Storage pouch for bile
C. Small opening in the duodenum in which the pancreatic and common bile duct enter to release secretions
D. Massive enlargement of the gallbladder
E. Tiny valves found within the cystic duct
F. Refers to common bile and hepatic ducts when cystic duct is not seen
G. Connects the gallbladder to the common hepatic duct
H. Central area of the liver where the portal vein, common duct, and hepatic artery enter
I. Small part of the gallbladder that lies near the cystic duct where stones may collect
J. Travels horizontally through the pancreas to join the common bile duct at the ampulla of Vater
K. Small muscle that guards the ampulla of Vater
L. Yellow pigment in bile formed by the breakdown of red blood cells
M. Removal of the gallbladder
N. Gallbladder variant in which part of the fundus is bent back on itself
O. Bile duct system that drains the liver into the common bile duct

Exercise 2
Match the following sonographic evaluation and pathology terms with their definitions.

1. __E__ adenomyomatosis
2. __C__ cholangitis
3. __K__ cholecystitis
4. __I__ cholecystokinin
5. __L__ choledochal cyst

A. Gallstones in the gallbladder
B. Calcification of the gallbladder wall
C. Inflammation of the bile duct
D. Excessive bilirubin accumulation causes yellow pigmentation of the skin; first seen in the whites of the eyes
E. Small polypoid projections from the gallbladder wall

6. ___O___ choledocholithiasis

7. ___A___ cholelithiasis

8. ___J___ cholesterolosis

9. ___D___ jaundice

10. ___M___ junctional fold

11. ___G___ Klatskin's tumor

12. ___P___ Murphy's sign

13. ___N___ polyp

14. ___B___ porcelain gallbladder

15. ___H___ sludge

16. ___F___ wall echo shadow (WES) sign

F. Sonographic pattern found when the gallbladder is packed with stones

G. Cancer at the bifurcation of the hepatic ducts; may cause asymmetric obstruction of the biliary tree

H. Low-level echoes found along the posterior margin of the gallbladder; move with change in position

I. Hormone secreted into the blood by the mucosa of the upper small intestine; stimulates contraction of the gallbladder and pancreatic secretion of enzymes

J. Variant of adenomyomatosis; cholesterol polyps

K. Inflammation of the gallbladder; may be acute or chronic

L. Dilation of the common duct that may cause obstruction

M. Small septum within the gallbladder, usually arising from the posterior wall

N. Small, well-defined soft tissue projection from the gallbladder wall

O. Stones in the bile duct

P. Positive sign implies exquisite tenderness over the area of the gallbladder upon palpation

ANATOMY AND PHYSIOLOGY

Exercise 3

Label the following illustrations.

1. Gallbladder and biliary system.

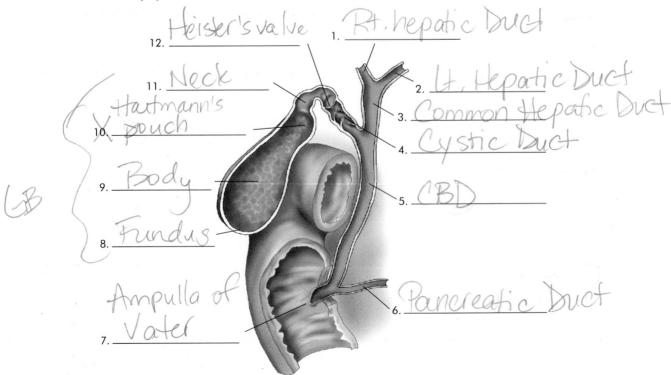

12. Heister's valve

11. Neck

10. Hartmann's pouch

9. Body

8. Fundus

7. Ampulla of Vater

1. Rt. hepatic Duct

2. Lt. Hepatic Duct

3. Common Hepatic Duct

4. Cystic Duct

5. CBD

6. Pancreatic Duct

2. Relationships within the porta hepatis.

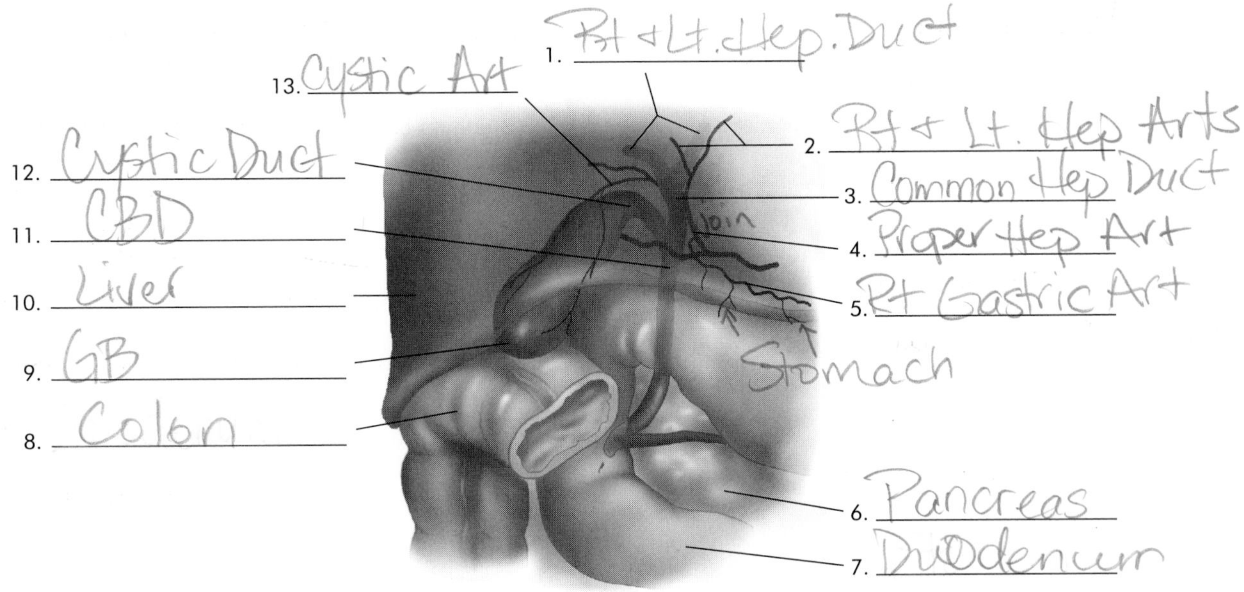

Handwritten labels:

1. Rt & Lt. Hep. Duct
13. Cystic Art
12. Cystic Duct
2. Rt & Lt. Hep Arts
11. CBD
3. Common Hep Duct
10. Liver
4. Proper Hep Art
9. GB
5. Rt Gastric Art
8. Colon
Join
Stomach
6. Pancreas
7. Duodenum

Exercise 4

Fill in the blank(s) with the word(s) that best completes the statements or provide a short answer about the anatomy and physiology of the gallbladder.

1. The gallbladder serves as a reservoir for __bile__ that is drained from the hepatic ducts in the liver.

2. The common hepatic duct is joined by the cystic duct to form the __CB__ duct.

3. The common bile duct is joined by the main pancreatic duct, and together they open through a small ampulla

   (the ampulla of __Vater__) into the duodenal wall.

4. The end parts of the common bile duct and main pancreatic duct and the ampulla are surrounded by circular muscle

   fibers known as the __Sphincter of Oddi.__

5. The arterial supply of the gallbladder is from the __cystic__ artery, which is a branch of the right hepatic artery.

6. List the two primary functions of the extrahepatic biliary tract.

   1) transportation of bile from liver to the intestine
   2) the regulation of its flow

Exercise 5

Fill in the blank(s) with the word(s) that best completes the statements or provide a short answer about the anatomy and physiology of the gallbladder.

1. Describe the normal function of the gallbladder during digestion.

_____

_____

_____

2. Bile is the principal medium for excretion of bilirubin and *cholesterol*

3. The *bile salts* from the small intestine stimulate the liver to make more bile. This activates intestinal and pancreatic enzymes.

4. The sign that indicates an extrahepatic mass compressing the common bile duct, which can produce an enlarged *(pancreatic)* *hydropic* gallbladder, is called *Courvoisier's sign*.

5. Sonographically, the common duct lies *anterior* and to the *right* of the portal vein in the region of the porta hepatis and gastrohepatic ligament.

6. The hepatic artery lies *anterior* and to the *left* of the portal vein. *left*

SONOGRAPHIC TECHNIQUE

Exercise 6

Fill in the blank(s) with the word(s) that best completes the statements about the sonographic techniques of the biliary system.

1. To ensure maximum dilation of the gallbladder, the patient should be given nothing to eat for at least

   8-12 hours before the ultrasound examination.

2. The patient is initially examined with ultrasound in full *inspiration*.

3. The patient should also be rolled into a steep *decubitus* or upright position (to ensure there are no stones within the gallbladder) in an attempt to separate small stones from the gallbladder wall or cystic duct.

4. The gallbladder may be identified as a *sonolucent* oblong structure located anterior to the right kidney, lateral to the head of the pancreas and duodenum.

5. The gallbladder commonly resides in a *fossa* on the medial aspect of the liver.

6. Because of *fat or fibrous* tissue within the main lobar fissure of the liver (which lies between the gallbladder and the right portal vein), this bright linear reflector is a reliable indicator of the location of the gallbladder.

7. A small *echogenic* fold has been reported to occur along the posterior wall of the gallbladder at the junction of the body and infundibulum. *(neck)*

8. On a transverse scan, the common duct, hepatic artery, and portal vein have been referred to as the

   "*Mickey Mouse* sign."

9. To obtain a cross-section of the portal triad, the transducer must be directed in a slightly *oblique* path from the left shoulder to the right hip.

10. On sagittal scans, the right branch of the hepatic artery usually passes *posterior* to the common duct.

11. The common duct is seen just *anterior* to the portal vein before it dips posteriorly to enter the head of the pancreas.

12. When the right subcostal approach is used, the common hepatic duct is seen as a tubular structure anterior to the portal vein. The right branch of the _hepatic_ artery can be seen between the duct and the portal vein as a small circular structure.

PATHOLOGY

Exercise 7

Fill in the blank(s) with the word(s) that best completes the statements or provide a short answer about the pathology of the gallbladder and biliary system.

1. The most classic symptom of gallbladder disease is _RUQ_ pain, usually occurring after ingestion of greasy foods.

2. A gallbladder attack may cause pain in the _right_ shoulder.

3. The normal wall thickness of the gallbladder is less than _3_ mm.

4. List the biliary causes of gallbladder wall thickening.

_____

_____

_____

5. Clinically the patient with acute cholecystitis presents with these symptoms:

_____

_____

_____

6. The _WES_ sign is described as a contracted bright gallbladder with posterior shadowing caused by a packed bag of stones.

7. A fairly rare complication of acute cholecystitis associated with the presence of gas-forming bacteria in the gallbladder wall and lumen with extension into the biliary ducts is called _emphysematous_

8. Clinically the patient falls under the five "F"s: _fat_ , _female_ , _40_ , _fertile_ , and _fair_ .

9. Explain why the patient position should be shifted during the ultrasound examination.

_____

_____

_____

10. Describe the factors that produce a shadow in the gallbladder.

_____

_____

_____

11. _____ may be the result of pancreatic juices refluxing into the bile duct because of an anomalous junction of the pancreatic duct into the distal common bile duct, causing duct wall abnormality, weakness, and out-pouching of the ductal walls.

12. A hyperplastic change in the gallbladder wall is _____.

13. The differential for a porcelain gallbladder would include a packed bag or _____ sign.

14. In carcinoma of the gallbladder, this is the most remarkable sonographic finding.

_____

_____

_____

15. The most common cause of biliary ductal system obstruction is the presence of a _____ or

_____ within the ductal system.

16. The job of the sonographer is to localize the level and cause of the obstruction. List the three primary areas where obstruction occurs.

_____

_____

_____

17. An uncommon cause for extrahepatic biliary obstruction as a result of an impacted stone in the cystic duct

creating extrinsic mechanical compression of the common hepatic duct is _____ syndrome.

18. _____ causes increasing pressure in the biliary tree with pus accumulation.

19. The majority of stones in the common bile duct have migrated from the gallbladder. Common duct stones are

usually associated with _____.

20. _____ within the duodenum may also give rise to a dirty shadow in the right upper quadrant.

21. On ultrasound, multiple cystic structures that converge toward the porta hepatis are seen in _____ disease.

Exercise 8

Provide a short answer for each question after evaluating the images.

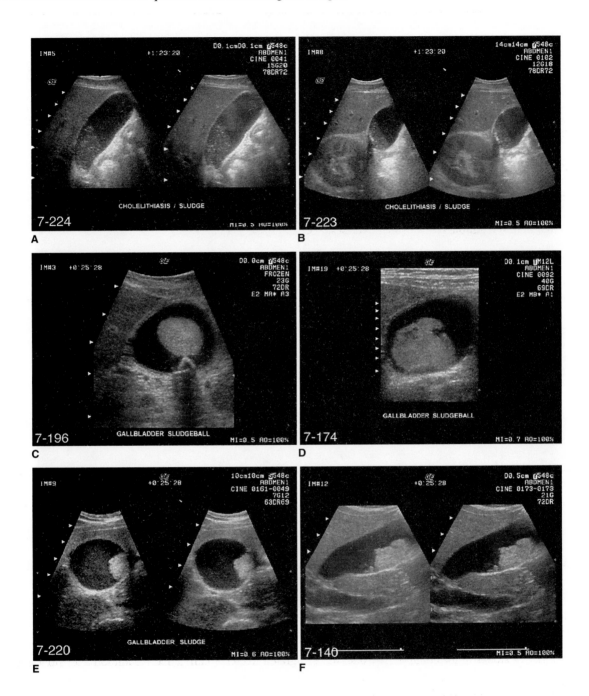

1. What maneuvers may be performed to be sure the sludge in the gallbladder is not a tumor?

_____

_____

_____

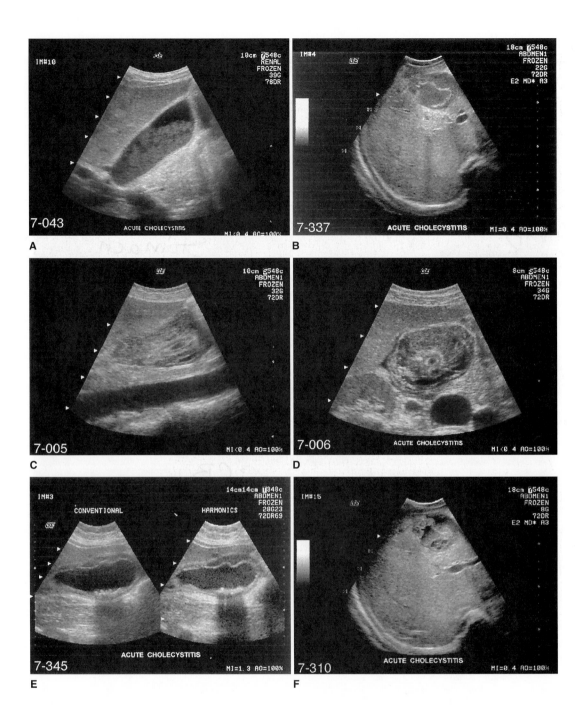

2. Describe the clinical signs and sonographic findings of the patient with acute cholecystitis as shown on these images. What complications should the sonographer be aware of?

_____

_____

_____

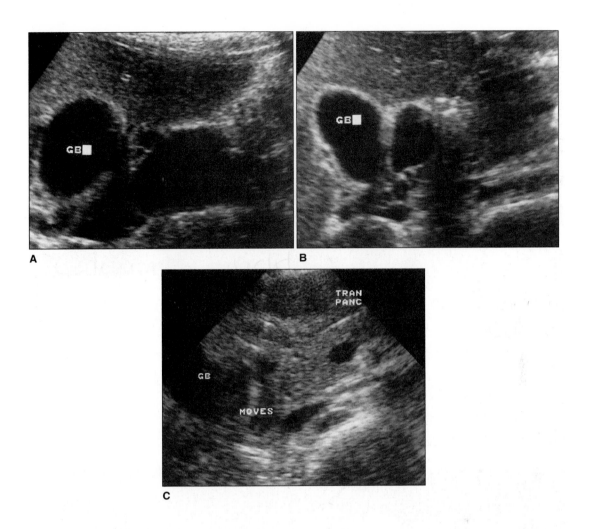

3. What anechoic structures surround the gallbladder that may lead to confusion during the examination?

_____

_____

_____

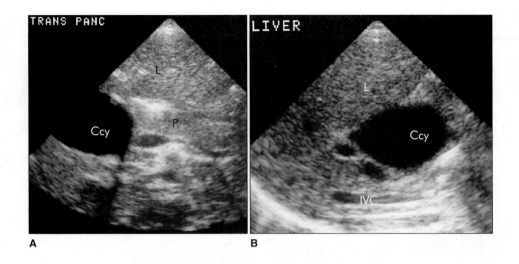

A

B

4. This scan over the right upper quadrant was made in a patient with a history of chronic pain. These sonographic images are representative of what disease?

_____

_____

_____

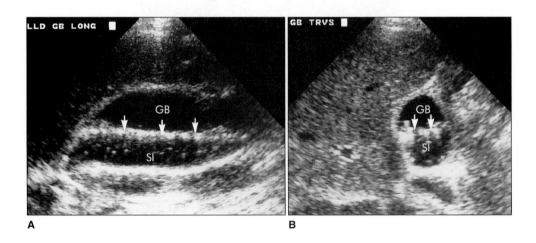

A

B

5. Describe what the arrows are pointing to in these two images of the gallbladder.

_____

_____

_____

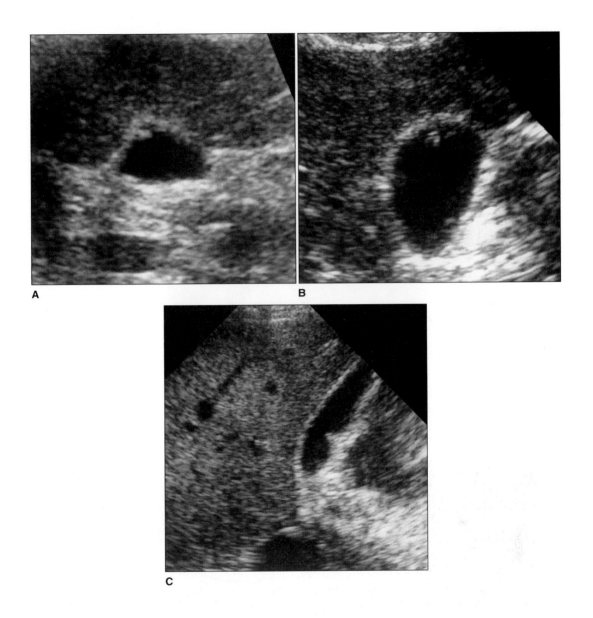

A

B

C

6. Describe the sonographic finding and position alteration that should be made with this patient.

_____

_____

_____

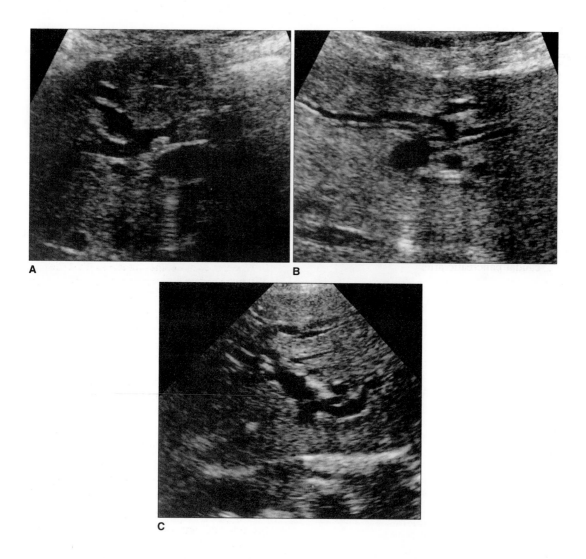

7. A 60-year-old female presents with a history of cholecystectomy several years ago. The patient was known to have had previous hepatic calculi and now presents with right upper quadrant pain. What questions should the sonographer ask before starting the examination? Describe the sonographic findings and what additional organ(s) should be imaged.

_____

_____

_____

8 The Pancreas

Exercise 1

Match the following anatomic terms with their definitions.

1. _____ body of the pancreas

2. _____ caudal pancreatic artery

3. _____ C-loop of the duodenum

4. _____ common hepatic artery

5. _____ dorsal pancreatic artery

6. _____ duct of Santorini

7. _____ duct of Wirsung

8. _____ head of the pancreas

9. _____ neck of the pancreas

10. _____ pancreaticoduodenal arteries

11. _____ portal-splenic confluence

12. _____ superior mesenteric artery

13. _____ superior mesenteric vein

14. _____ tail of the pancreas

15. _____ uncinate process

A. Branch of splenic artery that supplies the tail of the pancreas

B. Tapered end of the pancreas that lies in the left hypochondrium near the hilus of the spleen and upper pole of the left kidney

C. Junction of the splenic and main portal vein; posterior border of the body of the pancreas

D. Help supply blood to the pancreas along with the splenic artery

E. Lies in the midepigastrium anterior to the superior mesenteric artery and vein, aorta, and inferior vena cava

F. Small, curved tip of the pancreatic head that lies posterior to the superior mesenteric vein

G. Forms the lateral border of the head of the pancreas

H. Small area of the pancreas between the head and the body; anterior to the superior mesenteric vein

I. Lies posterior to the neck and/or body of the pancreas and anterior to the uncinate process of the gland

J. Forms the right superior border of the body and head of the gland and gives rise to the gastroduodenal artery

K. Largest duct of the pancreas that drains the tail, body, and head of the gland; it joins the common bile duct to enter the duodenum through the ampulla of Vater

L. Lies in the C-loop of the duodenum; the gastroduodenal artery is the anterolateral border, and the common bile duct is the posterolateral border

M. Serves as the posterior border to the body of the pancreas

N. Small accessory duct of the pancreas found in the head of the gland

O. Branch of the splenic artery that supplies the body of the pancreas

Exercise 2

Match the following physiology terms with their definitions.

1. _____ acinar cells

2. _____ amylase

3. _____ endocrine

4. _____ exocrine

5. _____ glucagons

6. _____ insulin

7. _____ islets of Langerhans

8. _____ lipase

9. _____ serum amylase

A. The endocrine function is production of the hormone insulin

B. Small cells that make up the endocrine portion of the pancreas for the production of insulin, glucagon, and somatostatin

C. Stimulates the liver to convert the glycogen to glucose; produced by alpha cells

D. Production and digestion of pancreatic juice; primary function of the pancreas

E. Pancreatic enzyme that is elevated during pancreatitis

F. Cells that perform exocrine function

G. Hormone that causes glycogen formation from glucose in the liver and allows cells within insulin receptors to take up glucose to decrease blood sugar

H. Pancreatic enzyme that breaks down fats; enzyme is elevated in pancreatitis and remains increased longer than amylase

I. Enzyme secreted by the pancreas to aid in the digestion of carbohydrates

Exercise 3

Match the following pathology terms with their definitions.

1. _____ Courvoisier's gallbladder

2. _____ cystic fibrosis

3. _____ hypercalcemia

4. _____ hyperlipidemia

5. _____ ileus

6. _____ leukocytosis

7. _____ lymphoma

8. _____ obstructive jaundice

9. _____ pancreatic ascites

10. _____ pancreatic pseudocyst

11. _____ pancreatitis

12. _____ pseudocyst

A. Congenital condition in which elevated fat levels cause pancreatitis

B. Excessive bilirubin in the bloodstream caused by an obstruction of bile from the liver; characterized by a yellow discoloration of the sclera of the eye, skin, and mucous membranes

C. A malignant neoplasm that arises from the lymphoid tissue

D. Dilated loops of bowel without peristalsis; associated with various abdominal problems, including pancreatitis, sickle cell crisis, and bowel obstruction

E. A space or cavity that contains fluid, but has no true endothelial lining membrane

F. Inflammation of the pancreas; may be acute or chronic

G. "Sterile abscess" collection of pancreatic enzymes that accumulate in the available space in the abdomen (usually in or near the pancreas)

H. An abnormal increase in white blood cells caused by infections

I. Enlargement of the gallbladder caused by a slow progressive obstruction of the distal common bile duct from an external mass (such as adenocarcinoma of the pancreatic head)

J. Elevated levels of calcium in the blood

K. Occurs when the pancreatic pseudocyst ruptures into the abdomen; free-floating pancreatic enzymes are very dangerous to surrounding structures

L. A hereditary disease that causes excessive production of thick mucus by the endocrine glands

Exercise 4

Label the following illustrations.
1. The aorta and inferior vena cava are the posterior landmarks of the pancreas.

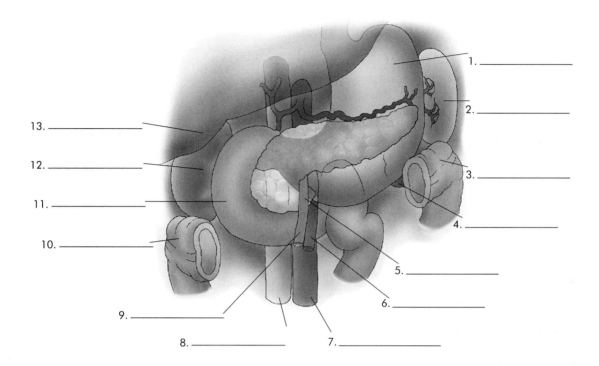

13. _____

12. _____

11. _____

10. _____

9. _____

8. _____

7. _____

1. _____

2. _____

3. _____

4. _____

5. _____

6. _____

2. Sagittal planes of the pancreas.

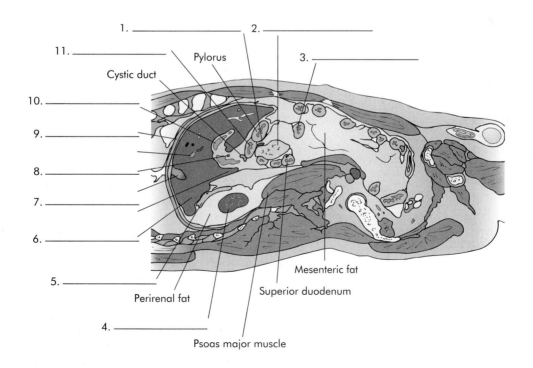

1. _____

2. _____

3. _____

11. _____

10. _____

9. _____

8. _____

7. _____

6. _____

5. _____

4. _____

Pylorus

Cystic duct

Mesenteric fat

Superior duodenum

Psoas major muscle

Perirenal fat

3. The portal venous system is the posterior border of the pancreas.

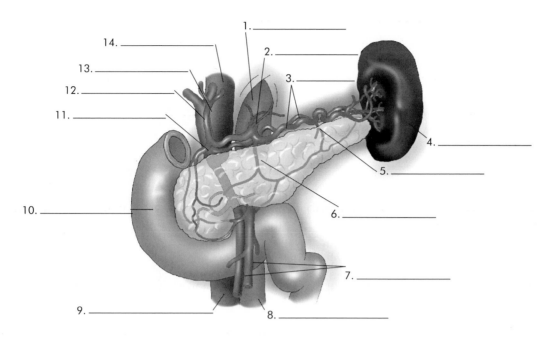

14. _____

13. _____

12. _____

11. _____

10. _____

9. _____

1. _____

2. _____

3. _____

4. _____

5. _____

6. _____

7. _____

8. _____

Exercise 5

Fill in the blank(s) with the word(s) that best completes the statements about the anatomy of the pancreas.

1. The pancreas is located in the _____ cavity posterior to the stomach, duodenum, and proximal jejunum of the small bowel.

2. The pancreatic gland appears sonographically _____ to slightly more _____ than the hepatic parenchyma.

3. The major posterior vascular landmarks of the pancreas are the _____ and _____.

4. The head of the pancreas lies _____ to the inferior vena cava.

5. The _____ crosses anterior to the uncinate process of the head of the gland and posterior to the neck and body.

6. The tortuous _____ is the superior border of the pancreas.

7. The tail of the pancreas is more difficult to image because it lies anterior to the left kidney and posterior to the left

    _____ and _____.

8. The _____ receives tributaries from lobules at right angles and enters the medial second part of the duodenum with the common bile duct at the ampulla of Vater.

9. The blood supply for the pancreas is from the _____ and _____ arteries.

10. The _____ artery is seen along the anterolateral border of the pancreas as it travels a short distance along the anterior aspect of the pancreatic head.

11. The _____ duct crosses the anterior aspect of the portal vein to the right of the proper hepatic artery.

12. The portal vein is _____ to the inferior vena cava.

Exercise 6

Fill in the blank(s) with the word(s) that best completes the statements about the physiology of the pancreas.

1. The pancreas is both a digestive (_____) and hormonal (_____) gland.

2. Failure of the pancreas to furnish sufficient insulin leads to _____.

3. Exocrine function is performed by _____ of the pancreas.

4. The _____ is a muscle surrounding the ampulla of Vater that relaxes to allow pancreatic juice and bile to empty into the duodenum.

5. The endocrine function is located in the _____ in the pancreas.

6. The beta cells are most prevalent and produce _____, a hormone that causes glycogen formation from glucose in the liver.

7. Alpha cells produce _____, a hormone that causes the cells to release glucose to meet the energy needs of the body.

8. Delta cells are the smallest composition of endocrine tissue and produce _____.

9. There are specific enzymes of the pancreas that may become altered in pancreatic disease, namely

   _____ and _____.

10. Both amylase and lipase rise at the same rate, but the elevation in _____ concentration persists for a longer period in pancreatitis.

11. _____ controls the blood sugar level in the body.

SONOGRAPHIC EVALUATION

Exercise 7

Provide a short answer that best completes the statements about the sonographic techniques of the pancreas.

1. Explain how fat influences the echogenicity of the pancreas on ultrasound.

_____

_____

_____

2. Name the structures that should be identified as landmarks to locate the pancreas.

_____

_____

_____

3. Describe the water technique used to image the pancreas with sonography.

_____

_____

_____

4. When the pancreas is enlarged, the anterior border of the _____ may depict a slight indentation.

PATHOLOGY

Exercise 8
Fill in the blank(s) with the word(s) that best completes the statements or provide a short answer about the pathology of the pancreas.

1. When the pancreas becomes damaged and malfunctions as a result of increased secretion and blockage of ducts,

   _____ occurs.

2. An acute attack of pancreatitis is commonly related to _____ and _____.

3. The patient with pancreatitis typically presents with moderate to severe tenderness in the _____ radiating to the _____.

4. When swelling does occur, the gland is hypoechoic to anechoic and is less echogenic than the liver because of the

   increased prominence of _____ and _____.

5. The pancreatic duct may be obstructed in acute pancreatitis as a result of:

   _____

   _____

   _____

6. Fluid collections around the pancreatic _____, along the _____ spaces, within the

_____ pouch, and around the _____ may be present in a patient with acute pancreatitis.

7. Patients with acute pancreatitis may develop complications, such as:

_____

_____

_____

8. Necrosis of the blood vessels results in the development of hemorrhagic areas referred to as _____ sign.

9. An inflammatory process that spreads along fascial pathways, causing localized areas of diffuse inflammatory

edema of soft tissue is known as _____.

10. The _____ become obstructed with a buildup of protein plugs with resultant calcifications along the

duct in _____ pancreatitis.

11. Briefly discuss the development of a pseudocyst.

_____

_____

_____

12. The most common location of a pseudocyst is in the _____ anterior to the pancreas and posterior to
the stomach.

13. A pseudocyst develops when pancreatic _____ escape from the gland and break down tissue to form a
sterile abscess somewhere in the abdomen.

14. The most common primary neoplasm of the pancreas is _____.

15. Name the clinical findings in a patient with carcinoma of the pancreas.

_____

_____

_____

16. The most frequent parapancreatic neoplasm is _____.

Exercise 9

Provide a short answer for each question after evaluating the images.

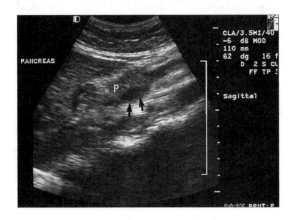

1. The arrows are pointing to which vascular structures?

_____

_____

_____

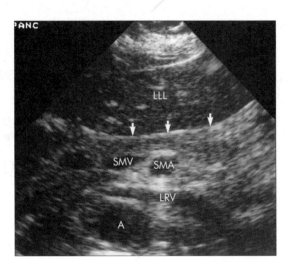

2. Identify whether the image is transverse or longitudinal. Also identify what the arrows are pointing to.

_____

_____

_____

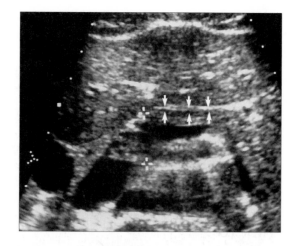

3. Identify what anatomic structure the arrows are pointing to.

_____

_____

_____

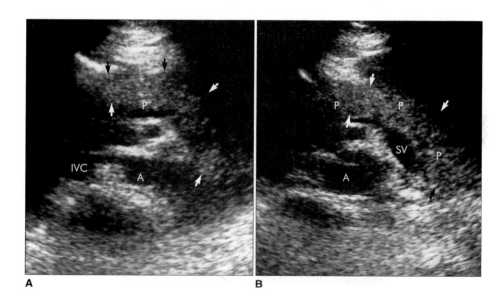

A   **B**

4. A 45-year-old male presents with midepigastric pain, elevated amylase and lipase levels, and tenderness. Identify the ultrasound findings.

_____

_____

_____

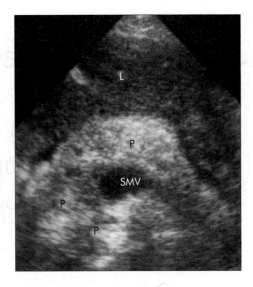

5. A patient with known acute pancreatitis presents with continued pain. Describe the sonographic findings.

_____

_____

_____

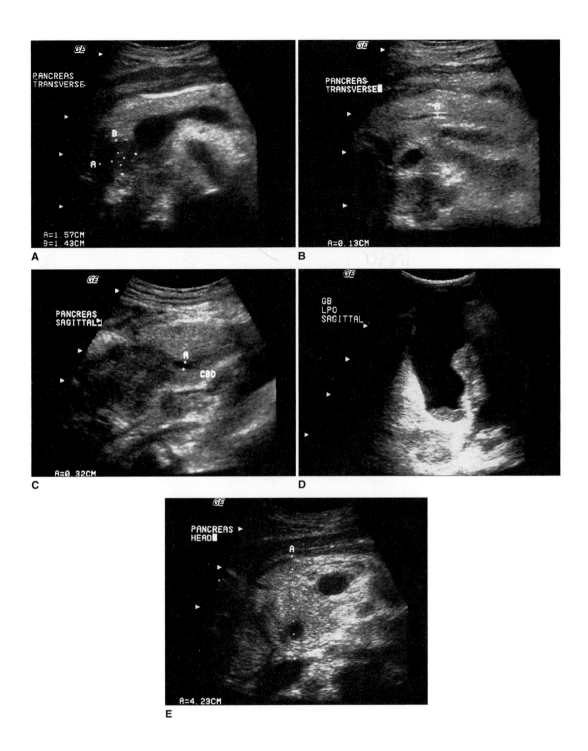

A

B

C

D

E

6. A 56-year-old male with a 1-week history of jaundice and pain has reported a 3-month history of nausea, vomiting, weight loss, and diarrhea. Based on the image above and the information provided, what are the sonographic findings?

_____

_____

_____

The Gastrointestinal Tract

KEY TERMS

Exercise 1

Match the following anatomic terms with their definitions.

1. _F_ alimentary canal or tract
2. _H_ cardiac orifice
3. _B_ duodenal bulb
4. _J_ gastrohepatic ligament
5. _D_ gastrophrenic, gastrosplenic, and lieno-renal ligaments
6. _C_ greater omentum
7. _M_ haustra
8. _A_ hepatic flexure
9. _N_ lesser omentum
10. _E_ mesentery
11. _I_ mesothelium
12. _I_ mucosa
13. _Q_ muscularis
14. _O_ pyloric canal
15. _S_ rugae
16. _P_ serosa
17. _K_ splenic flexure
18. _L_ submucosa
19. _R_ valvulae conniventes
20. _G_ villi

A. Ascending colon arises from the right lower quadrant to bend at this point to form the transverse colon
B. First part of the duodenum
C. Known as the "fatty apron" double fold of the peritoneum attached to the duodenum, stomach, and large intestine; helps support the greater curvature of the stomach
D. Helps support the greater curvature of the stomach
E. Projects from the parietal peritoneum and attaches to the small intestine anchoring it to the posterior abdominal wall
F. Also known as the digestive tract; includes the mouth, pharynx, esophagus, stomach, duodenum, and small and large intestine
G. Inner folds of the small intestine
H. Entrance of the esophagus into the stomach
I. First layer of bowel
J. Helps support the lesser curvature of the stomach
K. The transverse colon travels horizontally across the abdomen and bends at this point to form the descending colon
L. One of the layers of the bowel, under the mucosal layer; contains blood vessels and lymph channels
M. Normal segmentation of the wall of the colon
N. Suspends the stomach and duodenum from the liver; helps to support the lesser curvature of the stomach
O. Muscle that connects the stomach to the proximal duodenum
P. Fourth layer of bowel; thin, loose layer of connective tissue, surrounded by mesothelium covering the intraperitoneal bowel loops
Q. Third layer of bowel
R. Normal segmentation of the small bowel
S. Inner folds of the stomach wall
T. Fifth layer of bowel

Exercise 2

Match the following physiology and sonographic evaluation terms with their definitions.

1. __F__ abscess
2. __D__ absorption
3. __A__ cholecystokinin
4. __E__ gastrin
5. __C__ McBurney point
6. __B__ peristalsis
7. __G__ secretin

A. Hormone released by the presence of fat in the intestine; regulates gallbladder contraction and gastric emptying

B. Rhythmic dilatation and contraction of the gastrointestinal tract as food is propelled through it

C. Located by drawing a line from the right anterosuperior iliac spine to the umbilicus; at approximately the midpoint of this line lies the root of the appendix

D. Process of nutrient molecules passing through wall of intestine into blood or lymph system

E. Endocrine hormone released from the stomach (stimulates secretion of gastric acid)

F. Localized collection of pus surrounded by inflamed tissue

G. Released from small bowel as antacid; stimulates secretion of bicarbonate

Exercise 3

Match the following pathology terms with their definitions.

1. __J__ appendicolith
2. __H__ ascites
3. __L__ Crohn's disease
4. __B__ diverticulum
5. __A__ fecalith
6. __F__ hemorrhage
7. __C__ lymphoma
8. __G__ McBurney sign
9. __I__ Meckel's diverticulum
10. __D__ paralytic ileus
11. __K__ polyp
12. __E__ target sign

A. Calculus that may form around fecal material associated with appendicitis

B. A pouchlike herniation through the muscular wall of a tubular organ that occurs in the stomach, the small intestine, or most commonly, the colon

C. Malignancy of the lymph nodes, spleen, or liver

D. Dilated fluid-filled bowel loops without peristalsis

E. Characteristic of gastrointestinal wall thickening consisting of an echogenic center and a hypoechoic rim

F. Collection of blood

G. Site of maximal tenderness in the right lower quadrant; usually with appendicitis

H. Free fluid in the abdomen

I. Congenital sac or blind pouch found in the lower portion of the ileum

J. A fecalith or calcification located in the appendix

K. A small tumorlike growth that projects from a mucous membrane surface

L. Inflammation of the bowel, accompanied by abscess and bowel wall thickening

Exercise 4

Label the following illustrations.

1. The digestive system.

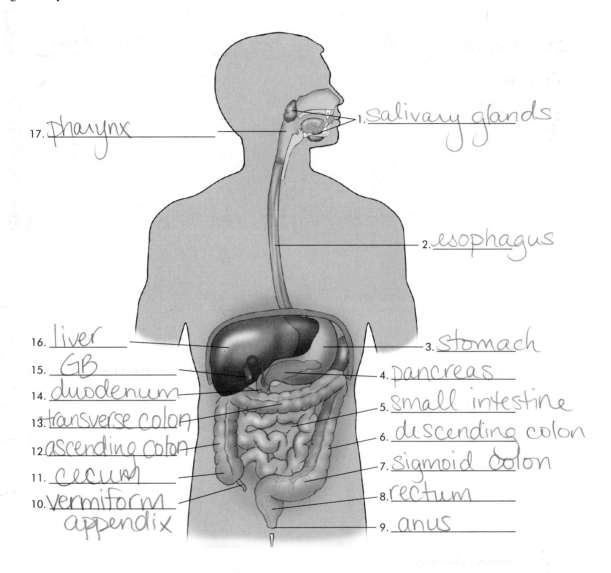

17. pharynx

1. salivary glands

2. esophagus

16. liver

15. GB

14. duodenum

13. transverse colon

12. ascending colon

11. cecum

10. vermiform appendix

3. stomach

4. pancreas

5. small intestine

6. descending colon

7. sigmoid colon

8. rectum

9. anus

2. The stomach.

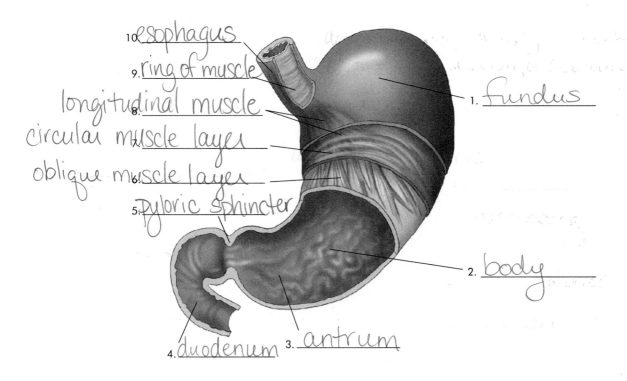

10. esophagus
9. ring of muscle
8. longitudinal muscle
7. circular muscle layer
6. oblique muscle layer
5. pyloric sphincter
4. duodenum
3. antrum
1. fundus
2. body

3. Vascular supply to the stomach.

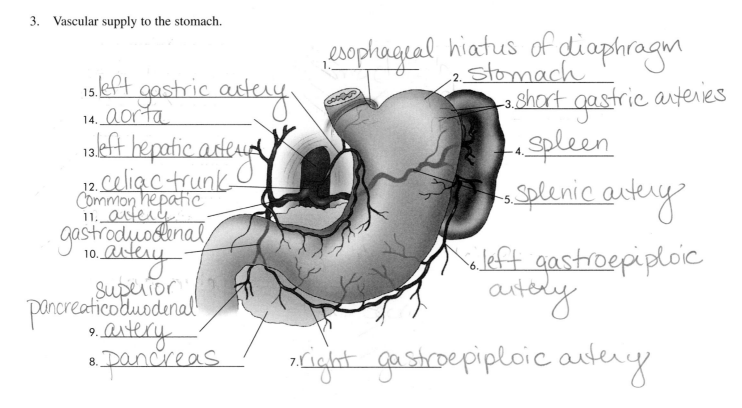

15. left gastric artery
14. aorta
13. left hepatic artery
12. celiac trunk
11. common hepatic artery
10. gastroduodenal artery
9. superior pancreaticoduodenal artery
8. pancreas

1. esophageal hiatus of diaphragm
2. stomach
3. short gastric arteries
4. spleen
5. splenic artery
6. left gastroepiploic artery
7. right gastroepiploic artery

4. The superior mesenteric artery.

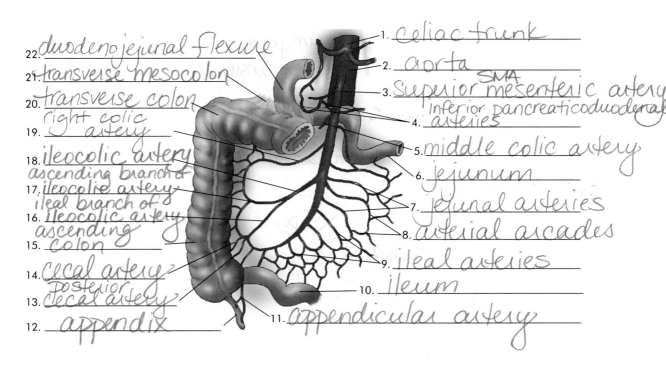

22. duodenojejunal flexure
21. transverse mesocolon
20. transverse colon
19. right colic artery
18. ileocolic artery
17. ascending branch of ileocolic artery
16. ileal branch of ileocolic artery
15. ascending colon
14. cecal artery
13. Posterior cecal artery
12. appendix

1. celiac trunk
2. aorta
3. superior mesenteric artery SMA
4. inferior pancreaticoduodenal arteries
5. middle colic artery
6. jejunum
7. jejunal arteries
8. arterial arcades
9. ileal arteries
10. ileum
11. appendicular artery

5. The inferior mesenteric artery.

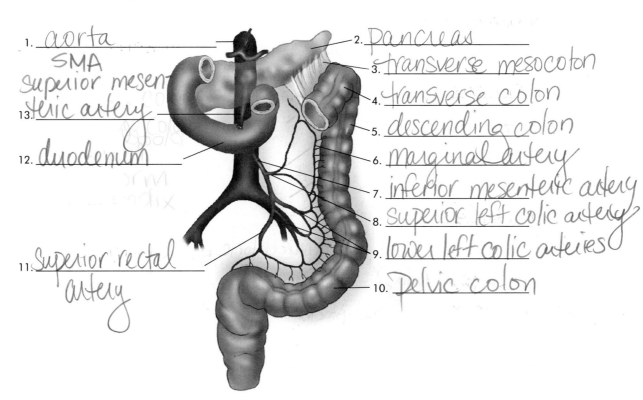

1. aorta
13. superior mesenteric artery SMA
12. duodenum
11. superior rectal artery

2. pancreas
3. transverse mesocolon
4. transverse colon
5. descending colon
6. marginal artery
7. inferior mesenteric artery
8. superior left colic artery
9. lower left colic arteries
10. pelvic colon

Exercise 5

Fill in the blank(s) with the word(s) that best completes the statements about the anatomy and physiology of the gastrointestinal tract.

1. List the sequential parts of the digestive system. _mouth, pharynx, esophagus, stomach, sm. int. (duodenum, jejunum, ileum), lg. int. (cecum, ascending colon, transverse colon, descending colon, rectum)_

2. The lower end of the esophagus is a circular muscle that acts as a sphincter, constricting the tube so that the entrance to the stomach, at the _cardiac orifice_, is generally closed. This helps to prevent gastric acid from moving up into the esophagus.

3. The pylorus is further subdivided into the _antrum_, the _pyloric_ canal, and the _pyloric_ sphincter.

4. The duodenum is subdivided into four segments: (1) _superior_, (2) _descending_, (3) _transverse_, and (4) _ascending_.

5. The duodenal bulb is peritoneal, supported by the hepatoduodenal ligament, and passes _anterior_ to the common bile duct, gastroduodenal artery, common hepatic artery, hepatic portal vein, and head of the pancreas.

6. The common bile duct joins the pancreatic duct to enter the _ampulla of Vater_.

7. The arteries that supply the esophagus include the inferior _thyroid_ branch of the _subclavian_ artery that supplies the upper esophagus, the descending _thoracic_ aorta that supplies the midesophagus, and the _gastric_ branch of the celiac axis and the left inferior _phrenic_ artery of the abdominal aorta that supplies the lower end of the esophagus.

8. The _mesentery_ outlines the small intestine and contains the superior mesenteric vessels, nerves, lymphatic glands, and fat between its two layers.

9. The nutrients are transported to the liver after they are absorbed by the _blood_; the liver processes and stores the nutrients.

10. The three layers of smooth muscle in the wall enable the stomach to mash and churn food and move it along with _peristalsis_.

11. Gastric glands secrete gastric juice containing _hydrochloric_ acid and _enzymes_.

12. The hormone _gastrin_, which is released by the stomach mucosa, stimulates gastric acid secretion.

13. Gastrointestinal hormones include _cholecystokinin_ and _secretin_.

14. _bacteria_ within the large intestine devour the chyme and in turn produce vitamins that can be absorbed and used by the body.

15. The most common laboratory data the sonographer may come across in a patient with gastrointestinal disease relate to the presence of _blood_ in the stool.

16. As a result of chronic blood loss, _anemia_ may be present.

SONOGRAPHIC EVALUATION

Exercise 6

Fill in the blank(s) with the word(s) that best completes the statements or provide a short answer about the sonographic techniques of the gastrointestinal tract.

1. Describe the technique used by sonographers to observe the upper gastrointestinal tract.

   See pg. 612

2. The _gastroesophageal_ junction is seen on the sagittal scan to the left of the midline as a bull's-eye or target-shaped structure anterior to the aorta, posterior to the left lobe of the liver, and inferior to the hemidiaphragm.

3. The gastric _antrum_ can be seen as a target shape in the midline.

4. Describe the measures that should be taken if a patient presents with a "cystic" mass in the left upper quadrant.

   _pg. 612_

5. The sonographer usually cannot see the small bowel with ultrasound; the valvulae conniventes may be seen as linear echo densities spaced 3 to 5 mm apart. This is called the "_keyboard sign_" and can be seen in the duodenum and jejunum.

6. The appendix is located on the abdominal wall under _McBurney's point_

PATHOLOGY

Exercise 7

Fill in the blank(s) with the word(s) that best completes the statements about the pathology of the gastrointestinal tract.

1. Movable intraluminal masses of congealed ingested materials that are seen on upper gastrointestinal radiographs are known as gastric _bezoars_.

2. A gastric _polyp_ is an outgrowth of tissue from the wall.

3. The most common tumor of the stomach is the _leiomyoma_

4. This is the result of luminal obstruction and inflammation, leading to ischemia of the vermiform appendix and is called _acute appendicitis_

5. The normal appendix can occasionally be visualized with gradual _compression_ on sonography.

6. The ultrasound pattern of acute appendicitis is characterized by a _target-shaped_ appearance of the appendix in transverse view.

7. A _mucocele_ designates gross enlargement of the appendix from accumulation of mucoid substance within the lumen.

8. _Crohn's disease_ is regional enteritis, a recurrent granulomatous inflammatory disease that affects the terminal ileum, colon, or both at any level.

Exercise 8

Provide a short answer for each question after evaluating the images.

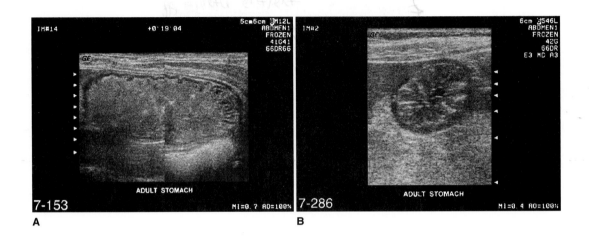

1. Identify the internal structures that are demonstrated in these images of the stomach.

    internal rugae of stomach

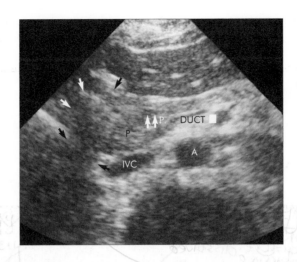

2. Identify the anatomic structure the arrows are pointing to.

fluid filled duodenum

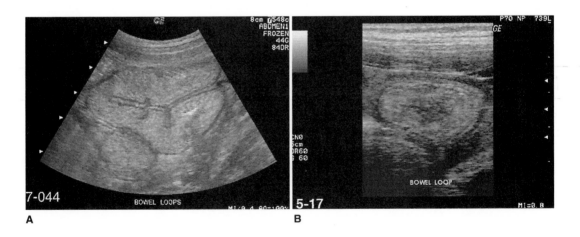

3. Describe the sonographic sign that is demonstrated in these images of the colon.

Target or bullseye sign
U/S images of prominent colon

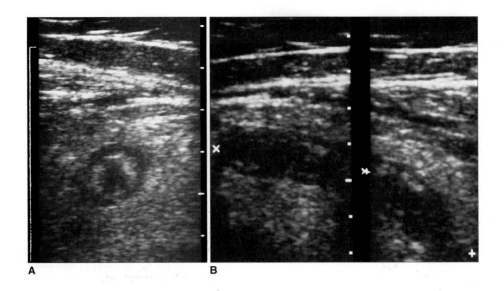

A   B

4. Identify the structure demonstrated in the images recorded over the right lower quadrant. Also identify the technique that should be used to further delineate this structure.

appendicitis – gradual compression should be used

10 The Urinary System

KEY TERMS

Exercise 1

Match the following anatomic terms with their definitions.

1. ___D___ afferent arteriole *into Glom*
2. ___H___ Bowman's capsule *part of filt contains H₂O, salts, gluc, urea, aas*
3. ___J___ cortex *outer parenc, corpuscle, prox+dist*
4. ___B___ Gerota's fascia *renal fascia w/ adrenals*
5. ___A___ hilus *where stuff ent + ext*
6. ___I___ major calyces *in b/t minors + pelvis*
7. ___E___ minor calyces *in b/t pyr's + majors*
8. ___C___ nephron *corp + tubule*
9. ___F___ renal corpuscle *consists of Bow + glom*
10. ___G___ renal pelvis *collects urine b4 ureter*
11. ___L___ retroperitoneum *space behind peritoneal lining*
12. ___K___ urethra *small membranous canal*

A. Area of kidney where vessels, ureter, and lymphatics enter and exit

B. Another term for the renal fascia; the kidney is covered by the renal capsule, perirenal fat, Gerota's fascia, and pararenal fat

C. Functional unit of the kidney; includes a renal corpuscle and a renal tubule

D. Carries blood into the glomerulus of the nephron

E. Receive urine from the renal pyramids; form the border of the renal sinus

F. Part of the nephron that consists of Bowman's capsule and the glomerulus

G. Area in the midportion of the kidney that collects urine before entering the ureter

H. Part of the filtration process; contains water, salts, glucose, urea, and amino acids

I. Receives urine from the minor calyces to convey to the renal pelvis

J. Refers to the outer parenchyma of the kidney that contains the renal corpuscle and proximal and distal convoluted tubules of the nephron

K. Small, membranous canal that excretes urine from the urinary bladder

L. Space behind the peritoneal lining of the abdominal cavity

Exercise 2

Match the following anatomic and physiologic terms with their definitions.

1. ___E___ arcuate arteries *vessels found at pyr. bases*
2. ___M___ blood urea nitrogen (BUN) *measures nit waste (along w/ creat)*
3. ___G___ calyx *part of collecting syst adj. to pyr + major calyx*
4. ___N___ creatinine *measures ability of kidneys to get rid of wastes*
5. ___K___ efferent arteriole *supplies peritubular cap st convoluted tubules*
6. ___H___ glomerulus *part of filt. syst.*

A. Portion of a renal tubule lying between the proximal and distal convoluted portions; reabsorption of fluid, sodium, and chloride occurs in the proximal convoluted tubule and the loop of Henle

B. Convey urine to the minor calyces

C. Retroperitoneal structures that exit the kidney to carry urine to the urinary bladder

D. Refers to the inner portion of the renal parenchyma that contains the loop of Henle

E. Small vessels found at the base of the renal pyramids

99

Chapter 10 The Urinary System

7. ___O___ homeostasis *maintenance*

8. ___A___ loop of Henle *b/t prox + dist reabs of water NaCl here*

9. ___D___ medulla *inner portion of parenc includes loop of H*

10. ___J___ Morison's pouch *rt. post subhepatic space loc'd ant to kid + inf to liver where fluid accumulat*

11. ___B___ pyramids *convey urine to calyces*

12. ___L___ renal hilum *where vessels + ureter ent/ext*

13. ___I___ renal sinus *central area inc. calyces,*
    ___P___ *pelvis, vessels, fat, nerves + lymph*

14. _____ specific gravity *measure dissolved material in urine*

15. ___C___ ureters *retroperitoneal structs that exit kid + carry urine to blad*

16. ___F___ urinary bladder *muscular retro- peritoneal org reservoir 4 urine*

F. Muscular retroperitoneal organ that serves as a reservoir for urine

G. Part of the collecting system adjacent to the pyramid that collects urine and is connected to the major calyx

H. Part of the filtration process in the kidney

I. Central area of the kidney that includes the calyces, renal pelvis, renal vessels, fat, nerves, and lymphatics

J. Right posterior subhepatic space located anterior to the kidney and inferior to the liver where fluid may accumulate

K. Blood from this structure supplies the peritubular capillaries, which also supply the convoluted tubules

L. Area in the midportion of the kidney where the renal vessels and ureter enter and exit

M. Measures amount of nitrogenous waste (along with creatinine); waste products accumulate in the blood when kidneys malfunction

N. One of the laboratory tests used to measure the ability of the kidney to get rid of waste; waste products accumulate in the blood when kidneys malfunction

O. Maintenance of normal body physiology

P. Laboratory tests that measure how much dissolved material is present in the urine

Exercise 3

Match the following physiologic, sonographic evaluations and pathologic terms with their definitions.

1. ___G___ columns of Bertin *bands of tis. separate pyramids*

2. ___A___ dromedary hump *bulge on lat border*

3. ___C___ ectopic kidney *not normal place usu in pelvis*

4. ___I___ horseshoe kidney *joined by isthmus at lower*

5. ___H___ hydronephrosis *dilation of renal colltg syst*

6. ___J___ renal agenesis *interruptn develpmt absence of kid*

7. ___E___ renal capsule *1st layer on kid tough fibrous covering*

8. ___F___ splaying *widening*

9. ___B___ tadpole sign *narrow bands of acoust. shadowing post to margins of cyst along lat borders of enhancement*

10. ___D___ urolithiasis → *stone in urin system*

A. Normal variant that occurs on the left kidney as a bulge on the lateral border

B. Seen as narrow bands of acoustic shadowing posterior to the margins of the cyst along the lateral borders of enhancement

C. Located outside of the normal position, most often in the pelvic cavity

D. Stone within the urinary system

E. First layer adjacent to the kidney that forms a tough, fibrous covering

F. Widening

G. Bands of cortical tissue that separate the renal pyramids; a prominent column of Bertin may mimic a renal mass on sonography

H. Dilation of the renal collecting system

I. Congenital malformation in which both kidneys are joined together by an isthmus, most commonly at the lower poles

J. Interruption in the normal development of the kidney resulting in absence of the kidney; may be unilateral or bilateral

medulla vs. sinus
hilus vs. renal hilum
hydro-Cecilia

ANATOMY AND PHYSIOLOGY

Exercise 4

Label the following illustrations.

1. The kidney cut longitudinally.

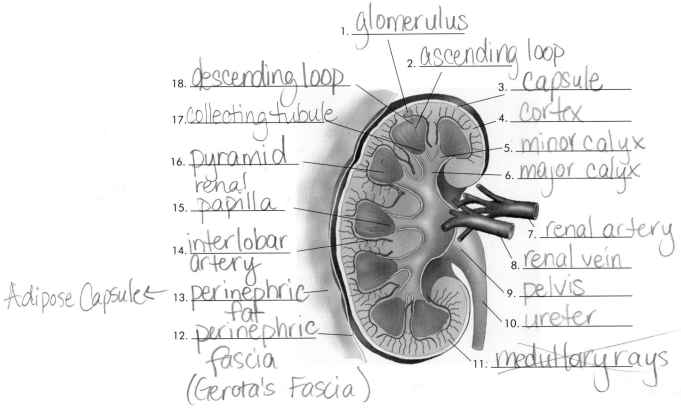

1. glomerulus
2. ascending loop
3. capsule
4. cortex
5. minor calyx
6. major calyx
7. renal artery
8. renal vein
9. pelvis
10. ureter
11. medullary rays
12. perinephric fascia (Gerota's Fascia)
13. perinephric fat — Adipose Capsule
14. interlobar artery
15. renal papilla
16. pyramid
17. collecting tubule
18. descending loop

2. Anatomic structures related to the anterior surfaces of the kidneys.

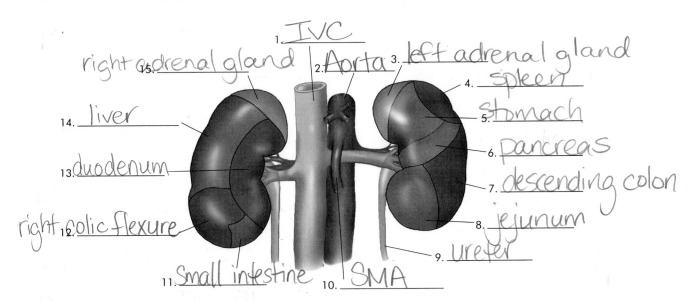

1. IVC
2. Aorta
3. left adrenal gland
4. spleen
5. stomach
6. pancreas
7. descending colon
8. jejunum
9. ureter
10. SMA
11. small intestine
12. right colic flexure
13. duodenum
14. liver
15. right adrenal gland

3. Vascular relationship of the great vessels and their tributaries to the kidneys.

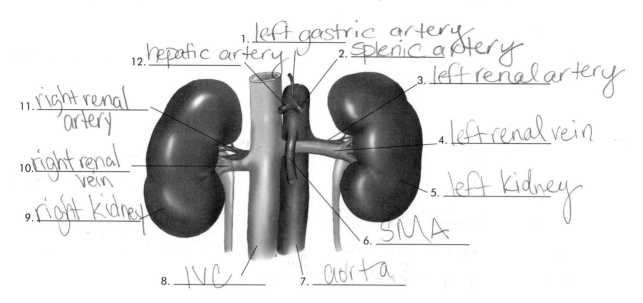

1. left gastric artery
12. hepatic artery
2. splenic artery
3. left renal artery
11. right renal artery
4. left renal vein
10. right renal vein
5. left kidney
9. right kidney
6. SMA
8. IVC
7. aorta

Exercise 5

Fill in the blank(s) with the word(s) that best completes the statements or provide a short answer about the anatomy of the kidney.

1. The urinary system has two principal functions: excreting _wastes_ and regulating the composition of _blood_.

2. The right kidney lies slightly _lower_ ~~more inferior~~ than the left kidney because the large right lobe of the _liver_ pushes it _inferiorly_.

3. The kidneys move with respiration; on deep inspiration, both kidneys move _down_ approximately 1 inch.

4. Within the hilus of the kidney are other _vascular_ structures, a ureter, and the _lymphatics_.

5. A fibrous capsule called the _true_ _renal capsule_ surrounds the kidney.

6. Outside of this fibrous capsule is a covering of ~~perirenal~~ _adipose capsule/ perirenal fat/perinephric_.

7. The ~~Gerota's~~ _Perinephric fascia_ fascia surrounds the perinephric fat and encloses the kidneys and adrenal glands.

8. The renal fascia, known as _Gerota's_ fascia, surrounds the true capsule and perinephric fat.

9. The medullary substance consists of a series of striated conical masses, called the renal _pyramids_.

10. A nephron consists of two main structures, a renal _corpuscle_ and a renal _tubule_.

11. Nephrons _filter_ the blood and produce _urine_.

12. The renal corpuscle consists of a network of capillaries, called the _glomerulus_, which is surrounded by a cuplike structure known as _Bowman's capsule_.

13. Blood flows into the glomerulus through a small _afferent_ arteriole and leaves the glomerulus through an _efferent_ arteriole.

14. There are three constrictions along the ureter's course:

   — _where ureter leaves renal pelvis_

   — _where it is kinked as it crosses the pelvic brim_

   — _where it pierces the bladder wall_

15. The main renal artery is a lateral branch of the aorta and arises just inferior to the _SM_ artery.

16. The renal vein drains into the _lateral walls_ of the inferior vena cava.

Exercise 6

Fill in the blank(s) with the word(s) that best completes the statements or provide a short answer about the physiology of the kidney.

1. The urinary system is located posterior to the peritoneum lining the abdominal cavity in an area called the _retroperitoneum_

2. The kidneys adjust the amounts of _water_ and _electrolytes_ leaving the body so that these equal the amounts of substances entering the body.

3. The principal metabolic waste products are _water_ , _CO_2_ , and nitrogenous wastes.

4. Both urea and uric acid are carried away from the liver into the kidneys by the _vascular_ system.

5. The presence of an acute infection causes _hematuria_ , _RBC's_ in the urine; pyuria causes _pus_ in the urine.

6. The pH refers to the strength of the urine as a partly _acidic_ or _alkaline_ solution.

7. The _specific gravity_ is the measurement of the kidney's ability to concentrate urine.

8. The specific gravity is especially _low_ in cases of renal failure, glomerular nephritis, and pyelonephritis.

9. A decreased _hematocrit_ occurs with acute hemorrhagic processes secondary to disease or blunt trauma.

10. Impairment of renal function and increased protein catabolism result in BUN _elevation_ that is relative to the degree of renal impairment and rate of urea nitrogen excreted by the kidneys.

SONOGRAPHIC EVALUATION

Exercise 7

Fill in the blank(s) with the word(s) that best completes the statements or provide a short answer about the sonographic techniques of the kidney.

1. The renal parenchyma surrounds the fatty central renal sinus, which contains the:

   1 _calyces_
   2 _infundibula_
   3 _pelvis_
   4 _vessels_
   5 _lymphatics_

2. Dilation of the collecting system has also been noted in _pregnant_ patients, especially the right kidney.

3. The _parenchyma_ is the area from the renal sinus to the outer renal surface.

4. The _arcuate_ and _interlobar_ arteries and are best demonstrated as intense specular echoes in cross-section or oblique section at the corticomedullary junction.

5. The _cortex_ generally is echo producing, whereas the medullary pyramids are _hypoechoic_.

6. The cortex and medullary pyramids are separated from each other by bands of cortical tissue, called _columns of Bertin_ that extend inward to the renal sinus.

7. The _crura_ lie posterior to the renal arteries and should be identified by their lack of pulsations and absence of Doppler flow.

8. The _apex_ of the pyramid points toward the sinus, and the _base_ lies adjacent to the renal cortex.

9. The _dromedary hump_ is a cortical bulge that occurs on the lateral border of the kidney, typically more on the left side.

10. A _junctional parenchymal defect /cortical junction defect_ is a triangular, echogenic area in the upper pole of the renal parenchyma that can be seen during normal scanning.

11. In a patient with a _horseshoe kidney_, there is fusion of the kidneys during fetal development that almost invariably involves the _lower_ poles.

12. A cystic mass presents sonographically with several characteristic features:

   -Smooth thin well-defined border, round or oval shape, sharp interface b/t cyst + renal parenchyma, anechoic + increased posterior acoustic enhancement

13. A cystlike enlargement of the lower end of the ureter is called _ureterocele._

Exercise 8

Fill in the blank(s) with the word(s) that best completes the statements or provide a short answer about the pathology of the kidney.

1. Sonographically, it is difficult to differentiate between a _Septated_ cyst and a small adjacent cortical cyst.

2. The parapelvic cyst is found in the _renal hilum_, but does not communicate with the renal collecting system.

3. There are four forms of autosomal recessive polycystic kidney disease:

   perinatal

   neonatal

   infantile

   juvenile

4. Discuss the characteristics of autosomal dominant polycystic kidney disease.

   bilateral, mult. cysts in cortex & medulla, present in 4th or 5th decade, by 6th - 50% will be in end stage renal disease; present w/ pain, HT, palpable mass, hematuria, H/A, UTI & renal insufficiency

5. Usually a(n) _abnormal_ renal contour is the first finding that a mass may be present and requires further investigation.

6. Define the characteristics of renal cell carcinoma.

   Most common of all renal tumors (85%), 2x more common in males esp. in 6th or 7th decade, hematuria, flank pain & palpable mass, usually unilateral, increased w/ von Hippel-Lindau & long term dialysis

7. One of the most common benign renal tumors is called _adenoma_.

8. An uncommon benign renal tumor composed mainly of fat cells and commonly found in the renal cortex is

   angiomyolipoma

9. _lipoma_ appears as a well-defined echogenic mass found more often in females.

10. Sonographic findings include one or more fluid spaces at the _corticomedullary_ junction that corresponds to the distribution of the renal pyramids.

11. Although the kidneys appear enlarged with a highly echogenic renal sinus, the intrarenal anatomy is preserved with uniform loss of renal tissue in patients with _renal atrophy_.

12. The most common medical renal disease that produces acute renal failure is _acute tubular nephrosis_.

13. Chronic renal disease is loss of renal _function_ as a result of disease, most commonly parenchymal disease.

14. There are three primary types of chronic renal failure: _nephron_, _vascular_, and _interstitial_ abnormalities.

15. _hydronephrosis_ is when the dilated pyelocalyceal system appears as separation of the renal sinus echoes by fluid-filled areas that conform anatomically to the infundibula, calyces, and renal pelvis.

16. A localized hydronephrosis occurs as a result of _strictures_, calculi, _focal masses_, or _duplicate collecting system_

17. Hydronephrosis with a dilated ureter and bladder indicates obstruction of the _ureterovesical_ junction or of the _urethra_.

18. If hydronephrosis is suspected, the sonographer should evaluate the _bladder_.

19. Name two conditions that might mimic a hydronephrosis.
extrarenal pelvis, peripelvic cyst,

20. Describe the sonographic findings in acute obstruction.
R.I greater than .70 for 48-72 hours no ureteral jet or decreased flow if only partially obstructed

21. Ureteral jets are best visualized by _color Doppler_ imaging.

22. This occurs when pus is found within the obstructed renal system and is known as _pyonephrosis_.

23. _Nephrocalcinosis_ is a diffuse foci of calcium deposits, which is usually located in the medulla and infrequently can also be seen in the renal cortex.

24. A renal _infarction_ occurs when part of the tissue undergoes necrosis after the cessation of the blood supply, usually as a result of artery occlusion.

Exercise 9

Fill in the blank(s) with the word(s) that best completes the statements or provide a short answer about renal transplantation.

1. The major problem encountered with renal transplantation is _____.

2. Early after surgery, a baseline sonographic examination is performed to determine _____,

   _____, and _____.

3. Perirenal fluid collections, such as _____, _____, _____, or

   _____, can be diagnosed reliably and differentiated from acute rejection.

4. _____ rejection occurs within hours of transplantation and is caused by vasculitis leading to thrombosis and usually the loss of the graft.

5. _____ rejection occurs within days to months after transplant.

6. _____ rejection causes include preformed antibodies, immune complexes, and cell-mediated responses.

7. _____ rejection can occur months after transplantation with gradual onset.

8. Sonographic findings in rejection include:

   _____

   _____

   _____

9. The incidence of ATN is usually higher in _____ transplants than in _____ transplants or in kidneys that undergo warm ischemia or prolonged preservation, kidneys with multiple renal arteries, or kidneys obtained from elderly donors.

10. Early signs of obstruction are _____ or severe _____ in a patient with satisfactory renal volumes.

11. Renal artery stenosis exhibits a _____ jet with distal turbulence.

12. This Doppler is not angle dependent and has a greater sensitivity to detect blood flow and is called

    _____.

Exercise 10

Fill in the blank(s) with the word(s) that best completes the statements or provide a short answer about urolithiasis and bladder pathology.

1. The initial clinical sign of a kidney stone is extreme _pain_, typically followed by cramping on the side that the stone is located on; nausea and vomiting may also occur.

2. Renal stones are very _echogenic_ foci with posterior acoustic shadowing.

3. If the stone causes obstruction, there will be _hydronephrosis_ and, depending upon the location of the stone, the ureter may be dilated _superior_ to the level of obstruction.

4. _Congenital diverticulum_ entails herniation of all layers of the bladder wall and is located in the posterior angle of the trigone.

5. _Acquired_ diverticula are herniations of only the two inner layers through the muscle layer.

6. _Cystitis_ is usually secondary to another condition that causes stasis of urine in the bladder.

7. The majority of bladder tumors in adults are _TC_ carcinoma.

Exercise 11

Provide a short answer for each question after evaluating the images.

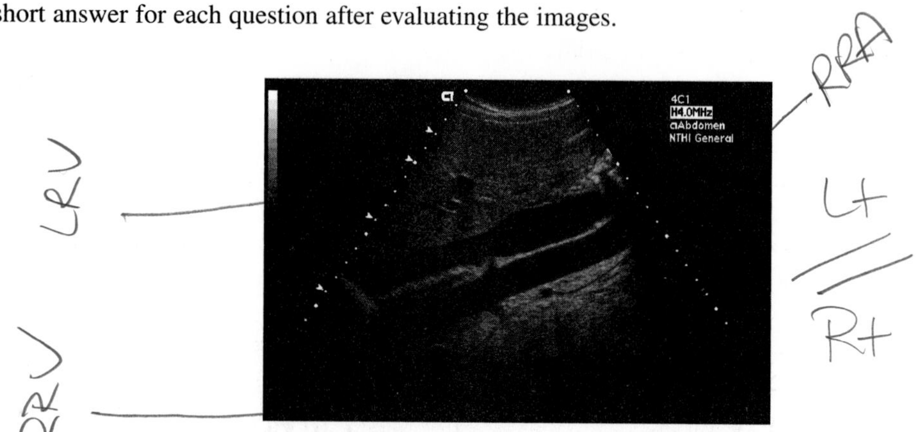

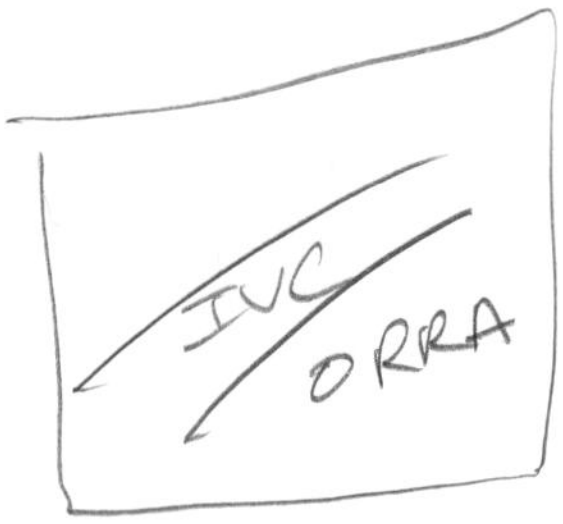

From Siemens Medical Solutions USA, Inc.

1. List the anatomic structures shown to arise from the inferior vena cava in this coronal image.

Renal veins branch off IVC

renal arteries off aorta inferior to SMA

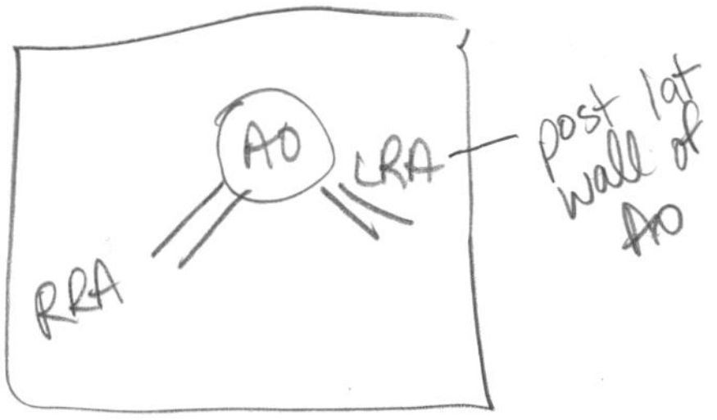

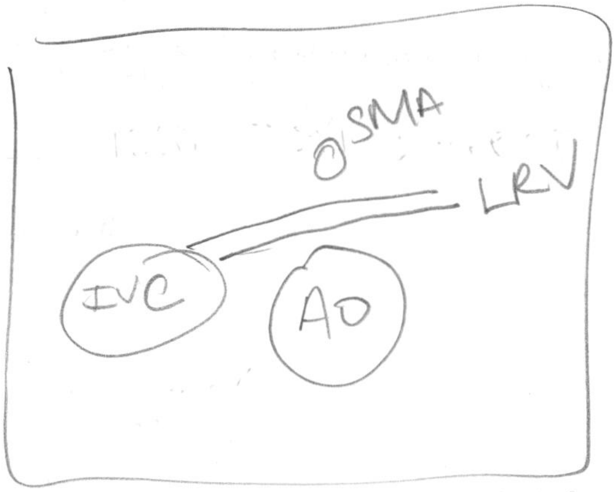

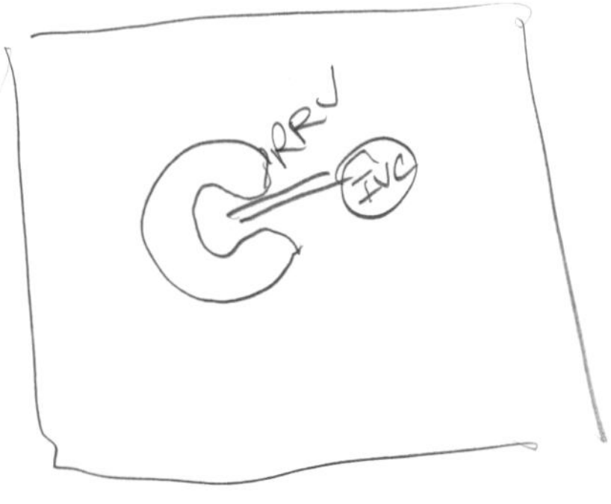

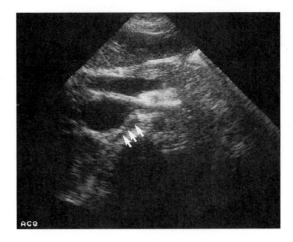

2. Identify the anatomic structure the arrows are pointing to.

   Crura of diaphragm

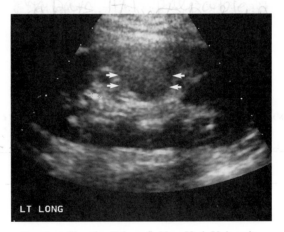

LT LONG

Courtesy Shpetim Telegrafi, New York University.

★ *Prominent*

3. Determine what anatomic variation of the kidney the arrows are pointing to.

   Column of Bertin° - check book

   almost looks like a mass

   Renal lobulations - irregular shaped border
   duplex collecting syst - 2 sinuses, faceless in trut
   double urethral jets
   Ren. Sinus lipomatosis - bright bigger sinus

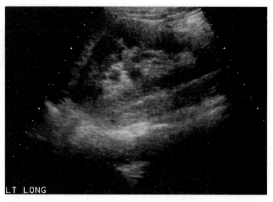

Courtesy Shpetim Telegrafi, New York University.

4. Identify the anatomic variant demonstrated in this image.

    Dromedary hump

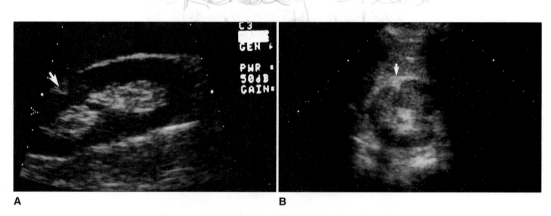

A   B

Courtesy Shpetim Telegrafi, New York University.

5. Name the structure that the arrow is pointing to along the anterior wall of the kidney.

    junctional parenchymal defect/
    cortical junction defect

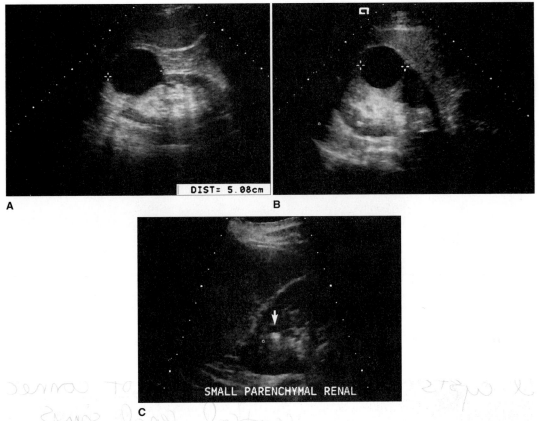

A   DIST= 5.08cm   **B**

C   SMALL PARENCHYMAL RENAL

Courtesy Shpetim Telegrafi, New York University.

6. A 75-year-old male was experiencing right upper quadrant pain. An incidental finding was seen on the right kidney, which most likely represents:

Right upper pole renal cyst - the incidental
Renal Stone - causing the pain

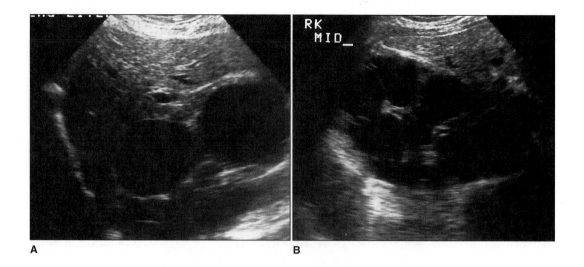

A   B

7. A 45-year-old female was in end-stage renal failure. Describe the pathology her ultrasound revealed. Explain how the sonographer can be certain that the lesion is not hydronephrosis.

enlarged kid
Polycystic Renal Disease
all cysts are distinct + do not connect w/
central renal sinus

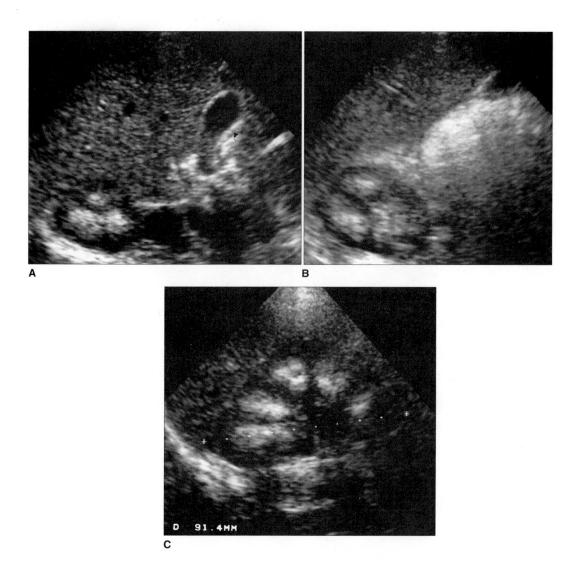

A

B

C

8. A 6-year-old male presents with multiple urinary tract infections. Describe what is demonstrated on the sonogram.

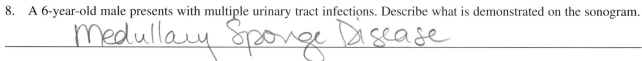

Medullary Sponge Disease

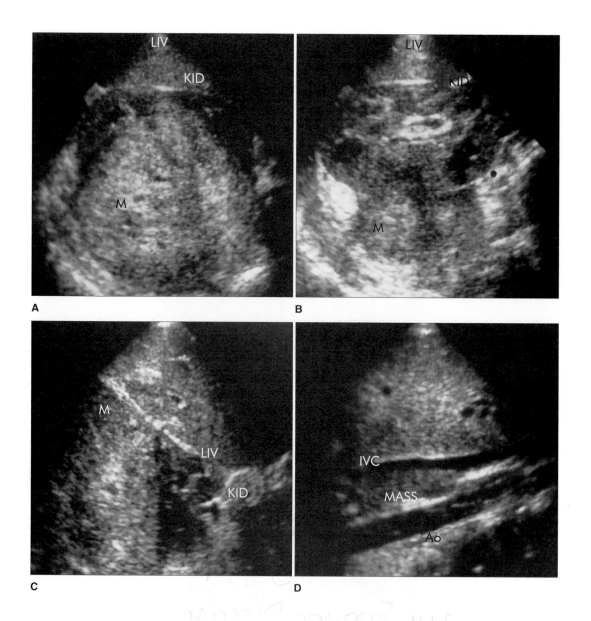

A

B

C

D

9. A 14-month-old child presents with a palpable right-sided mass, decreased appetite, and lethargy. The sonographic findings are:

Wilm's Tumor

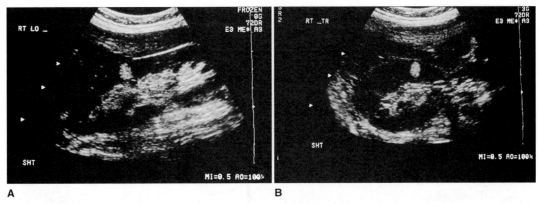

Courtesy Shpetim Telegrafi, New York University.

10. A 43-year-old female presented for an abdominal ultrasound examination. Name the abnormality that this image demonstrates.

angiomyolipoma

large hyperechoic fat that the debri

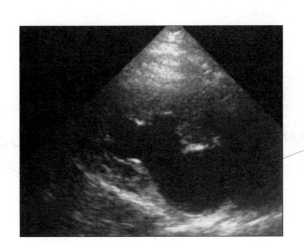

looks like cystic area

11. Does this patient have hydronephrosis? Explain why or why not.

extrarenal pelvis

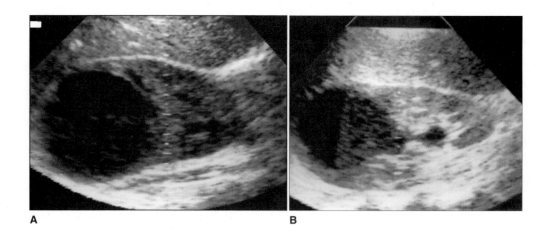

12. A middle-aged male presents with fever and flank pain for 1 week. The ultrasound shows:

Pyonephrosis

large complex mass w/ a fluid +/or debris level

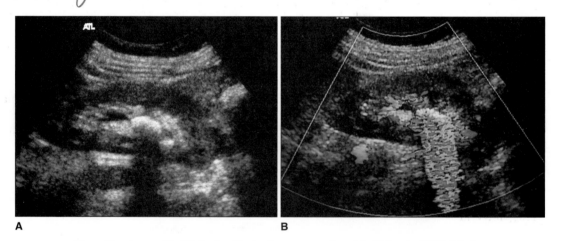

From Henningsen C: *Clinical guide to ultrasonography,* ed 1, St Louis, 2004, Mosby.

13. A 54-year-old female presents with right flank pain. The sonogram demonstrates:

Stone or renal calculi

11 | The Spleen

KEY TERMS

Exercise 1

Match the following anatomic terms with their definitions.

1. _____ accessory spleen

2. _____ gastrosplenic ligament

3. _____ intraperitoneal

4. _____ left hypochondrium

5. _____ lienorenal ligament

6. _____ lymph

7. _____ phrenocolic ligament

8. _____ polysplenia

9. _____ reticuloendothelial

10. _____ splenic agenesis

11. _____ splenic artery

12. _____ splenic hilum

13. _____ splenic vein

14. _____ wandering spleen

A. The ligament between the spleen and the colon

B. Within the peritoneal cavity

C. Complete absence of the spleen

D. Condition where there is more than one spleen

E. Results from the failure of fusion of separate splenic masses forming on the dorsal mesogastrium; most commonly found in the splenic hilum or along the splenic vessels or associated ligaments

F. Leaves the splenic hilum, travels transversely through the upper abdomen to join with the superior mesenteric vein to form the main portal vein; serves as the posterior medial border of the pancreas

G. Located in the middle of the spleen; site where vessels and lymph nodes enter and exit the spleen

H. Spleen that has migrated from its normal location in the left upper quadrant

I. One of the ligaments between the stomach and spleen that helps to hold the spleen in place

J. An alkaline fluid found in the lymphatic vessels

K. One of the ligaments that help to hold the spleen in its place (attachment of spleen to kidney)

L. Certain phagocytic cells (found in the liver and spleen) make up the reticuloendothelial system (RES); plays a role in the synthesis of blood proteins and hematopoiesis

M. Left upper quadrant of the abdomen that contains the left lobe of the liver, spleen, and stomach

N. Branch of the celiac axis; tortuous course towards the spleen; serves as the superior border of the pancreas

Exercise 2

Match the following physiologic terms with their definitions.

1. _____ culling
2. _____ erythrocyte
3. _____ hematopoiesis
4. _____ hemoglobin
5. _____ hemosiderin
6. _____ leukopenia
7. _____ malpighian corpuscles
8. _____ phagocytosis
9. _____ pitting
10. _____ red pulp
11. _____ splenic sinuses
12. _____ white blood cells
13. _____ white pulp

A. Found in the white pulp; lymph node in the spleen
B. Pigment released from hemoglobin process
C. Blood cell production
D. Defend the body by destroying invading microorganisms and their toxins
E. Consists of reticular cells and fibers (cords of Billroth), surrounds the splenic sinuses
F. Red blood cell
G. Abnormal decrease of white blood corpuscles; may be drug induced
H. Consists of lymphatic tissue and lymphatic follicles
I. Process by which the spleen removes nuclei from blood cells without destroying the erythrocytes
J. Process by which the spleen removes red blood cells as they pass through
K. Oxygen-binding protein found in red blood cells
L. Long irregular channels lined by endothelial cells or flattened reticular cells
M. Process by which the red pulp destroys the degenerating red blood cells

Exercise 3

Match the following pathologic terms with their definitions.

1. _____ amyloidosis
2. _____ autoimmune hemolytic anemia
3. _____ Gaucher's disease
4. _____ hemolytic anemia
5. _____ Hodgkin's disease
6. _____ infarction
7. _____ mononucleosis
8. _____ non-Hodgkin's lymphoma
9. _____ polycythemia
10. _____ polycythemia vera

A. An interruption in the blood supply to an area that may lead to necrosis of the area
B. Chronic, life-shortening condition of unknown cause involving bone marrow elements; characterized by an increase in red blood cell mass and hemoglobin concentration
C. An acute infection caused by the Epstein-Barr virus that most commonly affects teenagers and young adults; symptoms include fever, sore throat, enlarged lymph nodes, abnormal lymphocysts, and hepatosplenomegaly
D. A malignant disease of lymphoid tissue seen in increased frequency in individuals more than 50 years of age
E. Group of hereditary anemias occurring in Asian and Mediterranean populations
F. Condition in which erythrocytes assume a spheroid shape; hereditary
G. One of the storage diseases in which fat and proteins are deposited abnormally in the body

11. _____ sickle cell anemia

12. _____ sickle cell crisis

13. _____ spherocytosis

14. _____ splenomegaly

15. _____ thalassemia

H. An excess of red blood cells

I. A malignant disease that involves lymphoid tissue

J. Condition in sickle cell anemia in which the sickled cells interfere with oxygen transport, obstruct capillary blood flow, and cause fever and severe pain in the joints and abdomen

K. A metabolic disorder marked by amyloid deposits in organs and tissue

L. Enlargement of the spleen

M. Inherited disorder transmitted as an autosomal recessive trait that causes an abnormality of the globin genes in hemoglobin

N. Anemia resulting from hemolysis of red blood cells

O. Anemia caused by antibodies produced by the patient's own immune system

ANATOMY AND PHYSIOLOGY

Exercise 4

Label the following illustrations.

1. Sagittal plane of the spleen and left kidney.

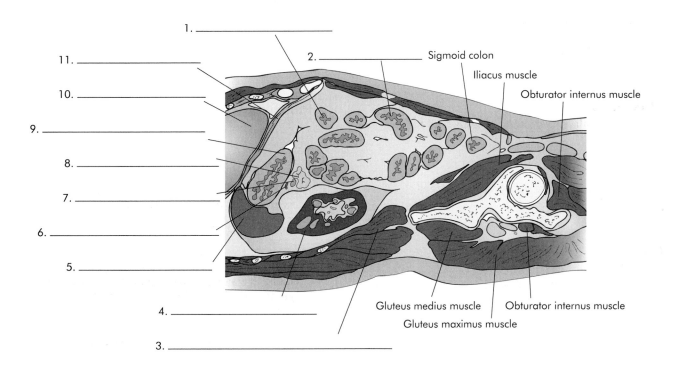

1. _____
2. _____ Sigmoid colon
Iliacus muscle
Obturator internus muscle
11. _____
10. _____
9. _____
8. _____
7. _____
6. _____
5. _____
4. _____
3. _____
Gluteus medius muscle   Obturator internus muscle
Gluteus maximus muscle

2. Anterior view of the spleen as it lies in the left hypochondrium.

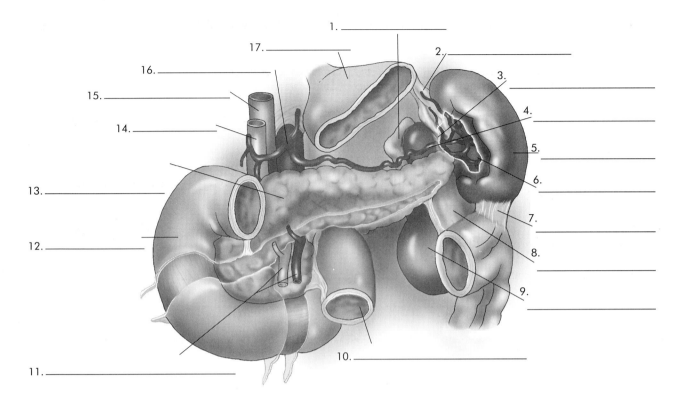

1. _____
17. _____
16. _____
15. _____
14. _____
13. _____
12. _____
11. _____
2. _____
3. _____
4. _____
5. _____
6. _____
7. _____
8. _____
9. _____
10. _____

3. The splenic vein leaves the hilum of the spleen.

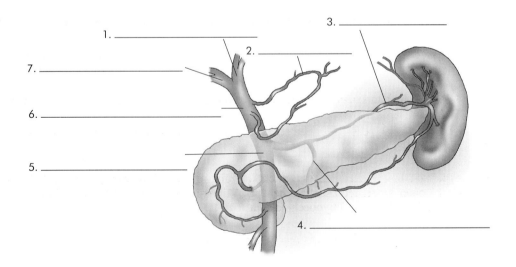

1. _____
7. _____
6. _____
5. _____
3. _____
2. _____
4. _____

Exercise 5

Fill in the blank(s) with the word(s) that best completes the statements about the anatomy and physiology of the spleen.

1. The spleen is part of the reticuloendothelial system and is the largest single mass of _____ tissue in the body.

2. The spleen is an _____ organ covered with peritoneum over its entire extent except for a small area at its hilum, where the vascular structures and lymph nodes are located.

3. The spleen is normally measured with ultrasound on a longitudinal image from the _____ margin to the

   _____ margin at the long axis.

4. _____ may occur as part of asplenic or polysplenia syndromes in association with complex cardiac malformations, bronchopulmonary abnormalities, or visceral heterotaxis.

5. An _____ is usually found near the hilum or inferior border of the spleen, but has been reported elsewhere in the abdominal cavity.

6. The _____ indicates the percentage of red blood cells per volume of blood.

7. The term _____ indicates bacteria in the bloodstream.

8. The increase in the number of white cells present in the blood that is usually a typical finding of infection

   is called _____.

SONOGRAPHIC EVALUATION

Exercise 6

Fill in the blank(s) with the word(s) that best completes the statements about the sonographic techniques of the spleen.

1. Sonographically the splenic parenchyma should have a fine homogeneous _____ as is seen within the liver parenchyma.

2. Systemic venous congestion is found in cardiac decompensation involving the _____ side of the heart.

3. In infants and children in crisis, the earlier stage of _____, the spleen is enlarged with marked congestion of the red pulp.

4. Patients with hepatosplenic _____ may show irregular masses within the spleen, the "wheels-within-wheels" pattern, with the outer wheel representing the ring of fibrosis surrounding the inner echogenic wheel of inflammatory cells and a central hypoechoic area.

5. If the patient has severe left upper quadrant pain secondary to trauma, a splenic _____ or

   _____ should be considered.

Exercise 7

Provide a short answer for each question after evaluating the images.

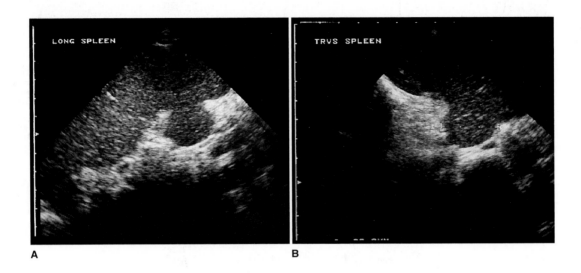

A   B

1. A young male with vague epigastric pain showed this anomaly on the ultrasound examination. In this scan over the left upper quadrant, the findings are:

_____

_____

_____

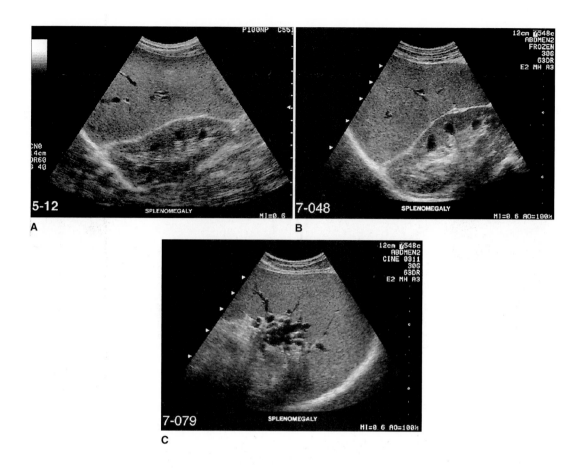

2. These images over the left upper quadrant demonstrate this feature.

_____

_____

_____

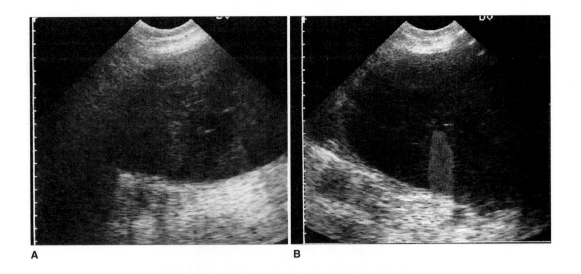

A   B

3. A patient with left upper quadrant pain and fever for 1 week had an ultrasound. The sonographic findings are:

_____

_____

_____

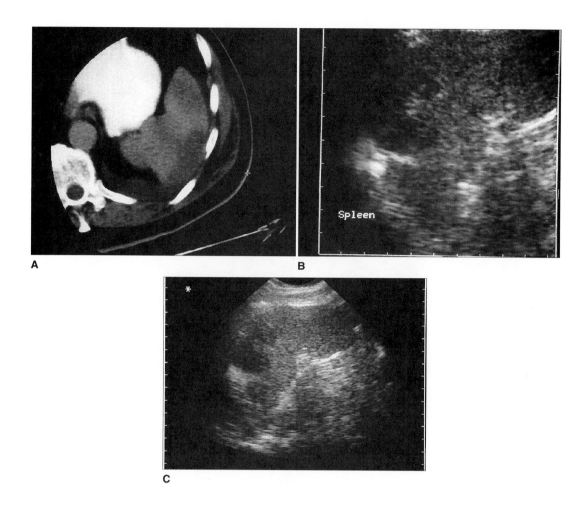

A

B

C

4. Describe the abnormality in the spleen in this patient with sickle cell anemia.

_____

_____

_____

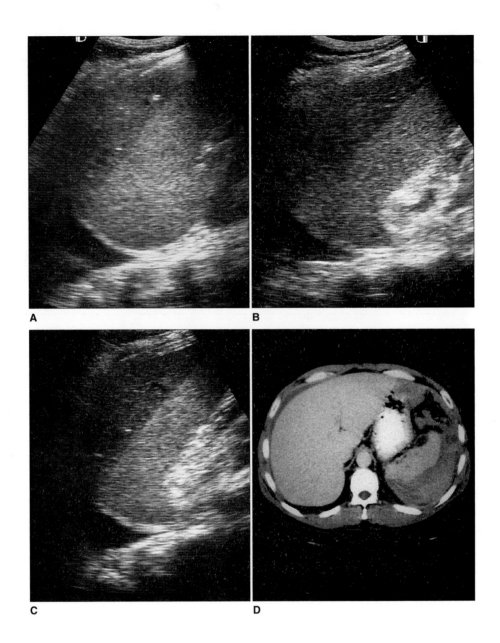

5.   A 20-year-old presents to the ER after a bicycle accident. Your findings are:

_____

_____

_____

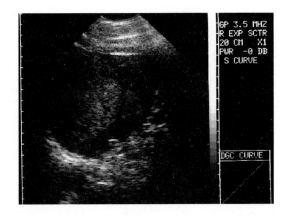

6. This benign finding in the spleen was present at the time of the abdominal scan for portal hypertension. The abnormality shown is:

_____

_____

_____

12 | The Retroperitoneum

KEY TERMS

Exercise 1
Match the following anatomic and physiologic terms with their definitions.

1. _____ Addison's disease

2. _____ adrenocorticotropic hormone (ACTH)

3. _____ cortex

4. _____ false pelvis

5. _____ hyperplasia

6. _____ medulla

7. _____ pheochromocytoma

A. Outer parenchyma of the adrenal gland that secretes steroid hormones, commonly called corticoids

B. Condition caused by hyposecretion of hormones from the adrenal cortex

C. Benign adrenal tumor that secretes hormones that produce hypertension

D. Portion of the pelvic cavity that is above the pelvic brim, bounded posteriorly by the lumbar vertebrae, laterally by the iliac fossae and iliacus muscles, and anteriorly by the lower anterior abdominal wall

E. Central tissue of the adrenal gland that secretes epinephrine and norepinephrine

F. A hormone secreted by the pituitary gland

G. Enlargement

Exercise 2
Match the following pathology terms to their definitions.

1. _____ adenoma

2. _____ adenopathy

3. _____ Cushing's syndrome

4. _____ lymphoma

5. _____ neuroectodermal tissue

6. _____ neuroblastoma

A. Multiple, enlarged lymph nodes

B. Malignant adrenal mass that is seen in pediatric patients

C. Early embryonic tissue that will eventually develop into the brain and spinal cord

D. Smooth, round, homogeneous benign tumor of the adrenal cortex associated with Cushing's syndrome

E. Malignancy that primarily affects the lymph nodes, spleen, or liver

F. Condition caused by hypersecretion of hormones from the adrenal cortex

Exercise 3

Label the following illustrations.

1. The psoas muscle extends from the mediastinum to the thigh.

13. _____

12. _____

11. _____

10. _____

9. _____

8. _____

1. _____

2. _____

3. _____

4. _____

5. _____

6. _____

7. _____

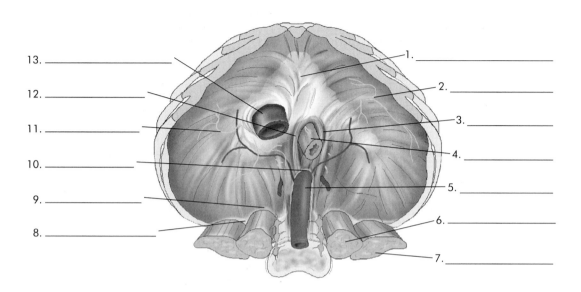

2. The quadratus lumborum muscle originates from the iliolumbar ligament.

7. _____

6. _____

1. _____

2. _____

3. _____

4. _____

5. _____

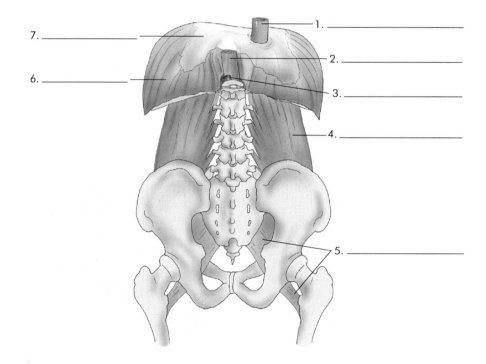

3. The iliacus muscle extends the length of the iliac fossa.

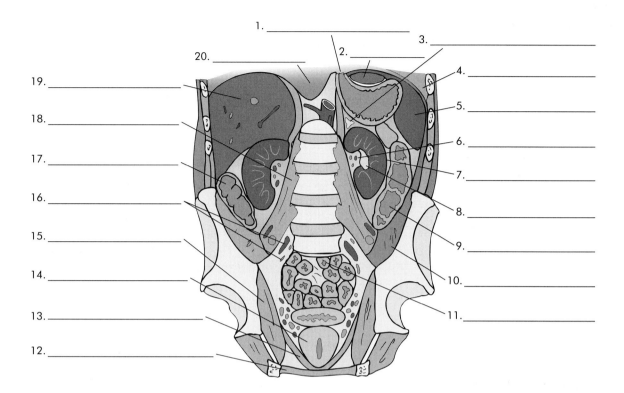

4. The right crus of the diaphragm passes posterior to the inferior vena cava.

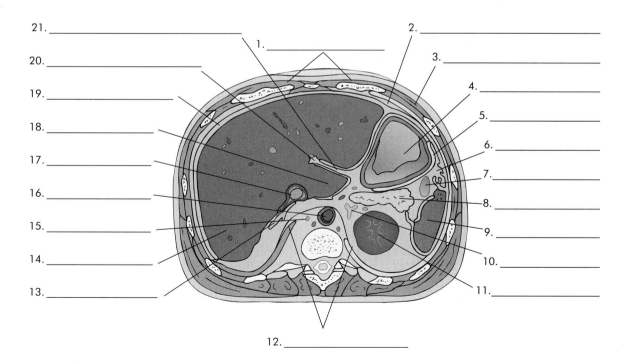

Exercise 4

Fill in the blank(s) with the word(s) that best completes the statements or provide a short answer about the anatomy of the retroperitoneum.

1. The retroperitoneal space is the area between the posterior portion of the _____ and the

   _____ abdominal wall muscles.

2. The retroperitoneal space is subdivided into three categories:

   _____

   _____

   _____

3. The _____ space surrounds the kidney, adrenal, and perirenal fat.

4. The _____ space includes the duodenum, pancreas, and ascending and transverse colon.

5. The _____ space includes the iliopsoas muscle, ureter, and branches of the inferior vena cava and their lymphatics.

6. The right adrenal is more _____ to the kidney, whereas the left adrenal is more _____ to the kidney.

7. The right renal artery crosses _____ to the crus and _____ to the inferior vena cava at the level of the right kidney.

8. The _____ muscle, the fascia of which merges with the posterior transversalis fascia, makes up the medial border of this posterior space.

Exercise 5

Fill in the blank(s) with the word(s) that best completes the statements about the physiology of the retroperitoneum.

1. The male sex hormones are _____, and the female sex hormones are _____.

2. Hypofunction of the adrenal cortex in humans is called _____ disease.

3. The steroids secreted by the adrenal cortex fall into the following three main categories: _____,

   _____, and _____.

4. _____ regulate electrolyte metabolism.

5. The principal mineralocorticoid is _____.

6. _____ play a principal role in carbohydrate metabolism.

7. The primary glucocorticoids are _____.

8. Adrenal tumors in women can promote secondary _____ characteristics.

9. The adrenal cortex is controlled by _____ hormone (ACTH) from the pituitary.

10. _____ elevate the blood pressure, the former working as an accelerator of the heart rate and the latter as a vasoconstrictor.

SONOGRAPHIC EVALUATION

Exercise 6

Fill in the blank(s) with the word(s) that best completes the statements or provide a short answer about the sonographic techniques of the retroperitoneum.

1. Describe the sonographic findings of the para-aortic lymph nodes.

_____

_____

_____

2. Explain how one can distinguish enlarged lymph nodes from bowel.

_____

_____

_____

3. Adrenal hemorrhages are more common in neonates, who experienced a traumatic delivery with:

_____

_____

_____

4. In pheochromocytoma, the clinical symptoms include: intermittent _____, severe _____,

   heart _____, and excess perspiration.

5. A _____ is a walled-off collection of extravasated urine that develops spontaneously after trauma, surgery, or a subacute or chronic urinary obstruction.

Exercise 7

Provide a short answer for each question after evaluating the images.

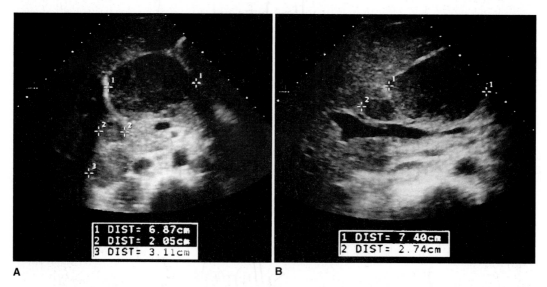

A   B

Courtesy Shpetim Telegrafi, New York University.

1. This is a 39-year-old female who presents for an abdominal ultrasound. She has a history of lymphoma. Describe the sonographic findings.

_____

_____

_____

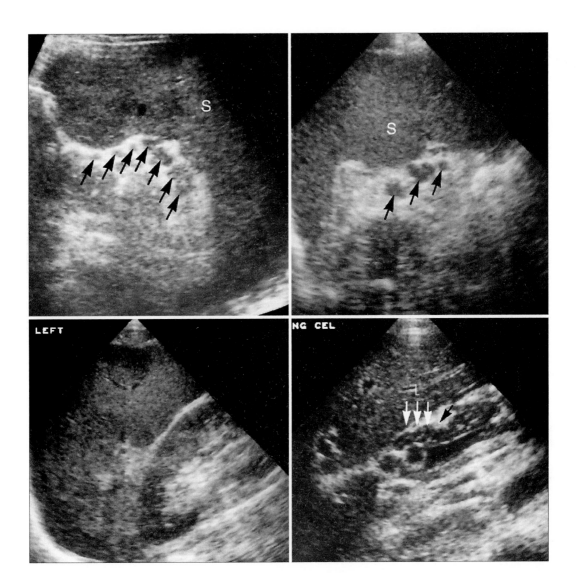

2. What are the arrows pointing to in this patient with splenomegaly? What should the sonographer do to be sure?

_____

_____

_____

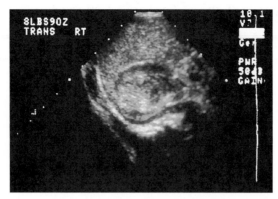

From Hoffman T, Weiler J, Albert Einstein Medical Center, Bronx, NY.

3. A 6-day-old premature infant with a change in hematocrit shows this abnormality on this right upper quadrant image.

_____

_____

_____

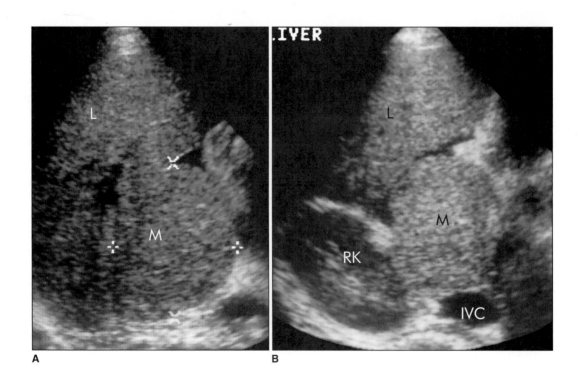

4. This patient presents with uncontrollable hypertension. Identify the anomaly shown in the sonogram.

_____

_____

_____

13 The Peritoneal Cavity and Abdominal Wall

KEY TERMS

Exercise 1

Match the following anatomic terms with their definitions.

1. _____ mesentery

2. _____ Morison's pouch

3. _____ omentum

4. _____ subhepatic

5. _____ subphrenic

A. The loops of the digestive tract are anchored to the posterior wall of the abdominal cavity by this large double fold of peritoneal tissue
B. Inferior to the liver
C. Pouchlike extension of the visceral peritoneum from the lower edge of the stomach, part of the duodenum, and the transverse colon
D. Below the diaphragm
E. Space anterior to the right kidney and posterior to the inferior border of the liver where ascites or fluid may accumulate or an abscess may develop

Exercise 2

Match the following pathology terms with their definitions.

1. _____ abscess

2. _____ ascites

3. _____ gutters

4. _____ hemorrhage

5. _____ leukocytosis

6. _____ peritonitis

7. _____ pyogenic

8. _____ sandwich sign

9. _____ sepsis

10. _____ septicemia

11. _____ urinoma

A. Condition that occurs when a vessel or organ is surrounded by a tumor on either side
B. Most dependent areas in the flanks of the abdomen and pelvis where fluid collections may accumulate
C. Inflammation of the peritoneum
D. Accumulation of serous fluid in the peritoneal cavity
E. Infection in the blood
F. Increase in the number of leukocytes (white blood cells)
G. Spread of an infection from its initial site to the bloodstream
H. Localized collection of pus
I. Pus producing
J. Cyst containing urine
K. Collection of blood

Exercise 3

Label the following illustrations.

1. Transverse view of the subphrenic spaces.

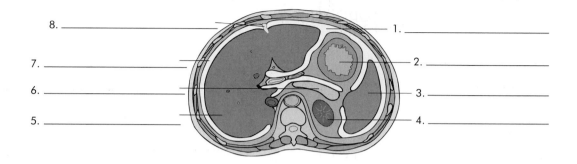

8. _____   1. _____

7. _____   2. _____

6. _____   3. _____

5. _____   4. _____

2. Transverse view of the retroperitoneal space.

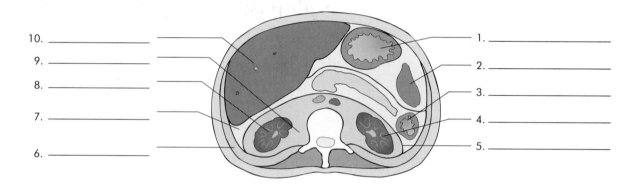

10. _____   1. _____

9. _____   2. _____

8. _____   3. _____

7. _____   4. _____

6. _____   5. _____

3. Transverse view of the subhepatic spaces and Morison's pouch.

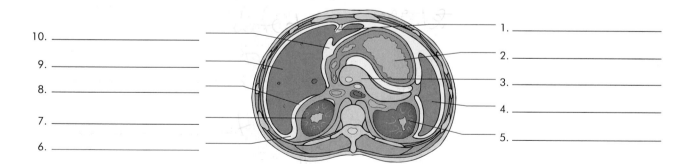

10. _____   1. _____

9. _____   2. _____

8. _____   3. _____

7. _____   4. _____

6. _____   5. _____

4. Sagittal view of the abdomen delineating the peritoneal cavity.

1. _____
22. _____
21. _____
20. _____
19. _____
18. _____
17. _____
16. _____
15. _____
14. _____
13. _____
12. _____
11. _____

2. _____
3. _____
4. _____
5. _____
6. _____
7. _____
8. _____
9. _____
10. _____

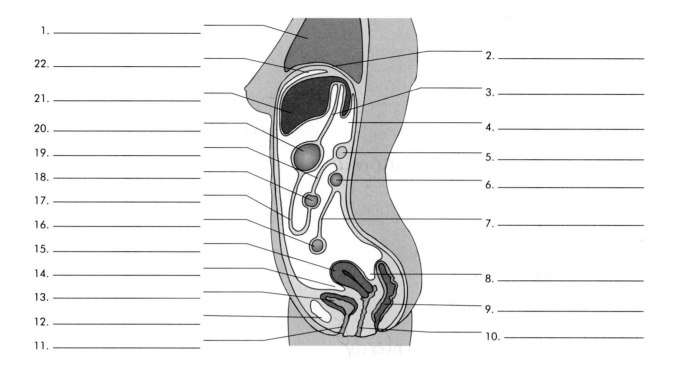

5. The muscles of the anterior and lateral abdominal walls.

12. _____
11. _____
10. _____
9. _____
8. _____

1. _____
2. _____
3. _____
4. _____
5. _____
6. _____
7. _____

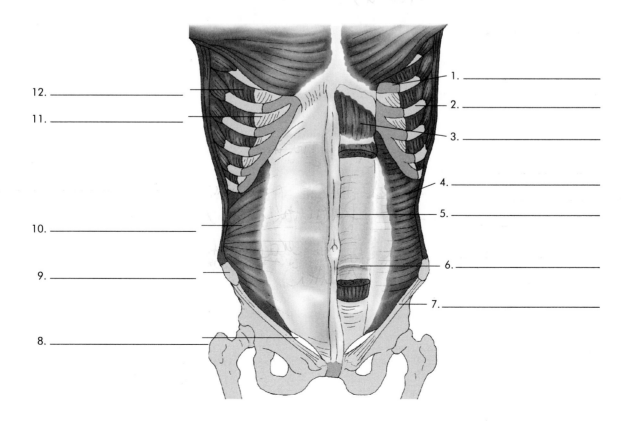

Exercise 4

Fill in the blank(s) with the word(s) that best completes the statements about the determination of intraperitoneal location.

1. Because of the ___Coronary___ ligament attachments, collections in the right posterior subphrenic space cannot extend between the bare area of the liver and the diaphragm.

2. The pleural fluid tends to distribute ___Posteromedially___ in the chest.

3. Subcapsular liver and splenic collections are seen when they are ___Inferior___ to the diaphragm unilaterally, and they conform to the shape of an organ capsule.

4. A mass is confirmed to be within the retroperitoneal cavity when anterior renal displacement or anterior displacement of the dilated ___ureters___ can be documented.

5. The mass interposed ___anteriorly___ or superiorly to kidneys can be located either intraperitoneally or retroperitoneally.

6. Fatty and collagenous connective tissues in the perirenal or anterior pararenal space produce echoes that are best demonstrated on ___Sagittal___ scans.

7. Retroperitoneal lesions displace echoes ___ventrally___ and cranially.

8. Hepatic and subhepatic lesions produce ___inferior___ and posterior displacement.

9. A large, right-sided retroperitoneal mass rotates the intrahepatic portal veins to the ___left___.

Exercise 5

Fill in the blank(s) with the word(s) that best completes the statements about the anatomy and sonographic evaluation of the peritoneal cavity and abdominal wall.

1. The peritoneal cavity is made up of multiple peritoneal ligaments and folds that connect the ___visceral___ to each other and to the abdominopelvic ___walls___.

2. Within the cavity are found the lesser and greater ___omentum___, the ___mesenteries, the ligs___ ligaments, and multiple fluid spaces (lesser sac, perihepatic and subphrenic spaces).

3. The ___peritoneum___ is a smooth membrane that lines the entire abdominal cavity and is reflected over the contained organs.

4. The part that lines the walls of the cavity is the ___parietal___ peritoneum, whereas the part covering the abdominal organs to a greater or lesser extent is the ___visceral___ peritoneum.

5. The general peritoneal cavity is known as the ___greater___ sac of the peritoneum.

6. With the development of the stomach and the spleen, a smaller sac, called the ___lesser___ sac (omental bursa), is the peritoneal recess posterior to the stomach.

7. This sac communicates with the greater sac through a small vertical opening known as the ___epiploic___ foramen.

8. When the patient is lying supine, the lowest part of the body is the ___pelvis___.

9. A double layer of peritoneum extending from the liver to the lesser curvature of the stomach is known as the _____lesser_____ omentum.

10. The _____greater_____ omentum is an apronlike fold of peritoneum that hangs from the greater curvature of the stomach.

11. Ligaments on the right side of the liver form the _____subphrenic_____ and _____subhepatic_____ spaces.

12. The subphrenic space is divided into right and left components by the _____falciform_____ ligaments.

13. The _____ligamentum teres_____ hepatis ascends from the umbilicus to the umbilical notch of the liver within the free margin of the falciform ligament before coursing within the liver.

14. The paired _____rectus_____ abdominis muscles are delineated medially in the midline of the body by the linea alba.

PATHOLOGY

Exercise 6

Fill in the blank(s) with the word(s) that best completes the statements or provide a short answer about the pathology of the peritoneal cavity.

1. The amount of intraperitoneal fluid depends on the _____location_____, _____volume_____, and patient _____position_____.

2. The ascitic fluid first fills the _____pouch of Douglas_____, then the lateral paravesical recesses before it ascends to both paracolic gutters.

3. The small bowel loops _____floats or sinks_____ in the surrounding ascitic fluid, depending on relative gas content and amount of fat in the mesentery.

4. Inflammatory or malignant ascites appears with _____fine or coarse internal_____ echoes: loculation; unusual distribution, matting, or clumping of bowel loops; and thickening of interfaces between the fluid and neighboring structures.

5. A cavity formed by necrosis within a solid tissue or a circumscribed collection of purulent material is a(n) _____abscess_____.

6. Name the five major pathways through which bacteria can enter the liver and cause abscess formation.
   1) thru the portal system
   2) by way of ascending cholangitis of the CBD (most common U.S. cause)
   3) via hep art 2ndary to bacteremia
   4) by direct extension from an infection
   5) by implantation of bacteria after trauma to abd'l wall

7. Extrahepatic loculated collections of bile that may develop because of iatrogenic, traumatic, or spontaneous rupture of the biliary tree are _____bilomas_____.

8. An abscess that forms within the renal parenchyma is a(n) _____renal carbuncle_____. Clinical symptoms vary from none to fever, leukocytosis, and flank pain.

9. The most common abdominal pathologic process is _____acute appendicitis_____, which requires immediate surgery.

Exercise 7

Fill in the blank(s) with the word(s) that best completes the statements or provide a short answer about the pathology of the mesentery, omentum, and peritoneum.

1. A mass or lesion within the mesentery and omentum may have solid or cystic characteristics, whereas a mass within the peritoneum may show a(n) _infiltrative_ pattern.

2. Mesenteric and omental cysts may be uniloculated or _multiloculated_ with smooth walls and thin internal septations.

3. An incomplete regression of the urachus during development is a(n) _urachal_ cyst.

4. An encapsulated collection of urine or _urinoma_ may result from a closed renal injury or surgical intervention or may arise spontaneously secondary to an obstructing lesion.

5. The most common primary sites of peritoneal metastases are the _ovaries_, _stomach_, and _colon_.

6. The "_sandwich sign_" of lymphoma represents a mass infiltrating the mesenteric leaves and encasing the superior mesenteric artery.

7. A key factor in determining if an abdominal wall mass is present is the _symmetry_ of the rectus sheath muscles.

8. A collection of fluid that occurs after surgery in the pelvis, retroperitoneum, or recess cavities is known as _lymphoceles_.

9. Extraperitoneal rectus sheath _hematomas_ are acute or chronic collections of blood lying either within the rectus muscle or between the muscle and its sheath.

10. An abdominal _hernia_ is the protrusion of a peritoneal-lined sac through a defect in the weakened abdominal wall.

11. A variant of the ventral hernia that is found more laterally in the abdominal wall is a(n) _Spigelian_ hernia.

12. List the sonographic criteria for a hernia.
    1) abd'l wall defect
    2) presence of bowel loops or mesenteric fat w/in a lesion
    3) exag. of lesion w/ strain/Vasalva
    4) reducibility of lesion w/ gentle pressure

Exercise 8

Provide a short answer for each question after evaluating the images.

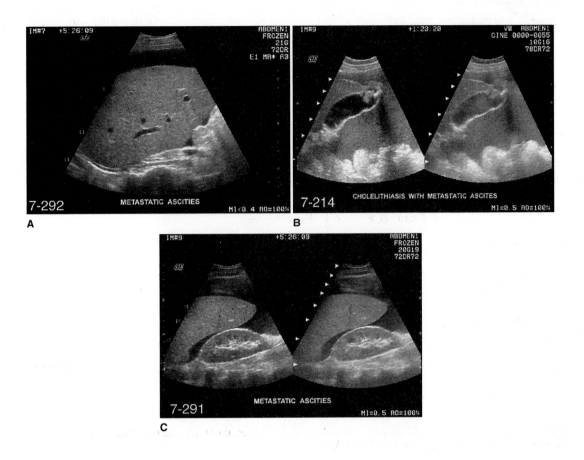

1. Identify which image demonstrates ascites in Morison's pouch.

Morrison's pouch ascites

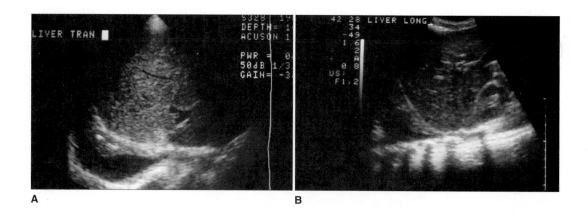

A   B

2. These transverse (**A**) and longitudinal (**B**) images demonstrate this abnormality in this patient with dyspnea.

pleural effusion

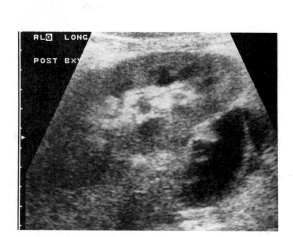

3. A patient 2 days after surgery for a renal transplant was imaged for a baseline study. Describe what this image shows and what the differential considerations are.

fluid collection post to renal transplant = postop urinoma

Diffs = hematoma, lymphocele, abscess, seroma

14 Abdominal Applications of Ultrasound Contrast Agents

KEY TERMS

Exercise 1

Match the following ultrasound terms to their definitions.

1. _____ acoustic emission

2. _____ contrast-enhanced sonography

3. _____ tissue-specific ultrasound contrast agent

4. _____ first-generation agents

5. _____ grayscale harmonic imaging

6. _____ harmonic imaging

7. _____ induced acoustic emission

8. _____ intravenous injection

9. _____ mechanical index

10. _____ second-generation agents

11. _____ molecular imaging agents

12. _____ ultrasound contrast agents

13. _____ vascular ultrasound contrast agents

A. An index that defines the low acoustic output power that can be used to minimize the destruction of microbubbles by energy in the acoustic field

B. Agents containing room air

C. After the injection of the tissue-specific UCA Sonazoid, the reflectivity of the contrast-containing tissue increases; when the right level of acoustic energy is applied to tissue, the contrast microbubbles eventually rupture, resulting in random Doppler shifts; these shifts appear as a transient mosaic of colors on the color Doppler display; masses that have destroyed or replaced normal Kupffer cells will be displayed as color-free areas

D. Agent used to reduce or eliminate some of the current limitations of ultrasound imaging and Doppler blood flow detection color flow imaging

E. A type of ultrasound contrast agent whose microbubbles are contained in the body's vascular spaces

F. Agents include Optison, Definity, Imagent, Levovist, and SonoVue

G. Allows detection of contrast-enhanced blood flow and organs with grayscale ultrasound

H. Agents that can be administered intravenously to evaluate blood vessels, blood flow, and solid organs

I. Occurs when an appropriate level of acoustic energy is applied to the tissue; the microbubbles first oscillate and then rupture

J. A hypodermic injection into a vein for the purpose of injecting a contrast medium

K. In the HI mode, the ultrasound system is configured to receive only echoes at the second harmonic frequency, which is twice the transmit frequency

L. Agents containing heavy gasses

M. A type of contrast agent whose microbubbles are removed from the blood and are taken up by specific tissues in the body

Exercise 2

Match the following clinical application terms to their definitions.

1. _____ acute tubular necrosis

2. _____ focal nodular hyperplasia

3. _____ hepatocellular carcinoma

4. _____ renal artery stenosis

5. _____ TIPS

A. Liver tumors with an abundance of Kupffer cells

B. Transjugular intrahepatic portosystemic shunt

C. Acute damage to the renal tubules; usually caused by ischemia associated with shock

D. A common liver malignancy related to cirrhosis

E. Narrowing of the renal artery

ULTRASOUND CONTRAST AGENTS

Exercise 3

Identify the abbreviations used in contrast agents for ultrasound.

1. AE _____

2. CES _____

3. CFI _____

4. GSHI _____

5. HI _____

6. IAE _____

7. MI _____

8. PDI _____

9. UCA _____

Exercise 4

Instructions: Answer the following review questions regarding ultrasound contrast agents.

1. Most of the research and development of ultrasound contrast agents has centered on creating agents that can:
   a. enhance the detection of stationary blood.
   b. be administered by intraarterial injection.
   c. be administered intravenously.
   d. enhance the detection of tumors in solid organs.
   e. be used for therapeutic applications.

2. Vascular ultrasound contrast agents enhance Doppler flow signals by:
   a. increasing the velocity of blood flow.
   b. adding more and better acoustic scatterers to the bloodstream.
   c. increasing the number of red blood cells in the vessel being evaluated.
   d. decreasing the speed of sound through tissue.
   e. a and b above.

3. For a vascular ultrasound contrast agent to be clinically useful, it should be:
   a. nontoxic.
   b. with microbubbles that are small enough to traverse the pulmonary capillary beds.
   c. stable enough to provide multiple recirculations.
   d. all of the above.
   e. high in viscosity.

4. What type of substance does the microbubble of a "first-generation" ultrasound contrast agent contain?
   a. a heavy gas, such as a perfluorocarbon
   b. a fluid that has low solubility in blood
   c. room air
   d. a fluid that has acoustic properties that are drastically different from human blood
   e. albumin

5. Depending on the clinical application, vascular ultrasound contrast agents may be administered via:
   a. intravenous bolus injection.
   b. oral ingestion.
   c. intravenous infusion.
   d. all of the above.
   e. a and c above.

6. The microbubbles of tissue-specific ultrasound contrast agents:
   a. are significantly larger than red blood cells.
   b. are significantly larger than liver cells (hepatocytes).
   c. are taken up by or have an affinity toward specific tissue.
   d. are toxic to the targeted tissue.
   e. decrease the echogenicity of targeted tissue.

7. When in harmonic imaging mode, the ultrasound system is configured to receive:
   a. only echoes that are at one half the frequency of the transmitted frequency.
   b. only echoes that are high in amplitude.
   c. only echoes arising from contrast microbubbles.
   d. only echoes at the second harmonic frequency, which is twice the transmit frequency.
   e. only echoes arising from stationary tissue.

8. When insonating microbubble-based ultrasound contrast agents, the energy present within the acoustic field:
   a. has no effect on the microbubbles.
   b. can have a detrimental effect on the contrast microbubbles.
   c. usually results in increasing the microbubble size.
   d. usually results in the creation of more microbubbles.
   e. c and d above.

9. Ultrasound contrast agents have shown the potential to improve the accuracy of hepatic sonography, including:
   a. enhanced detection of hepatic masses.
   b. enhanced characterization of hepatic masses.
   c. improved detection of intrahepatic and extrahepatic blood flow.
   d. a and c above.
   e. a, b, and c above.

10. Vascular ultrasound contrast agents can be useful in the evaluation of patients with suspected renal artery stenosis because they:
    a. increase the ability to visualize blood flow using color flow imaging.
    b. increase the velocity of blood flow to the kidneys.
    c. improve the intensity of spectral Doppler flow signals.
    d. a and c above.
    e. all of the above.

CLINICAL APPLICATIONS

Exercise 5

Fill in the blank(s) with the word(s) that best completes the statements or provide a short answer about the clinical applications.

1. The current limitations of ultrasound imaging and Doppler blood flow detection include:

   _____

   _____

   _____

2. The limitations of the sonographic detection of blood flow are:

   _____

   _____

   _____

3. Vascular or blood pool ultrasound contrast agents enhance Doppler (color and spectral) flow signals by adding

   more and better acoustic _____ to the bloodstream.

4. Some vascular agents also improve grayscale ultrasound visualization of flowing blood and demonstrate changes

   to the _____ of tissue.

5. For an agent to be clinically useful, it should be:

   _____

   _____

   _____

6. Agents containing room air are commonly referred to as _____ contrast agents, whereas agents con-

   taining heavy gasses are referred to as _____ agents.

7. Describe how tissue-specific ultrasound contrast agents differ from vascular agents.

   _____

   _____

   _____

8. The rupture of the _____ results in random Doppler shifts appearing as a transient mosaic of colors on a color Doppler display.

9. Currently, tissue-specific agents that are taken up by the _____ system appear to be most useful in the assessment of patients with suspected liver abnormalities, including the ability to both detect and characterize liver tumors using contrast enhanced sonography.

10. In harmonic imaging mode, the ultrasound system is configured to receive only echoes at the _____ harmonic frequency, which is twice the transmit frequency.

11. When using a microbubble-based ultrasound contrast agent, the microbubbles _____ (i.e., they get larger and smaller) when subjected to the acoustic energy present in the ultrasound field with grayscale ultrasound.

12. In the harmonic imaging mode, the echoes from the oscillating microbubbles have a higher _____ ratio than would be provided by using conventional US so that regions with microbubbles (e.g., blood vessels and organ parenchyma) are more easily appreciated visually.

13. Wide-band grayscale harmonic imaging provides a way to better differentiate areas with and without contrast

    and has the potential to demonstrate real-time grayscale blood pool imaging or _____.

14. Although ultrasound is usually sensitive for the detection of medium to large hepatic lesions, it is limited in its

    ability to detect _____, isoechoic, and/or peripherally located lesions, particularly in obese patients or patients with diffuse liver disease.

15. Hepatic ultrasound blood flow studies are limited by _____ velocity blood flow (e.g., in cases of portal hypertension) or for the detection of flow in the intrahepatic artery branches.

15 Ultrasound-Guided Interventional Techniques

KEY TERMS

Exercise 1
Match the following terms with their definitions.

1. _____ alpha fetoprotein

2. _____ coagulopathy

3. _____ fine-needle aspiration

4. _____ international normalized ratio

5. _____ pneumothorax

6. _____ prostate-specific antigen

7. _____ prothrombin time (PT)

8. _____ partial thromboplastin time (PTT)

9. _____ thoracentesis

10. _____ vasovagal

A. A defect in blood-clotting mechanisms

B. Surgical puncture of the chest wall for removal of fluids; usually done by using a large-bore needle

C. Laboratory test used to detect clotting abnormalities of the extrinsic pathway; measured against a control sample, PT tests the time it takes for a blood sample to coagulate after thromboplastin and calcium are added to it

D. Laboratory test that can be used to evaluate the effects of heparin, aspirin, and antihistamines on the blood clotting process; PTT detects clotting abnormalities of the intrinsic and common pathways

E. A laboratory test that measures levels of alpha fetoprotein in blood serum; an elevated level could indicate a liver lesion

F. Concerning the action of stimuli from the vagus nerve on blood vessels

G. A collection of air or gas in the pleural cavity

H. Use of a fine-gauge needle to obtain cells from a mass

I. Laboratory test that measures levels of the protein prostate-specific antigen in the body; elevated levels could indicate prostate cancer

J. A method developed to standardize PT results among laboratories by accounting for the different thromboplastin reagents used to determine PT

Exercise 2
Spell out the following acronyms.

1. AFP _____

2. FNA _____

3. INR _____

4. PSA _____

5. PT _____

6. PTT _____

Exercise 3

Fill in the blank(s) with the word(s) that best completes the statements or provide a short answer about the ultrasound-guided procedures.

1. Describe the main advantage of using ultrasound for biopsy guidance.

   _____

   _____

   _____

2. List the limitations of ultrasound guidance.

   _____

   _____

   _____

3. The most common indication for a biopsy is to confirm _____ in a mass.

4. Identify the contraindications of a biopsy.

   _____

   _____

   _____

5. The effects of heparin, aspirin, and antihistamines on the blood clotting process can be evaluated using

   _____.

6. Biopsies are used to confirm if a mass is _____, _____, or _____.

7. A _____ uses an automated, spring-loaded device, termed a biopsy gun, to provide a core of tissue for histologic analysis.

8. FNA uses a _____ needle procedure to obtain cells from a mass.

9. One method is called the _____ technique and is performed without the use of a needle guide on the transducer.

10. Identify the benefits of using a needle guide.

_____

_____

_____

11. The patient must be informed of the potential _____, alternate methods of obtaining the same information, and what would be the course of the disease if the biopsy was not performed and the correct treatment could not be planned.

12. The new national patient safety standards (www.jcaho.org) mandate that a "timeout" be performed before

beginning any procedure. Explain what timeout implies. _____

13. Complications from an ultrasound-guided biopsy are usually minor and may include _____,

_____ reactions, and _____.

14. It is important to determine how much the mass moves with _____ and also how well and how long the patient can hold his or her breath.

15. Describe how to see the needle tip in ultrasound.

_____

_____

_____

16. Whenever possible, a _____ approach should be used to prevent the possibility of a pneumothorax or damage to the intercostal arteries.

17. Typically the _____ pole of the kidney is biopsied to prevent possible lacerations of the main renal vessels and ureter.

18. Patients may be marked for a thoracentesis or have the procedure under sonographic guidance. Patients should be

scanned in the _____ position as the procedure will be performed in, which is usually in an upright position, through the back.

16 Emergent Abdominal Ultrasound Procedures

KEY TERMS

Exercise 1

Match the following abdominal ultrasound terms with their definitions.

1. _____ extracorporeal shock wave lithotripsy

2. _____ focused assessment with sonography for trauma

3. _____ hemoperitoneum

4. _____ incarcerated hernia

5. _____ intravenous urography

6. _____ peritoneal lavage

7. _____ pseudodissection

8. _____ reducible hernia

9. _____ strangulated hernia

A. Collection of bloody fluid in the abdomen or pelvis secondary to trauma or surgical procedure

B. Capable of being replaced in a normal position; the visceral contents can be returned to normal intraabdominal location

C. A procedure that breaks up kidney stones

D. Invasive procedure that is used to sample the intraperitoneal space for evidence of damage to viscera and blood vessels

E. Limited examination of the abdomen or pelvis to evaluate free fluid or pericardial fluid

F. An incarcerated hernia with vascular compromise

G. Procedure used in radiography wherein contrast is administered intravenously to help visualize the urinary system

H. Condition seen in a patient with aortic dissection

I. Imprisonment or confinement of a part of the bowel; the visceral contents cannot be reduced

Exercise 2

Label the following illustrations.

1. The two common sites for peritoneal lavage.

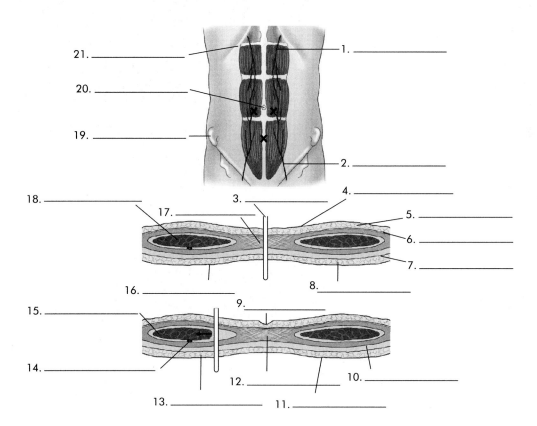

2. Transverse view of the perihepatic space and Morison's pouch.

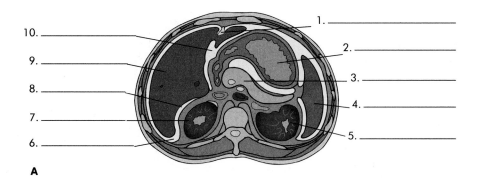

A

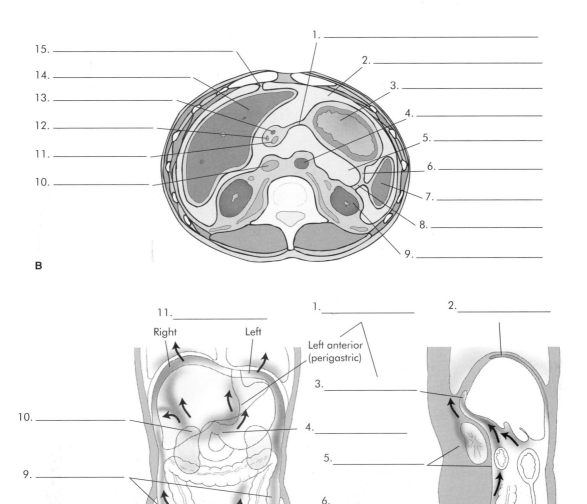

B

11. _____

Right   Left

10. _____

9. _____

8. _____

C

1. _____

Left anterior
(perigastric)

3. _____

4. _____

5. _____

6. _____

7. _____

2. _____

D

EMERGENT ABDOMINAL ULTRASOUND PROCEDURES

Exercise 3

Fill in the blank(s) with the word(s) that best completes the statements or provide a short answer about emergent abdominal ultrasound procedures.

1. This procedure, called _____, is used to sample the intraperitoneal space for evidence of damage to the viscera and blood vessels.

2. Peritoneal lavage is usually used as a diagnostic technique in certain cases of _____ abdominal trauma.

3. Peritoneal lavage carries a risk of organ injury and decreases the specificity of subsequent ultrasonography or

   computed tomography (CT) because of the introduction of _____ fluid and air.

4. The _____ scan in the emergency department is a limited examination of the abdomen and/or pelvis to evaluate free fluid or pericardial fluid.

5. In the context of traumatic injury, free fluid is usually a result of _____ and contributes to the assessment of the circulation.

6. The FAST scan area of evaluation is widespread, extending from the pericardial sac to the urinary bladder and includes the _____ area (including Morison's pouch), _____ region (including splenorenal recess), _____, and _____.

7. Accessibility and _____ of performance are critical in the trauma setting.

8. The goal is to scan the _____ quadrants, _____ sac, and cul-de-sac for the presence of free fluid or hemoperitoneum.

9. Hemorrhage in the peritoneal cavity collects in the most _____ area of the abdomen.

10. _____ lacerations or contusions are more easily detected with ultrasound than any other visceral abdominal injury.

11. A brisk intraparenchymal hemorrhage may be identified as a(n) _____ region within the abnormal parenchyma, whereas a global parenchymal injury may project into the liver as a widespread architectural disruption with absence of the normal vascular pattern.

12. In female patients of reproductive age with trauma, free fluid isolated to the cul-de-sac is likely _____.

13. If the patient is female with symptoms of right upper quadrant pain, fever, and leukocytosis, _____ should be ruled out.

14. The most common cause of acute cholecystitis is _____ with a cystic duct obstruction.

15. Midepigastric pain that radiates to the back is characteristic of _____.

16. Sonographic findings in acute pancreatitis show a normal to edematous gland that is somewhat _____ to normal texture.

17. Flank pain caused by _____ is a common problem in patients presenting to the emergency department.

18. If the stone completely obstructs the ureter, no _____ will be present.

19. When obstruction occurs, ultrasound is very effective in demonstrating the secondary sign of _____.

20. With the bladder distended, the color Doppler is an excellent tool to image the presence of ureteral jets into the bladder; the transducer should be angled in a _____ presentation through the distended urinary bladder.

21. The pulse repetition frequency should be _____ to assess the low velocity of the ureteral jet flow.

22. A _____ is a condition in which a propagating intramural hematoma actually dissects along the length of the vessel, stripping away the intima, and in some cases, part of the media.

23. Most aortic dissections will occur at one of three sites:

_____

_____

_____

24. Most aortic dissections are located in the _____ aorta.

25. _____ hypertension is nearly always associated with aortic dissection.

26. The most typical presentation of an aortic dissection is that of a sudden onset of severe, tearing _____ pain radiating to the arms, neck, or back.

27. With appendicitis, the patient will usually have rebound tenderness, "_____ sign," associated with peritoneal irritation.

28. Sonographic findings use a _____ compression technique over the right lower quadrant.

29. A _____ forms when the abdominal wall muscles are weakened, thus allowing the viscera to protrude into the weakened abdominal wall.

30. Sonography allows visualization of the _____ movement of the bowel during Valsalva maneuvers and determines the presence or absence of vascular flow within the defect.

31. Most paraumbilical hernias contain _____, _____, and _____.

32. The patient should be instructed to perform a _____ maneuver to determine the site of wall defect and confirm the presence of the protruding hernia.

Exercise 4

Provide a short answer for each question after evaluating the images.

1. Identify what abnormality is visible in the images of the right upper quadrant.

_____

_____

_____

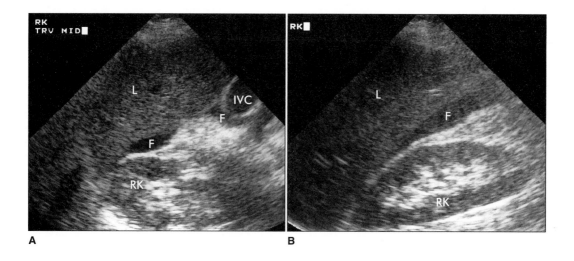

A   B

2. A trauma patient demonstrated fluid in the right upper quadrant in the area of Morison's pouch. Identify the other areas where the sonographer should look for fluid.

_____

_____

_____

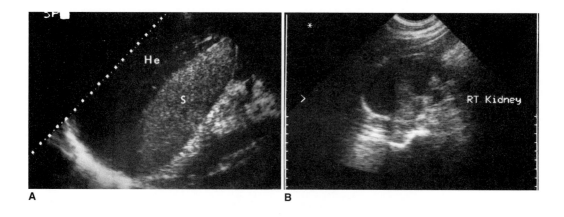

A   B

3. After evaluating the images above, determine whether this patient has an acute or chronic bleed.

_____

_____

_____

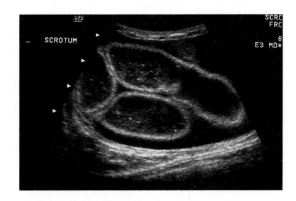

4. Describe what the sonographer should look for in this herniated scrotal sac.

_____

_____

_____

17 The Breast

KEY TERMS

Exercise 1
Match the following terms with their definitions.

1. _____ acinus (acini)

2. _____ anechoic

3. _____ areola

4. _____ axilla

5. _____ breast

6. _____ breast cancer (breast carcinoma)

7. _____ breast cancer screening

8. _____ Cooper's ligaments

9. _____ cyst aspiration

10. _____ gynecomastia

11. _____ mammary layer

12. _____ retromammary layer

13. _____ subcutaneous layer

14. _____ tail of Spence

15. _____ terminal ductal lobular unit (TDLU)

A. Connective tissue septa that connect perpendicularly to the breast lobules and extend out to the skin

B. Most superficial of the three layers of the breast identified on breast ultrasound

C. Armpit

D. Involves two main types of cells (ductal and lobular)

E. Glandular (milk-producing) component of the breast lobule

F. Middle layer of the breast tissue that contains the ductal, glandular, and stromal portions of the breast

G. Smallest functional portion of the breast involving the terminal duct and its associated lobule containing at least one acinus

H. Hypertrophy of residual ductal elements that persist behind the nipple in the male

I. Without echoes

J. Differentiated apocrine sweat gland with a functional purpose of secreting milk during lactation

K. Deepest of the three layers of the breast noted on breast ultrasound

L. The pigmented skin surrounding the breast nipple

M. A normal extension of breast tissue into the axillary or armpit region

N. Screening for breast cancer involves annual screening mammography, monthly breast self-examination, and regular clinical breast examination

O. Common breast procedure; involves placing a needle through the skin of the breast into a cystic mass and pulling fluid out of the cystic mass through the needle

Exercise 2

Match the following breast evaluation terms with their definitions.

1. _____ antiradial
2. _____ asymptomatic
3. _____ breast imaging reporting and data system
4. _____ breast self-examination
5. _____ clinical breast examination
6. _____ diagnostic breast imaging
7. _____ fremitus
8. _____ juxtathoracic
9. _____ Paget's disease
10. _____ palpable
11. _____ peau d'orange
12. _____ radial
13. _____ sentinel node
14. _____ spiculation

A. Plane of imaging on ultrasound of the breast
B. Part of breast cancer screening
C. Plane of imaging on ultrasound of the breast that is perpendicular to the radial plane of imaging
D. Surface erosion of the nipple (reddened area with flaking and crusty areas) that results from direct invasion of the skin of the nipple from underlying breast cancer
E. A type of breast imaging examination more intensive than routine screening mammography
F. Fingerlike extension of a malignant tumor
G. Near the chest wall
H. Part of breast cancer screening
I. Represents the first lymph node along the axillary node chain
J. Refers to vibrations produced by phonation and felt through the chest wall during palpation
K. Without symptoms
L. Can be felt on clinical examination
M. Trademark system created by the American College of Radiology (ACR) to standardize mammographic reporting terminology, categorize breast abnormalities according to the level of suspicion for malignancy, and facilitate outcome monitoring
N. French term for skin thickening of one breast that, on clinical breast examination, resembles the skin of an orange

Exercise 3

Match the following pathology terms with their definitions.

1. _____ adenosis
2. _____ apocrine metaplasia
3. _____ atypical ductal hyperplasia
4. _____ atypical hyperplasia
5. _____ atypical lobular hyperplasia
6. _____ cyst
7. _____ epitheliosis
8. _____ fibroadenoma
9. _____ fibrocystic condition

A. Echo texture that is less echogenic than the surrounding tissue
B. Abnormal proliferation of cells with atypical features involving the TDLU, with an increased likelihood of evolving into breast cancer
C. Not considered a true cancer or treated as such
D. Most common benign solid tumor of the breast, consisting primarily of fibrous and epithelial tissue elements
E. Cannot be felt on clinical examination
F. Fluid-filled sac
G. Overgrowth of the acini within terminal ductal lobular unit (TDLU) of the breast
H. Cancer of the lobular epithelium of the breast, arises at the level of the TDLU
I. Breast cancer occurring in more than one site within the same quadrant of the same ductal system of the breast

10. _____ hyperechoic

11. _____ hypoechoic

12. _____ infiltrating ductal carcinoma

13. _____ infiltrating lobular carcinoma

14. _____ isoechoic

15. _____ lobular carcinoma in situ

16. _____ lobular neoplasia

17. _____ multicentric breast cancer

18. _____ multifocal breast cancer

19. _____ nonpalpable

J. Condition that represents many different tissue processes within the breast that are all basically normal processes that in some patients become exaggerated to the point of raising concern for breast cancer

K. The pathologist recognizes some, but not all, of the features of ductal carcinoma in situ.

L. Breast cancer occurring in different quadrants of the breast at least 5 cm apart

M. Shows some, but not all, of the features of lobular carcinoma in situ

N. Echo texture that resembles the surrounding tissue

O. Form of fibrocystic change in which the epithelial cells of the acini undergo alteration

P. Cancer of the ductal epithelium; most common general category of breast cancer, accounting for approximately 85% of all breast cancers

Q. Overgrowth of the cells lining the small ducts of the TDLU

R. A term preferred by many authors to replace LCIS and atypical hyperplasia

S. Echo texture that is more echogenic than the surrounding tissue

ANATOMY AND PHYSIOLOGY

Exercise 4

Label the following illustrations.

1. Breast anatomy.

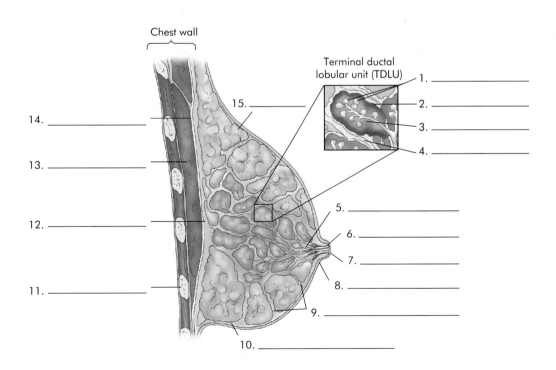

2. Description of right breast anatomy.

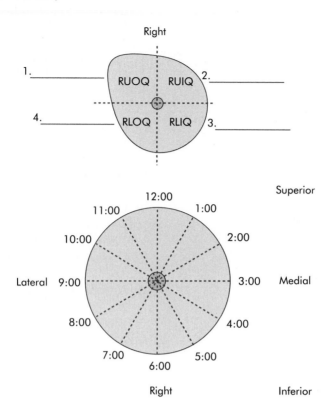

3. Description of left breast anatomy.

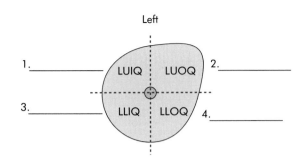

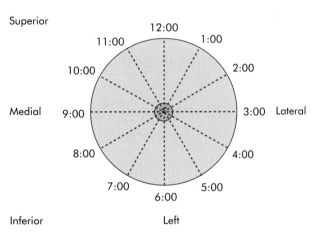

Exercise 5

Fill in the blank(s) with the word(s) that best completes the statements or provide a short answer about the anatomy of the breast.

1. The breast is a modified _____ gland located in the superficial fascia of the anterior chest wall.

2. Sonographically the breast is divided into three layers located between the skin and the pectoralis major muscle on the anterior chest wall. These layers include the:

   _____

   _____

   _____

3. Fat is the least _____ tissue within the breast.

4. The fatty tissue appears _____, whereas the ducts, glands, and supporting ligaments appear echogenic.

5. The _____ quadrant of the breast contains the highest concentration of lobes.

6. Each lobule contains _____ (milk-producing glands) that are clustered on the terminal ends of the ducts like grapes on a vine.

7. The _____ muscle lies posterior to the retromammary layer.

8. The _____ tissue can situate itself in and among the areas of glandular tissue and in some scanning planes, mimic isoechoic or hypoechoic masses.

9. Sonographically, cancers can be difficult to differentiate in the fatty breast because most cancers appear

_____ and can be difficult to differentiate from the normal breast tissue.

10. The main arterial supply to the breast comes from the internal _____ and the lateral

_____ artery.

11. Lymphatic drainage from all parts of the breast generally flows to the _____ lymph nodes.

Exercise 6

Fill in the blank(s) with the word(s) that best completes the statements or provide a short answer about the physiology of the breast.

1. The primary function of the breast is for _____ transport.

2. The _____ system is critical in the transport of fluids within the breast, and they are also a source for ductal pathologic conditions.

3. An important function during the reproductive years is for the breast to make _____ from nutrients and water taken from the bloodstream.

4. Milk is produced within the _____ and carried to the nipple by the ducts.

5. Breast development begins before _____ and continues until the patient is approximately 16 years old.

6. During this time of development, the ductal system proliferates under the influence of _____.

7. During pregnancy, acinar development is accelerated to enable milk production by estrogen, _____, and prolactin.

8. The hormone produced by the pituitary gland that stimulates the acini to produce and excrete milk is called

_____.

9. The expulsion of the placenta after the birth of a baby causes a drop in circulating progesterone, initiating

_____ production within the breasts.

10. The physical stimulation of suckling by the baby initiates the release of _____ (produced by the hypothalamus and released by the pituitary gland), which further incites prolactin secretion, stimulating additional milk production.

11. Full maturation of the acini occurs during lactation and is thought to be mildly protective against the development

of breast _____.

Exercise 7

Fill in the blank(s) with the word(s) that best completes the statements or provide a short answer about the sonographic techniques of the breast.

1. Ultrasound may be used for screening purposes in _____ breasts that are difficult to penetrate by mammography, to evaluate palpable masses that are not visible on a mammogram, and to image the deep juxtathoracic tissues not normally visible by mammography.

2. Ultrasound is also useful in _____ structures within uniformly dense breast tissue where mammography is limited (e.g., in differentiating solid, round masses from fluid-filled cysts and visualizing tissue adjacent to implants or other structures that limit visualization by mammography).

3. A _____ aspiration can be performed to determine whether the lesion is a complex cyst or truly a solid mass.

4. The sonographer must have basic clinical information regarding any patient who is referred for breast ultrasound. List the pertinent clinical information necessary.

   _____

   _____

   _____

5. Pertinent clinical information that should be provided by the referring physician includes size and location of the

   lump, when it was noticed, and its relation to the _____.

6. A dominant cyst is frequently _____ or _____ (long axis toward nipple), smooth, soft (some cysts under tension can be firm and are usually very tender), and easily movable.

7. Fibroadenomas are usually similar in shape, but are often quite firm and rubbery in consistency and

   _____ on ultrasound.

8. Breast cancer is usually lobular or _____ in shape, uneven in surface contour (sometimes gritty in texture), and fixed or poorly movable.

9. Most breast masses that arise during the adolescent years are _____.

10. A(n) _____ implant rupture occurs when there is a breach of the membrane surrounding an implant, but the silicone that leaks out is still confined within the fibrous scar tissue that forms a "capsule" around the implant.

11. As the implant collapses and the membrane folds inward, a series of discontinuous echogenic lines parallel to the

    face of the transducer may be seen and are referred to as the "stepladder sign" or "_____ sign."

12. The use of the _____ positions is unique to the breast and can often pick up subtle abnormalities extending toward the nipple along the ductal system from the mass.

13. _____ tend to grow within the ducts and will often follow the ductal system in a radial plane, toward the convergence at the nipple.

14. To be considered a simple cyst, a lesion must meet several criteria on ultrasound:

_____

_____

_____

15. Discuss the disruption of breast architecture with benign and malignant tumors of the breast.

_____

_____

_____

16. A rounded or oval shape is usually associated with _____ lesions, whereas sharp, angular margins are associated with _____.

17. The normal tissue planes of the breast are _____ oriented.

18. Benign lesions tend to grow within the normal tissue planes, and their long axis lies _____ to the chest wall.

19. Malignant lesions are able to grow through the connective tissue and may have a _____ orientation when imaging the breast from anterior to posterior.

20. If a mass measures longer in the anteroposterior dimension (_____) than in either transverse or sagittal planes (_____), the mass has a vertical orientation that is usually described as being "taller than wide" and is suspicious for malignancy.

21. Malignant masses will often demonstrate increased _____ within the lesion and often have a feeder vessel, which can be identified with careful evaluation.

PATHOLOGY

Exercise 8

Fill in the blank(s) with the word(s) that best completes the statements about the abnormalities of the breast.

1. Lesions more common to younger women are _____ disease and fibroadenomas.

2. Older or postmenopausal women are more likely to have _____ papillomas, duct ectasia, and cancer.

3. Skin dimpling or ulceration and nipple retraction nearly always result from _____.

4. Benign tumors are rubbery, _____, and well delineated (as seen in a fibroadenoma), whereas malignant tumors are often stone hard and irregular with a gritty feel.

5. Clinical signs and symptoms of _____ include the lumps and pain that the patient feels that fluctuate with every monthly cycle. In most cases both breasts are equally involved.

6. The growth of a fibroadenoma is stimulated by _____.

7. Sonographically, fat necrosis appears as an irregular, complex mass with low-level echoes, may mimic a

   _____ lesion, and may appear as fat, but is separate and different from the rest of the breast
   parenchyma.

8. _____ may result from infection, trauma, mechanical obstruction in the breast ducts, or from other
   conditions. It often occurs during lactation, beginning in the lactiferous ducts and spreading via the lymphatics or
   blood.

9. An intraductal papilloma is a small, _____ tumor that grows within the acini of the breast.

10. In _____ tissue, most cancer growth occurs along the borders.

11. _____ and _____ are frequently used as pathways for new tumor development.

12. If the tumor is _____, it continues to grow in one area, compressing and distorting the surrounding
    architecture.

13. Most cancer originates in the _____ ductal lobular units, whereas a smaller percentage originates in
    the glandular tissue.

14. _____ refers to breast tumors that arise from the epithelium, in the ductal and glandular tissue, and
    usually have tentacles.

15. Breast carcinomas are generally categorized by two factors—where the cancer cells originate (_____

    or _____) and whether the cancer is prone to spreading (_____ or _____).

16. Carcinomas that do not normally spread outside of the duct or lobule are called noninvasive, noninfiltrating, or

    _____ cancers, whereas cancers that spread into nearby tissue are said to be invasive or infiltrating.

Exercise 9

Provide a short answer for each question after evaluating the images.

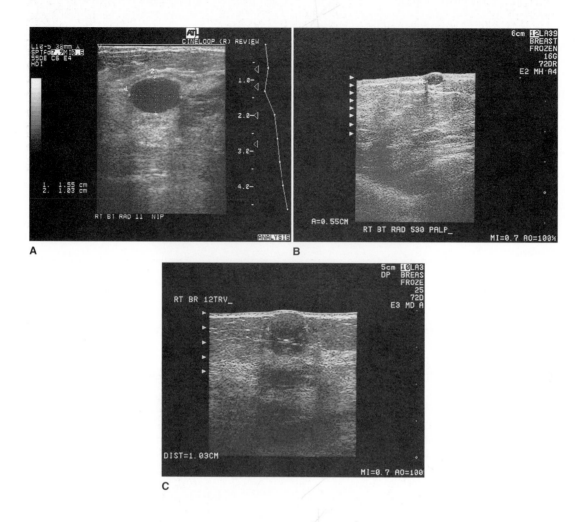

A

B

C

1. Identify which figure clearly identifies a simple cyst of the breast.

_____

_____

_____

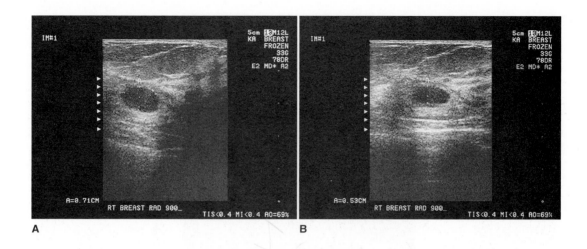

A   B

2. Would you suspect this breast lesion to be benign or malignant? (**A**) without compression and (**B**) with compression.

_____

_____

_____

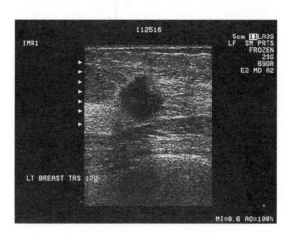

3. Would you suspect this breast lesion to be benign or malignant?

_____

_____

_____

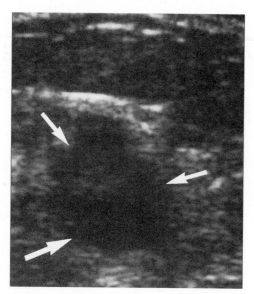

From Rumack C, Wilson S, Charboneau W: *Diagnostic ultrasound,* ed 3, St Louis, 2005, Mosby.

4.   This mass was described as a large tumor with necrosis in a 45-year-old female. The differential is:

_____

_____

_____

18 The Thyroid and Parathyroid Glands

KEY TERMS

Exercise 1

Match the following anatomic and physiologic terms with their definitions.

1. __D__ calcitonin
2. __K__ euthyroid
3. __G__ fine-needle aspiration
4. __N__ hyperthyroidism
5. __E__ hypophosphatasia
6. __B__ hypothyroidism
7. __L__ isthmus
8. __I__ longus colli muscles
9. __C__ microcalcifications
10. __J__ parathyroid hormone
11. __O__ pyramidal lobe
12. __F__ serum calcium
13. __M__ sternocleidomastoid muscles
14. __A__ strap muscles
15. __H__ thyroid-stimulating hormone

A. Group of three muscles (sternothyroid, sternohyoid, omohyoid) that lie anterior to the thyroid
B. Underactive thyroid hormones
C. Tiny echogenic foci within a nodule that may or may not shadow
D. A thyroid hormone that is important for maintaining a dense, strong bone matrix and regulating the blood calcium level
E. Low phosphate level, which can be seen with hyperparathyroidism
F. Laboratory value that is elevated with hyperparathyroidism
G. Invasive procedure used to obtain a small specimen from a specific lesion
H. A hormone secreted by the pituitary gland that stimulates the thyroid gland to secrete thyroxine and triiodothyronine
I. Wedge-shaped muscle posterior to the thyroid lobes
J. A hormone that is secreted by parathyroid glands, which regulates serum calcium levels
K. Refers to a normal functioning thyroid gland
L. Small piece of thyroid tissue that connects the right and left lobes of the gland
M. Large muscles anterolateral to the thyroid
N. Oversecretion of thyroid hormones
O. Present in small percentage of patients; extends superiorly from the isthmus

Exercise 2

Match the following pathology terms with their definitions.

1. __J__ adenoma
2. __G__ adenopathy
3. __O__ anaplastic carcinoma
4. __M__ branchial cleft cyst
5. __F__ cystic hygroma
6. __D__ de Quervain's thyroiditis
7. __C__ diffuse nontoxic goiter (colloid goiter)
8. __R__ follicular carcinoma
9. __T__ goiter
10. __E__ Graves' disease
11. __Q__ Hashimoto's thyroiditis
12. __N__ hyperparathyroidism
13. __U__ medullary carcinoma
14. __H__ multinodular goiter
15. __A__ nodular hyperplasia
16. __K__ papillary carcinoma
17. __S__ parathyroid hyperplasia
18. __I__ primary hyperparathyroidism
19. __P__ secondary hyperparathyroidism
20. __B__ thyroiditis
21. __L__ thyroglossal duct cyst

A. Degenerative nodules within the thyroid
B. Inflammation of the thyroid
C. Occurs as a compensatory enlargement of the thyroid gland resulting from thyroid hormone deficiency
D. Viral infection of the thyroid that causes inflammation
E. Autoimmune disorder of diffuse toxic goiter characterized by bulging eyes
F. Cystic neck mass caused by malformations of the cervical thoracic lymphatic system
G. Enlargement of the lymph nodes
H. Nodular enlargement of the thyroid associated with hyperthyroidism
I. Oversecretion of parathyroid hormone, usually from a parathyroid adenoma
J. Benign thyroid neoplasm characterized by complete fibrous encapsulation
K. Most common form of thyroid malignancy
L. Congenital anomalies that present in midline of the neck anterior to the trachea
M. Remnant of embryonic development that appears as a cyst in the neck
N. Disorder associated with elevated serum calcium level, usually caused by a benign parathyroid adenoma
O. Rare, undifferentiated carcinoma occurring in middle age
P. Enlargement of parathyroid glands in patients with renal failure or vitamin D deficiency
Q. Chronic inflammation of the thyroid gland caused by the formation of antibodies against normal thyroid tissue
R. Occurs as a solitary malignant mass within the thyroid gland
S. Enlargement of the multiple parathyroid glands
T. Enlargement of the thyroid gland that can be focal or diffuse; multiple nodules may be present
U. Neoplastic growth that accounts for 10% of thyroid malignancies

Exercise 3

Label the following illustrations.

1. Anterior view of the thyroid and parathyroid glands.

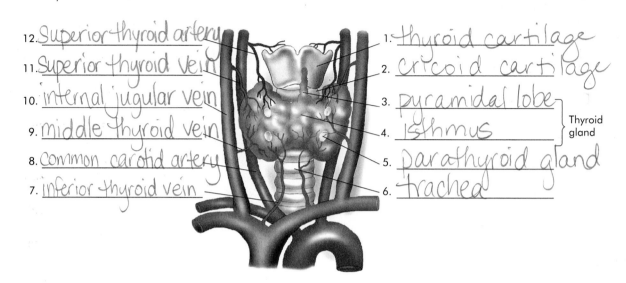

12. Superior thyroid artery
11. Superior thyroid vein
10. internal jugular vein
9. middle thyroid vein
8. common carotid artery
7. inferior thyroid vein

1. thyroid cartilage
2. cricoid cartilage
3. pyramidal lobe
4. isthmus   } Thyroid gland
5. parathyroid gland
6. trachea

2. Cross-section of the thyroid region.

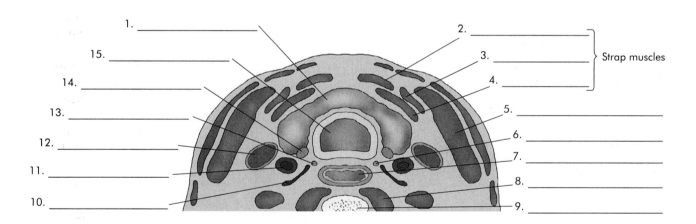

1. _____
15. _____
14. _____
13. _____
12. _____
11. _____
10. _____

2. _____
3. _____   } Strap muscles
4. _____
5. _____
6. _____
7. _____
8. _____
9. _____

THE THYROID AND PARATHYROID GLANDS

Exercise 4

Fill in the blank(s) with the word(s) that best completes the statements about the thyroid and parathyroid glands.

1. The thyroid straddles the trachea anteriorly, whereas the paired lobes extend on either side bounded laterally by the

   _____ arteries and _____ veins.

2. Along the anterior surface of the thyroid gland lie the _____ muscles, including the sternothyroid, omohyoid, sternohyoid, and sternocleidomastoid muscles.

3. The parathyroid glands are normally located on the _____ surface of the thyroid gland.

175

4. The parathyroid glands are the _____ organs in the body.

5. The parathyroid glands produce _____ and monitor the serum calcium feedback mechanism.

6. When the serum calcium level _____, the parathyroid glands are stimulated to release PTH.

7. PTH acts on _____, _____, and intestine to enhance calcium absorption.

8. Primary hyperparathyroidism is characterized by _____, hypercalciuria, and low serum levels of phosphate.

9. Primary hyperparathyroidism occurs when increased amounts of PTH are produced by an _____, primary hyperplasia, or, rarely, carcinoma located in the parathyroid gland.

10. A chronic hypocalcemia caused by renal failure, vitamin D deficiency (rickets), or malabsorption syndromes is

_____ hyperparathyroidism.

Exercise 5
Fill in the blank(s) with the word(s) that best completes the statements about the thyroid and parathyroid glands.

1. The thyroid gland is the part of the endocrine system that maintains body _____, _____,

and _____ through the synthesis, storage, and secretion of thyroid hormones.

2. These hormones include triiodothyronine (_____), thyroxine (_____),

and _____.

3. The mechanism for producing thyroid hormones is _____ metabolism.

4. When thyroid hormone is needed by the body, it is released into the bloodstream by the action of thyrotropin, or

thyroid-stimulating hormone (_____), which is produced by the pituitary gland.

5. The secretion of TSH is regulated by thyrotropin-releasing factor, which is produced by the _____.

6. The concentration of calcium in the blood is decreased by _____, which first acts on the bone to inhibit its breakdown.

7. Low intake of iodine (goiter) in the body may cause _____, or the inability of the thyroid to produce the proper amount of thyroid hormone, or a problem in the pituitary gland that does not control the thyroid production.

8. The metabolic rate is dramatically increased by _____; clinical signs include weight loss, increased appetite, high degree of nervous energy, tremor, excessive sweating, heat intolerance, and palpitations, and many patients show signs of exophthalmos (protruding eyes).

9. The function of the thyroid is determined by _____.

10. An enlargement of the thyroid gland is _____, which is often visible on the anterior neck.

11. One of the most common forms of thyroid disease is _____.

12. _____ is characterized by a triad of the following findings: hypermetabolism, diffuse toxic goiter, exophthalmos (inflammatory infiltration of the orbital tissue resulting in proptosis, or bulging of the eyes), and cutaneous manifestations (thickening of the dermis of the pretibial areas and the dorsum of the feet).

13. A benign thyroid neoplasm characterized by complete fibrous encapsulation is a(n) _____.

14. The most common of the thyroid malignancies is _____ of the thyroid and is the preponderant cause of thyroid cancer in children.

Exercise 6
Fill in the blank(s) with the word(s) that best completes the statements about the thyroid and parathyroid glands.

1. The normal thyroid gland has a fine _____ echotexture that is more echogenic than the surrounding muscle structure.

2. _____ of the neck results from congenital modification of the lymphatics.

3. A normal lymph node is oval in shape with a _____ texture with a central core echo complex.

4. The _____ muscle is posterior and lateral to each thyroid lobe and appears as a hypoechoic triangular structure adjacent to the cervical vertebrae.

PATHOLOGY

Exercise 7
Provide a short answer for each question after evaluating the images.

1. Identify the structure that the arrows are pointing to.

_____

_____

_____

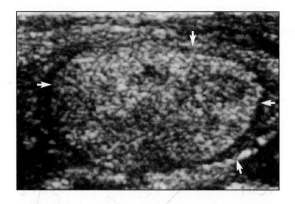

2. A young woman presents with a palpable mass in her neck. Describe what the ultrasound shows and what the arrows are pointing to.

_____

_____

_____

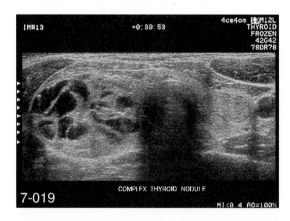

3. An asymptomatic female patient appeared with a mass in her neck. Identify the ultrasound findings.

_____

_____

_____

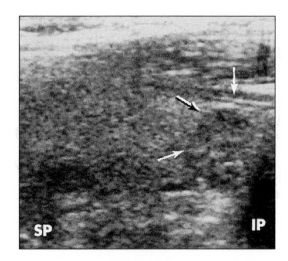

4. A 64-year-old male presents with a palpable mass in his neck. Identify the ultrasound findings.

_____

_____

_____

19 The Scrotum

KEY TERMS

Exercise 1
Match the following anatomic terms with their definitions.

1. __F__ centripetal artery
2. __N__ dartos
3. __A__ ejaculatory ducts
4. __J__ epididymis
5. __L__ mediastinum testis
6. __C__ pampiniform plexus
7. __H__ pudendal artery
8. __O__ septa of testis
9. __B__ seminal vesicles
10. __Q__ spermatic cord
11. __E__ testicle
12. __K__ testicular artery
13. __P__ tunica albuginea
14. __G__ tunica vaginalis
15. __M__ urethra
16. __I__ vas deferens
17. __D__ verumontanum

A. Connect the seminal vesicle and the vas deferens to the urethra at the verumontanum
B. Reservoirs for sperm located posterior to the bladder
C. Plexus of veins in the spermatic cord that drain into the right and left testicular veins
D. Junction of the ejaculatory ducts with the urethra
E. Male gonad that produces hormones that induce masculine features and spermatozoa
F. Terminal intratesticular arteries arising from the capsular arteries
G. Membrane consisting of a visceral layer and a parietal layer lining the inner wall of the scrotum
H. Partially supply the scrotal wall and epididymis and occasionally the lower pole of the testis
I. Tube that connects the epididymis to the seminal vesicle
J. Anatomic structure formed by the network of ducts leaving the mediastinum testis that combine into a single, convoluted epididymal tubule
K. Artery arising from the aorta just distal to each renal artery
L. Central linear structure formed by the convergence of multiple, thin septations within the testicle; the septations are invaginations of the tunica albuginea
M. Tubular structure that extends from the bladder to the end of the penis
N. Layer of muscle underneath the scrotal skin
O. Multiple septa formed from the tunica albuginea that course toward the mediastinum testis and separate the testicle into lobules
P. Inner fibrous membrane surrounding the testicle
Q. Structure made up of vas deferens, testicular artery, cremasteric artery, and pampiniform plexus that suspends the testis in the scrotum

inside testis
250-400 conical lobules containing seminif tubules which converge at ape of lobule + join to become rete testis (in mediastinum)
Rt goes thru efferent ductules to epididymis → vas deferens

Exercise 2

Match the following vascular supply terms with their definitions.

1. ___D___ cremasteric artery
2. ___A___ cremaster muscle
3. ___C___ deferential artery
4. ___E___ recurrent rami
5. ___B___ testicular vein

A. An extension of the internal oblique muscle that descends to the testis with the spermatic cord

B. The pampiniform plexus forms each testicular vein.

C. Arises from the vesicle artery and supplies the vas deferens and epididymis

D. Small artery arising from the inferior epigastric artery, which supplies the peritesticular tissue, including the cremasteric muscle

E. Terminal ends of the centripetal arteries that curve backward toward the capsule

Exercise 3

Match the following pathology terms with their definitions.

1. ___G___ cryptorchidism
2. ___C___ epididymal cyst
3. ___F___ epididymitis
4. ___J___ hematocele
5. ___D___ hydrocele
6. ___H___ pyocele
7. ___I___ rete testis ?
8. ___A___ scrotum
9. ___E___ spermatocele
10. ___B___ varicocele

A. Sac containing the testes and epididymis

B. Dilated veins in the pampiniform plexus

C. Cyst filled with clear, serous fluid located in the epididymis

D. Fluid formed between the visceral and parietal layers of the tunica vaginalis

E. Cyst in the vas deferens containing sperm

F. Inflammation of the epididymis

G. Testicles remain within the abdomen or groin and fail to descend into the scrotal sac

H. Pus located between the visceral and parietal layers of the tunica vaginalis

I. Network of the channels formed by the convergence of the straight seminiferous tubules in the mediastinum testis

J. Blood located between the visceral and parietal layers of the tunica vaginalis

ANATOMY AND PHYSIOLOGY

Exercise 4

Fill in the blank(s) with the word(s) that best completes the statements about the anatomy and physiology of the scrotum.

1. The testes are symmetric, oval-shaped glands residing in the _Scrotum_.

2. These tubules converge at the apex of each lobule and anastomose to form the _rete testis_ in the mediastinum.

3. The largest part of the epididymis is the _head_, measuring 6 to 15 mm in width.

4. The ductus epididymis becomes the _Vas deferens_ and continues in the spermatic cord.

5. The testis is completely covered by a dense, fibrous tissue termed the _tunica albuginea_

6. The _mediastinum_ supports the ducts coursing within the testis.

7. The space between the layers of the tunica vaginalis is where _hydroceles_ form.

8. The _vas deferens_ is a continuation of the ductus _epididymis_.

9. The vas deferens dilates at the terminal portion near the _seminal vesicles_.

10. Right and left testicular arteries arise from the _abd'l aorta_ just below the level of the renal arteries.

11. Venous drainage of the scrotum occurs through the veins of the _pampiniform_ plexus.

12. Power Doppler is often used as a way to quickly get to a sensitive setting that will demonstrate _slow_ flow.

PATHOLOGY

Exercise 5

Fill in the blank(s) with the word(s) that best completes the statements or provide a short answer about the pathologic conditions of the scrotum.

1. The most important goal of the ultrasound examination in testicular trauma is to determine if _rupture_ has occurred.

2. An acute hematocele is _echogenic_ with numerous, highly visible echoes that can be seen to float or move in real time.

3. The most common cause of acute scrotal pain in adults is _Epididymo-orchitis_ infection of the epididymis and testis.

4. The normal epididymis shows _little_ flow with color Doppler.

5. With epididymitis, Doppler waveforms demonstrate _increased_ velocities in both systole and diastole. A low resistance waveform pattern is present.

6. Hydroceles are found around the _anterolateral_ aspect of the testis.

7. _Torsion_ of the spermatic cord occurs as a result of abnormal mobility of the testis within the scrotum.

8. The _bell clapper_ anomaly occurs when the tunica vaginalis completely surrounds the testis, epididymis, and distal spermatic cord, allowing them to move and rotate freely within the scrotum.

9. Torsion is the most common cause of acute scrotal pain in _adolescents_.

10. An _absence_ of perfusion in the symptomatic testis with normal perfusion demonstrated in the asymptomatic side is considered to be diagnostic of torsion.

11. Extratesticular cysts are found in the tunica _albuginea_ or epididymis.

12. _Varicoceles_ are usually caused by incompetent venous valves within the spermatic vein.

13. Omental hernias appear _brightly echogenic_ because of the omental fat.

14. A _hydrocele_ contains serous fluid and is the most common cause of painless scrotal swelling.

15. Testicular cancer occurs most frequently between the ages of _20-34_ years.

16. Patients with _undescended_ testes are 2.5 to 8 times more likely to develop cancer.

17. These masses called _non-germ cell tumors_ *extratesticular/* are usually benign, whereas _germ cell tumors/intratesticular_ masses are more likely to be malignant.

18. The term _cryptorchidism_ describes a condition in which the testis has not descended into the scrotum and cannot be brought into the scrotum with external manipulation.

Exercise 6

undescended testicle

Provide a short answer for each question after evaluating the images.

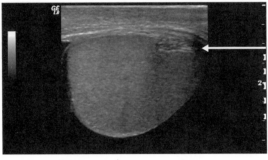

1. The arrow is pointing to this anatomic structure.

    rete testis

    testis mediastinum

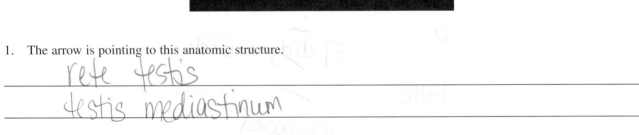

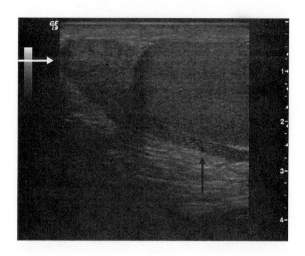

2. Identify the parts of the epididymis at the black arrow and white arrow.

white -(head)   black-body

or upper pole

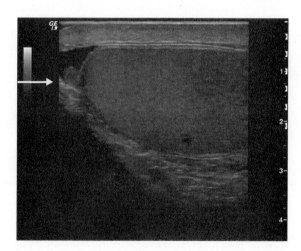

3. Identify the structure (arrow) superior to the normal testis.

appendix testis

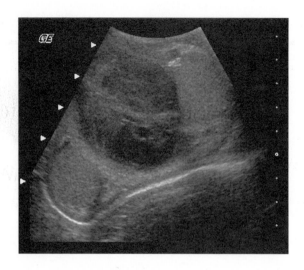

4. A young hemophilic patient experienced a recent bike trauma. The image of the left testis demonstrates:

Complex hematoma

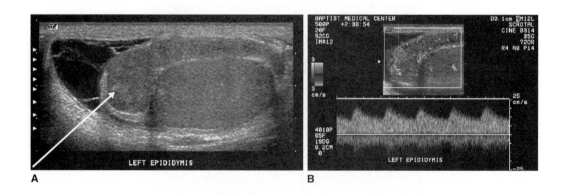

A   B

5. A young male presents with exquisite pain and tenderness over the left testis. These images demonstrate this abnormality:

Severe epididymitis w/ enlarged epididymis w/ a heterogeneous echo pattern. Focal hyperechoic areas w/ in epididymis may represent hemorrhage. A complex hydrocele w/ numerous septations is seen near the epididymal head. Doppler shows increased diastolic flow associated w/ inflammation.

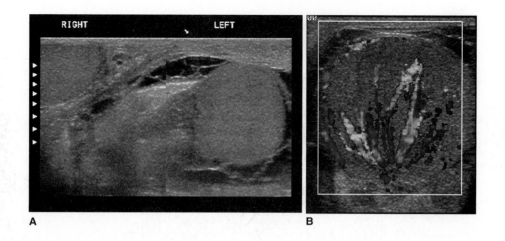

A   B

6. A young male presents with severe scrotal pain and swelling. The sonogram demonstrates:

enlarged left + normal right. complex hydrocele around left. Marked skin thickening on left. Hyperemic flow

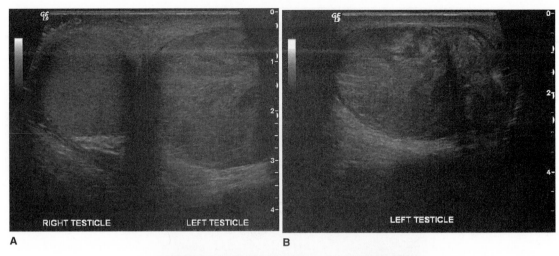

A

B

C

7. A young adolescent with a history of scrotal pain of duration greater than 24 hours had an ultrasound examination. The findings are:

Lt spermatic cord torsion. Lt testis is enlarged & heterogeneous. The infarcted testis has a mixed echo pattern caused by hemorrhage, necrosis + vascular congestion b/c more than 24 hrs. No flow shown in Lt.

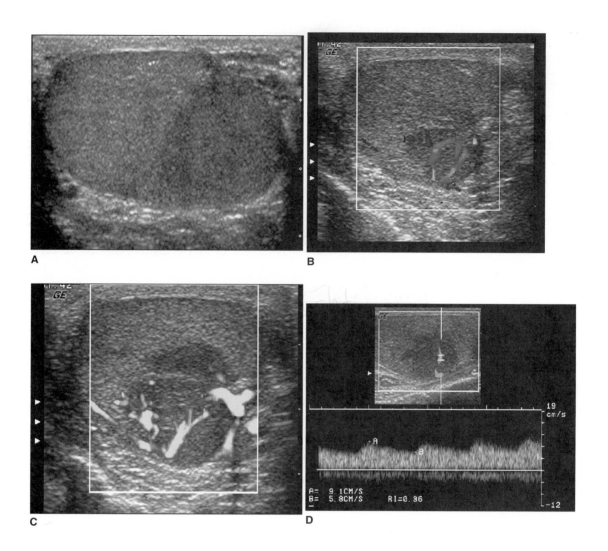

A   B

C   D

8. A young male with a recent history of a scrotal mass. The ultrasound shows:

Germ cell testicular tumor. Testis is heterogeneous b/c hypoechoic area. B shows distortion of normal vessel architecture. C-power doppler shows distorted vasculature of testis w/ in the mass. D-low resistance Dop flow pattern w/ prominent end diast, velocities characteristic of tumor flow

20 The Musculoskeletal System

KEY TERMS

Exercise 1
Match the following anatomic terms with their definitions.

1. _____ aponeurosis

2. _____ bursa

3. _____ epineurium

4. _____ fasciculi

5. _____ ligament

6. _____ muscle

7. _____ myelin

8. _____ perineurium

9. _____ pennate

10. _____ synovial sheath

11. _____ tendon

12. _____ volar

A. A type of tissue consisting of contractile cells or fibers that affects movement of an organ or part of the body

B. The covering of a nerve that consists of connective tissue

C. Membrane surrounding a joint, tendon, or bursa that secretes a viscous fluid called synovia

D. The surrounding connective tissue of muscle

E. Bandlike flat tendons connecting the process of the scapula

F. Fibrous band of tissue connecting bone or cartilage to bone that aids in stabilizing a joint

G. Fibrous tissue connecting muscle to bone

H. A saclike structure containing thick fluid that surrounds areas subject to friction, such as the interface between bone and tendon

I. Substance forming the sheath of Schwann cells

J. The anterior portion of the body when in the anatomic position

K. Term describing a small bundle of muscles, nerves, and tendons

L. Featherlike pattern of muscle growth

Exercise 2
Match the following artifact, sonography, and pathology terms with their definitions.

1. _____ acromioclavicular joint

2. _____ anisotropy

3. _____ cartilage interface sign

4. _____ comet tail artifact

5. _____ dorsiflexion

6. _____ Guyon's canal or tunnel

A. Echogenic line on the anterior surface of the cartilage surrounding the humeral head

B. A fibrous tunnel that contains the ulnar artery and vein, ulnar nerve, and some fatty tissue

C. Accumulation of serous fluid within tissue

D. The joint found in the shoulder that connects the clavicle to the acromion process of the scapula

E. Pointing of the toes toward the plantar surface of the foot

F. The quality of comprising varying values of a given property when measured in different directions

7. _____ plantar flexion

8. _____ refractile shadowing

9. _____ seroma

10. _____ tendonitis

11. _____ Thompson test

G. The bending of the sound beam at the edge of a circular structure, resulting in the absence of posterior echoes

H. A test used to evaluate the integrity of the Achilles tendon that involves plantar flexion with squeezing of the calf

I. Upward movement of the hand and foot

J. Inflammation of the tendon

K. Posterior linear equidistant artifact created when sound reverberates between two strong reflectors, such as air bubbles, metal, and glass

ANATOMY

Exercise 3

Label the following illustrations.

1. Different types of muscle.

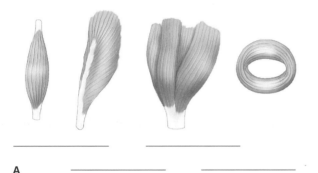

_____   _____

A   _____   _____

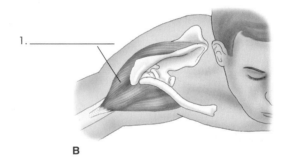

1. _____

B

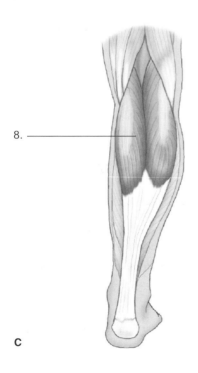

8. _____

C

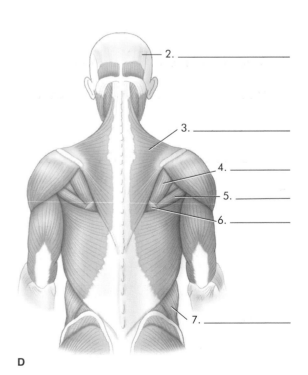

2. _____

3. _____

4. _____

5. _____

6. _____

7. _____

D

2. The subscapularis, biceps tendon, and the acromioclavicular joint image.

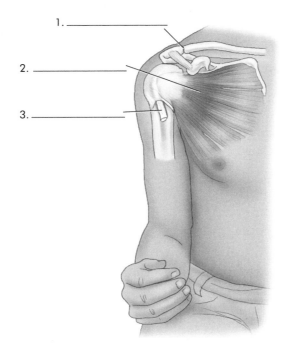

1._____

2._____

3._____

Exercise 4

Fill in the blank(s) with the word(s) that best completes the statements about the anatomy of the musculoskeletal system.

1. Skeletal muscle contains long organized units called muscle _____.

2. The characteristic long fibers are under voluntary control, allowing us to contract a _____ and move a joint.

3. A _____ muscle has a division of several featherlike sections in one muscle, and the _____ is the convergence of fibers to a central tendon.

4. The attachment of the muscle that occurs at the proximal and distal portion of the bundle is called

   a _____.

5. Tendons occur with or without a _____ sheath.

6. The sheath surrounding a tendon has two layers. The fluid separates the layers in this part of the body:

   _____, _____, _____, and _____.

7. Short bands of tough fibers that connect bones to other bones are _____.

8. The saclike structure surrounding joints and tendons that contains a viscous fluid is the _____.

9. The knee joint has _____ bursa.

10. A loose areolar connective tissue that fills the fascial compartment of the tendon lacking a synovial sheath is

   _____.

11. The dense _____ is another layer of connective tissue that closely adjoins the tendon.

12. Interwoven and interconnected collagen fibers found in the tendon run in a _____ path.

13. The _____ (transverse and/or longitudinal) imaging of the ligament is the only method to image injury.

14. The proximal portion of the muscle is considered the _____, whereas the _____ is the distal end.

15. The normal nerve has a _____ appearance when compared with muscle, but is _____ to tendons.

16. The minute amount of viscous fluid contained within the bursa helps reduce _____ between the moving parts of the joint.

17. A Baker's cyst is an example of a _____ (communicating and/or noncommunicating) bursa in the medial popliteal fossa.

18. The loss of definition of the curved upper pole of the right kidney is an example of _____ phenomenon.

19. The bending of the transmitted sound beam to an oblique path occurs often and is seen as an _____ artifact on the sonographic image.

20. The angles formed from the retracted tendon cause _____ shadowing.

21. _____ artifacts occur when the returning sound wave has passed between two tissues with markedly different speeds of sound.

SIGNS AND TESTS

Exercise 5

Match the following musculoskeletal signs and tests with their definitions.

1. _____ Barlow's test

2. _____ cartilage interface sign

3. _____ clapper-in-the-bell sign

4. _____ comet tail artifact (ring down)

5. _____ naked tuberosity sign

6. _____ Ortolani test

7. _____ Phalen sign

A. An increase in wrist compression caused by hyper-flexion of the wrist for 60 seconds; this test is done with the patient holding the forearms upright and pressing the ventral side of the hands together

B. Posterior linear equidistant artifact created when sound reverberates between two strong reflectors, such as air bubbles, metal, and glass

C. Infant hip dislocation occurring with flexion, adduction, and posterior force upon the 90-degree flexed infant hip while the examiner's thumbs are placed on the medial proximal thigh and the fingers placed over the greater trochanter

D. Pins and needles type of tingling felt distally to a percussion site and either a normal or abnormal occurrence (e.g., hitting the elbow creates a tingling in the distal arm)

8. _____ refractile shadowing (edge artifact)

9. _____ Thompson test

10. _____ Tinel's sign

E. The deltoid muscle is on the humeral head; seen with a full-thickness tear of the rotator cuff

F. A test used to evaluate the integrity of the Achilles tendon that involves plantar flexion with squeezing of the calf

G. Hypoechoic hematoma found at the end of a completely retracted muscle fragment

H. Reduction of the infant hip through abduction and anterior traction of the thigh; confirmation of reduction is through the palpable and occasionally audible clunk of the femoral head returning to the acetabulum

I. Echogenic line on the anterior surface of the cartilage surrounding the humeral head

J. The bending of the sound beam at the edge of a circular structure resulting in the absence of posterior echoes

SONOGRAPHIC EVALUATION

Exercise 6

Fill in the blank(s) with the word(s) that best completes the statements or provide a short answer about the sonographic techniques of the musculoskeletal system.

1. To begin the examination of the biceps, place the patient with a slight _____ rotation of the shoulder.

2. When facing the patient and imaging the right shoulder, the lateral anatomy displays on the _____ side of the image and the medial anatomy on the _____ side of the screen.

3. The groove located between the greater and lesser tuberosities, coupled with the overlying transverse ligament, maintains the _____ tendon location.

4. Using the biceps tendon as a landmark, angle the transducer _____ to locate the subscapularis tendon.

5. The bandlike tendon that has a medium level echotexture is the _____ tendon and originates from the greater tuberosity of the humerus.

6. A good landmark to help find the anteriorly located infraspinatus tendon is the posterior _____.

7. Fluid imaged _____ to the infraspinatus tendon indicates bursal fluid, whereas _____ fluid indicates joint effusion.

8. The carpal tunnel is located between the _____ bones and the _____ retinaculum on the palmar side of the wrist.

9. The ulnar artery and veins indicate the medial border of the carpal tunnel, whereas the most lateral structure is the _____ artery and veins.

10. The tendon that connects the gastrocnemius and soleus muscles to the calcaneus is the _____ tendon.

11. The dislocation of the biceps tendon from the bicipital groove may be due to a problem with:

_____

_____

_____

12. The _____ thickness tear involves either the bursal or articular cuff surface or the intrasubstance material.

13. The presence of large amounts of fluid in the subacromial-subdeltoid bursa raises the chance of a nonvisualized

_____ tear.

14. The normal tendon cannot be compressed; however, the injured tendon _____ as the torn edges move apart.

15. Joint effusion around the biceps tendon combined with subacromial-subdeltoid bursitis results in the

_____ sign.

16. Acute tendonitis involves not only the tendon but the surrounding _____ sheath.

17. The normal synovial sheath appears as a hypoechoic _____ around the tendon.

18. The abrupt stretching of the muscle beyond the maximum length results in a _____ tear.

19. External force resulting in a crush injury is considered a _____ tear.

PATHOLOGY

Exercise 7
Provide a short answer for each question after evaluating the images.

1. The arrow is pointing to this mildly hyperechoic structure in the shoulder.

_____

_____

_____

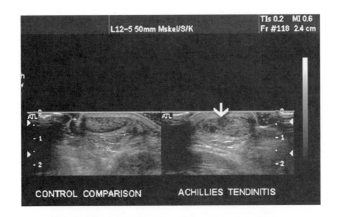

CONTROL COMPARISON   ACHILLIES TENDINITIS

2. The comparison of the normal with the injured Achilles tendon may show this abnormality.

_____

_____

_____

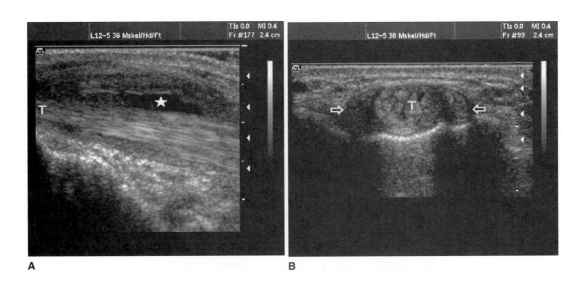

A   B

3. De Quervain's tendonitis is identified in this patient. The sonographic findings are:

_____

_____

_____

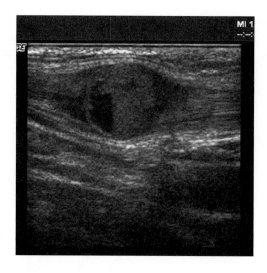

4. A soccer player experienced intense pain in his calf after a sudden blow in a championship game. The sonographic findings are:

_____

_____

_____

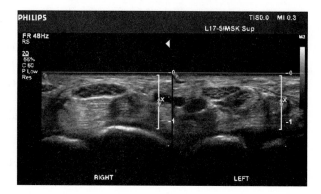

5. This sonographic image demonstrates this abnormality that may be seen in carpal tunnel syndrome.

_____

_____

_____

21 Neonatal Echoencephalography

KEY TERMS

Exercise 1

Match the following embryology and anatomic terms with their definitions.

1. _____ asphyxia

2. _____ atrium (trigone) of the lateral ventricles

3. _____ brain stem

4. _____ caudate nucleus

5. _____ cavum septum pellucidum

6. _____ cerebellum

7. _____ cerebrum

8. _____ choroid plexus

9. _____ cistern

10. _____ corpus callosum

11. _____ falx cerebri

12. _____ fontanelle

13. _____ hypoxia

14. _____ meninges

15. _____ sulcus

16. _____ tentorium cerebelli

17. _____ thalamic-caudate groove

18. _____ thalamus

A. Echogenic cluster of cells important in the production of cerebrospinal fluid that lies along the atrium of the lateral ventricles

B. Three membranes enclosing the brain and spinal cord

C. Echogenic fibrous structure that separates the cerebral hemispheres

D. Composed of the midbrain, pons, and medulla oblongata

E. Prominent structure best seen in the midline filled with cerebrospinal fluid in the premature infant

F. The region at which the thalamus and caudate nucleus join

G. Two equal hemispheres; largest part of the brain

H. Prominent group of nerve fibers that connect the right and left sides of the brain

I. Severe hypoxia or inadequate oxygenation

J. Decrease oxygen in the body

K. Forms the lateral borders of the anterior horns, anterior to the thalamus

L. Echogenic "V-shaped/tent" structure in the posterior fossa that separates the cerebellum from the cerebrum

M. Lies posterior to the brain stem below the tentorium

N. Two ovoid brain structures located midbrain, situated on either side of the third ventricle superior to the brain stem

O. The ventricle is measured at this site on the axial view

P. Groove on the surface of the brain that separates the gyri

Q. Soft space between the bones

R. Reservoir for cerebrospinal fluid

Exercise 2

Match the following neonatal echoencephalography terms with their definitions.

1. _____ aqueductal stenosis

2. _____ Chiari malformation

3. _____ coronal plane

4. _____ Dandy-Walker malformation

5. _____ extracorporeal membrane oxygenation

6. _____ holoprosencephaly

7. _____ neonatal

8. _____ periventricular leukomalacia

9. _____ sagittal plane

10. _____ subependyma

11. _____ subependymal cyst

12. _____ ventriculitis

A. Transducer is perpendicular to the anterior fontanelle in the coronal axis of the head

B. Perpendicular to the coronal plane with the transducer in the anterior fontanelle

C. Abnormal single ventricular cavity with some form of thalami fusion

D. Congenital defect in which the cerebellum and brain stem are pulled toward the spinal cord (banana sign)

E. Cyst that occurs at the site of a previous bleed in the germinal matrix

F. Echogenic white matter necrosis best seen in the posterior aspect of the brain or adjacent to the ventricular structures

G. Congenital blockage of the aqueduct connecting the third and fourth ventricles causing dilation of the third and fourth ventricles

H. Early newborn period

I. Inflammation/infection of the ventricles, which appears as echogenic linear structures along the gyri

J. Term used for the treatment of infants with severe respiratory failure who have not responded to maximal conventional ventilatory support

K. Area beneath the ependyma

L. Abnormal development of the fourth ventricle, often accompanied by hydrocephalus

ANATOMY AND PHYSIOLOGY

Exercise 3

Label the following illustrations.

1. Lateral view of an embryo at 23 days.

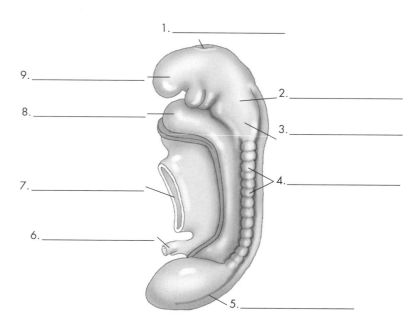

1. _____
9. _____
8. _____
2. _____
3. _____
4. _____
7. _____
6. _____
5. _____

2. Development of the brain and the ventricular system at 10 weeks.

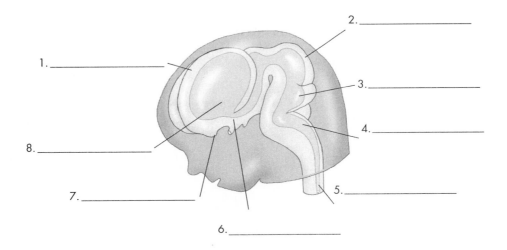

1. _____

2. _____

3. _____

4. _____

5. _____

6. _____

7. _____

8. _____

3. Neonatal skull showing the sutures and open anterior fontanelle (Fig. 21-4).

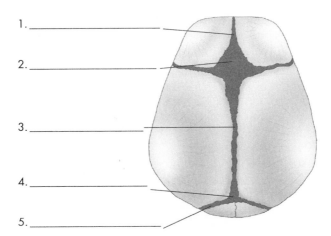

1. _____

2. _____

3. _____

4. _____

5. _____

4. Sagittal view of the ventricular system.

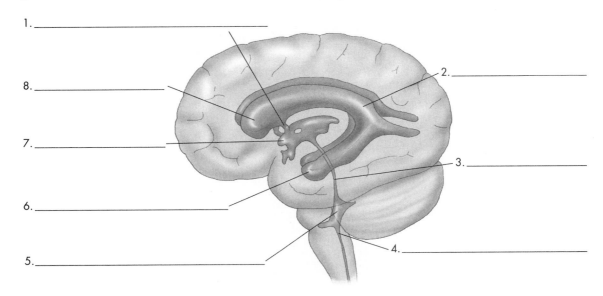

1. _____

2. _____

3. _____

4. _____

5. _____

6. _____

7. _____

8. _____

5. Anterior view of the ventricles.

8. _____

7. _____

6. _____

5. _____

1. _____

2. _____

3. _____

4. _____

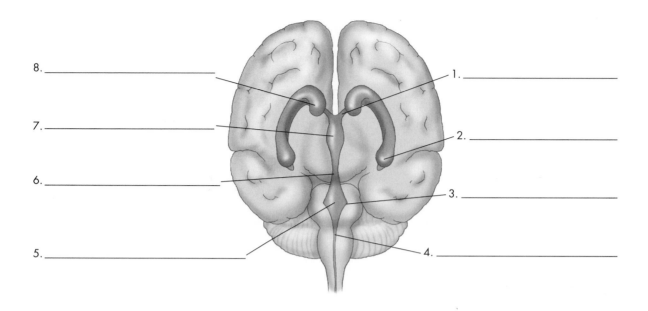

6. Sagittal view of choroid plexus and cisterns of the ventricular system.

9. _____

8. _____

7. _____

6. _____

1. _____

2. _____

3. _____

4. _____

5. _____

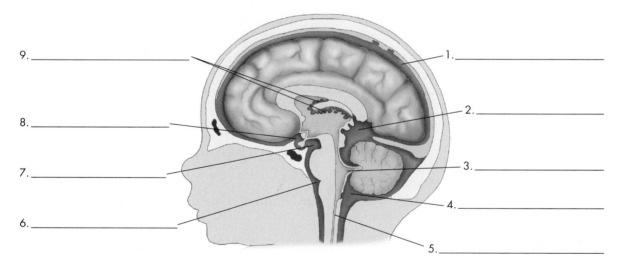

7. Sagittal view of cerebral cortex.

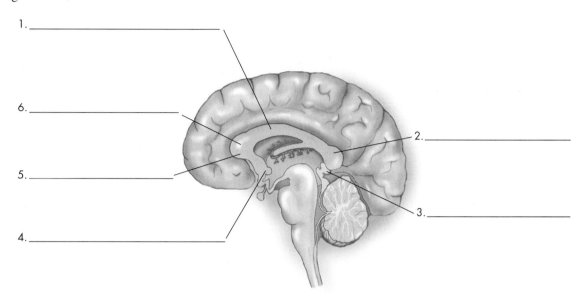

1._____

6._____

2._____

5._____

3._____

4._____

8. Axial view of cerebral cortex and corpus callosum.

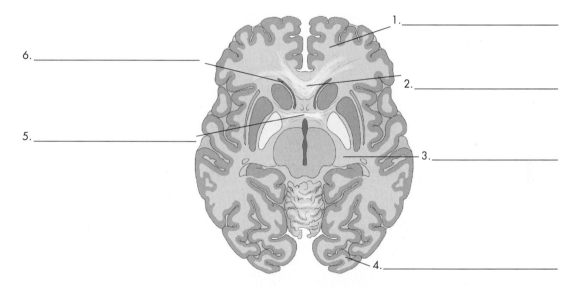

1._____

6._____

2._____

5._____

3._____

4._____

9. Coronal view of cerebral lobes, corpus callosum, and sylvian fissure.

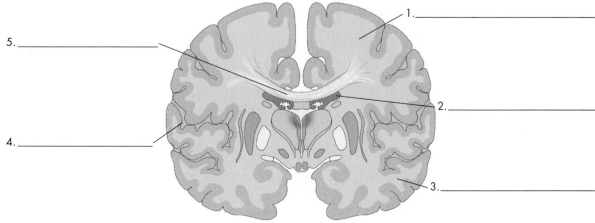

1._____

5._____

2._____

4._____

3._____

10. Lateral and axial view of the basal ganglia.

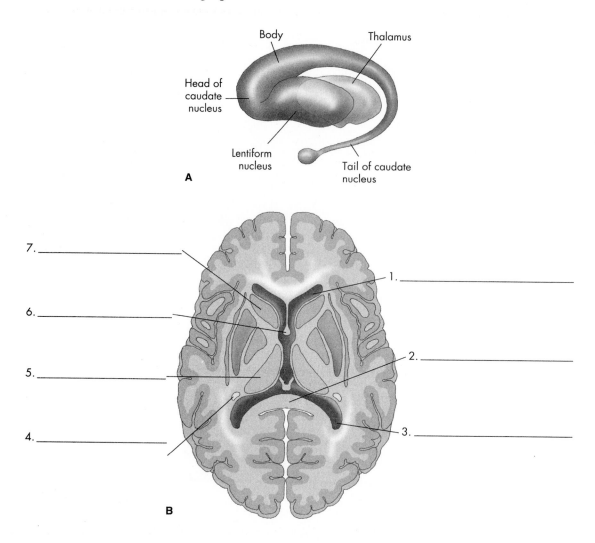

Body

Thalamus

Head of
caudate
nucleus

Lentiform
nucleus

Tail of caudate
nucleus

A

7.

6.

5.

4.

1.

2.

3.

B

11. Coronal view of the medulla oblongata.

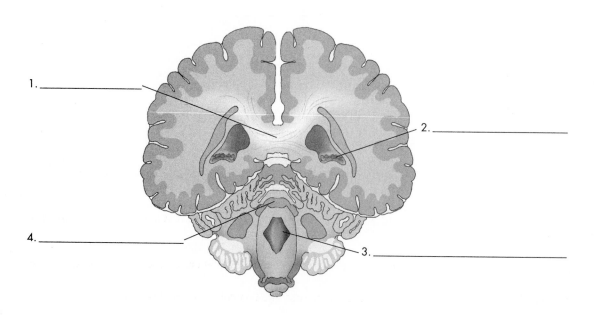

1.

2.

4.

3.

Exercise 4

Fill in the blank(s) with the word(s) that best completes the statements about the anatomy of the neural axis.

1. The central nervous system develops from the _____ plate.

2. Consisting of both the brain and the spinal cord, the _____ differentiates into the central nervous system.

3. The thalami fuse in the midline and form a fusion called the _____.

4. Along the choroidal fissure, the medial wall of the developing cerebral hemisphere becomes thin. Invaginations of vascular pia form the _____ of the lateral ventricles at this site.

5. As the mesenchyme is trapped in the midline with the growth of the hemispheres the _____ is formed.

6. The _____ forms from the cavity of the hindbrain and also contains choroid plexus like the lateral and third ventricles.

7. The spaces between the bones of the skull are _____.

8. The _____ fontanelle is located at the top of the neonatal head and may be easily felt as the "soft spot."

9. A double layered outer membrane that forms the toughest barrier is the _____.

10. The " V-shaped" echogenic structure, also known as the _____, separates the cerebrum and the cerebellum; it is an extension of the falx cerebri.

11. The _____ ventricles communicate with the third ventricle through the interventricular foramen of Monro.

12. The cavum septum pellucidum forms the medial wall and the _____ forms the roof.

13. The _____ touches the inferior lateral ventricular wall and the body of the caudate _____ borders the superior wall.

14. The third and fourth ventricles are connected by the _____.

15. The lateral angles of the fourth ventricle form the foramen of _____.

16. The _____ surrounds and protects the brain and spinal cord from physical impact.

17. The mass of special cells that regulate the intraventricular pressure by secretion or absorption of cerebral spinal fluid is the _____

18. The _____ is located along the lateralmost aspect of the brain and is the area where the middle cerebral artery is located.

19. The _____ borders the third ventricle and connects through the middle of the third ventricle by the massa intermedia.

20. The _____ extends from the pons to the foramen magnum where it continues as the spinal cord.

21. Three pairs of nerve tracts, the _____, connect the cerebellum to the brain stem.

Exercise 5

Fill in the blank(s) with the word(s) that best completes the statements about the sonographic techniques of neonatal encephalography.

1. Both cerebral hemispheres, the basal ganglia, the lateral and third ventricles, the interhemispheric fissure, and the

   subarachnoid space surrounding the hemispheres are shown in _____ studies.

2. The cerebellum, the brain stem, the fourth ventricle, and the basal cisterns are visualized in _____ studies.

3. Technically a _____ view is 90 degrees to Reid's baseline.

4. When the transducer is angled _____, the frontal horns of the lateral ventricles appear as slit-like hypoechoic to cystic formations.

5. As the transducer is angled _____, the ventricles acquire a comma-like shape.

6. Ultrasound depicts the choroid plexus as a very _____ structure inside the ventricular cavities surrounding the thalamic nuclei.

7. In premature infants the caudate nuclei may have _____ echogenicity than the rest of the brain parenchyma.

8. The _____ ventricle appears in the midline as a small anechoic space approximately 2 to 3 mm wide, located anteriorly to the vermis.

PATHOLOGY

Exercise 6

Fill in the blank(s) with the word(s) or provide a short answer that best completes the statements about the pathology of the neonatal head.

1. A congenital anomaly associated with spina bifida is a _____ malformation in which the cerebellum and brain stem are pulled toward the spinal cord and secondary hydrocephalus develops.

2. Chiari malformation is frequently associated with myelomeningocele, _____, dilation of the third ventricle, and absence of the septum pellucidum.

3. _____ is characterized by a grossly abnormal brain in which there is a common large central ventricle.

4. Dandy-Walker syndrome is a congenital anomaly in which a huge _____ ventricle cyst occupies the area where the cerebellum usually lies, with secondary dilation of the third and lateral ventricles.

5. A Dandy-Walker variant is present when there is an enlarged _____ communicating with the fourth ventricle in the presence of a normal or hypoplastic cerebellar vermis.

6. Complete absence of the _____ is distinguished by narrow frontal horns, as well as marked separation of the anterior horns and bodies of the lateral ventricles associated with widening of the occipital horns and the third ventricle.

7. Any condition in which enlargement of the ventricular system is caused by an imbalance between production and

reabsorption of cerebrospinal fluid (CSF) is referred to as _____.

8. The CSF pathways are open within the ventricular system in _____ hydrocephalus but there is decreased absorption of CSF.

9. The most common cause of congenital hydrocephalus is _____.

10. The most common hemorrhagic lesions in preterm newborn infants are _____ hemorrhages.

11. Subependymal hemorrhages (SEHs) are caused by capillary bleeding in the _____ .

12. Studies from the anterior fontanelle may not detect small IVHs, since intraventricular blood tends to "settle out" in

the _____ horns.

13. Intraparenchymal hemorrhages appear as very _____ zones in the white matter adjacent to the lateral ventricles.

14. _____ can result from a variety of insults including respiratory failure, congenital heart disease, and sepsis.

15. White matter ischemia leads to white matter volume loss or _____ leukomalacia.

16. The chronic stage of WMN is identified with ultrasound when _____ develop in the echogenic white matter.

17. A common complication of purulent meningitis in newborn infants is _____.

18. _____ occurs when the ependyma become thickened and hyperechoic as a result of irritation from hemorrhage within the ventricle.

Provide a short answer for each question after evaluating the images.

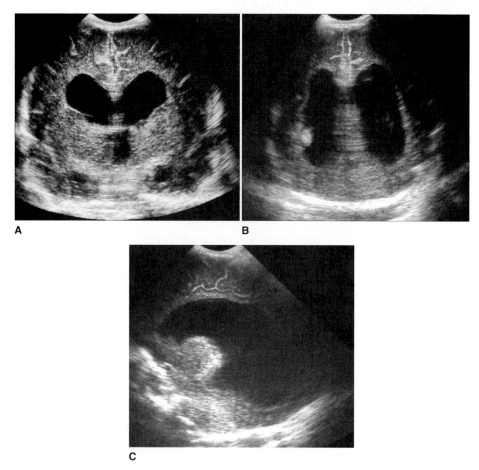

A   B

C

From Henningsen C: *Clinical guide to ultrasonography*, St. Louis, 2004, Mosby.

1. An infant was delivered by cesarean section at 39 weeks gestation for a thoracic spina bifida. What are the sonographic findings in the head?

_____

_____

_____

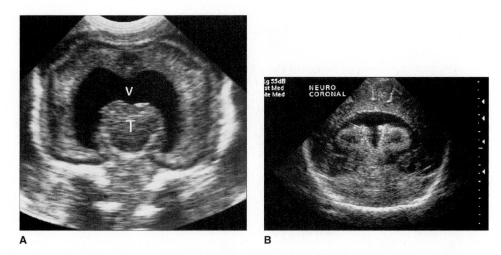

A

B

From Henningsen C: *Clinical guide to ultrasonography*, St. Louis, 2004, Mosby.

2. Describe the difference between the two types of holoprosenecephaly shown in these two images.

_____

_____

_____

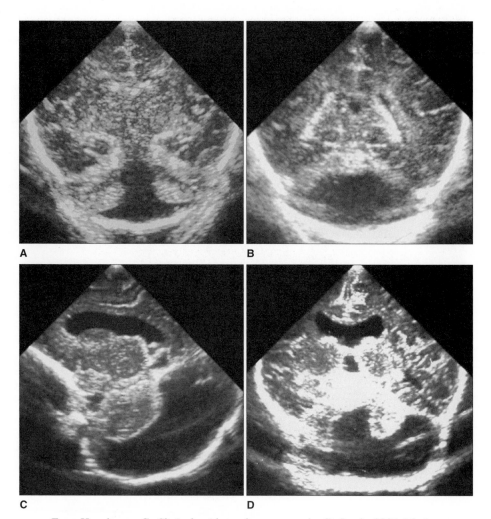

From Henningsen C: *Clinical guide to ultrasonography*, St. Louis, 2004, Mosby.

3. A female infant was delivered at 37 weeks gestation. What are the sonographic findings?

_____

_____

_____

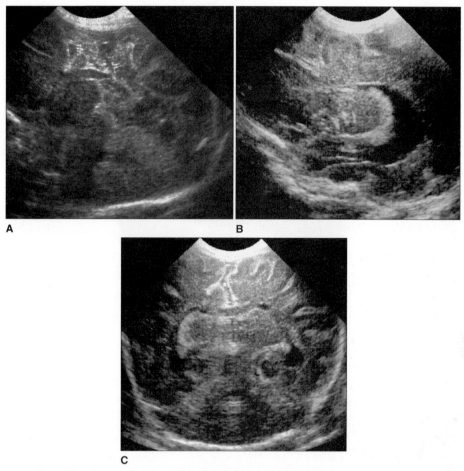

A   B

C

From Henningsen C: *Clinical guide to ultrasonography*, St. Louis, 2004, Mosby.

4. These sonographic images are typical of what abnormality of the neonatal head?

_____

_____

_____

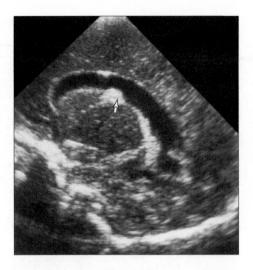

5. The arrow points to what abnormality in this premature infant?

_____

_____

_____

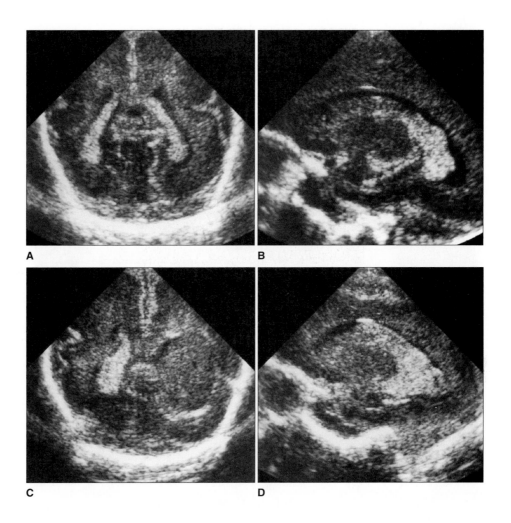

A

B

C

D

6. What bleed classification would you consider for this premature infant?

_____

_____

_____

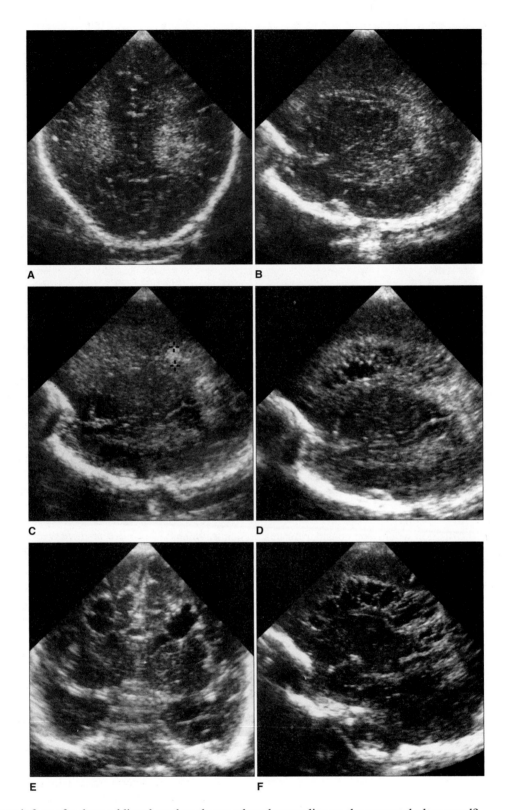

A   B

C   D

E   F

7. Premature infant of a drug-addicted mother shows what abnormality on the neonatal ultrasound?

_____

_____

22 The Pediatric Abdomen: Jaundice and Common Surgical Conditions

KEY TERMS

Exercise 1

Match the following pathology terms with their definitions.

1. _____ Beckwith-Wiedemann syndrome

2. _____ biliary atresia

3. _____ choledochal cyst

4. _____ hemihypertrophy

5. _____ hypertrophic pyloric stenosis

6. _____ inspissated

7. _____ intussusception

8. _____ neuroblastoma

9. _____ neonate

10. _____ projectile vomiting

11. _____ pyloric canal

12. _____ scintigraphy

13. _____ target (donut) sign

14. _____ Wilms' tumor

A. Thickened by absorption, evaporation, or dehydration

B. The excessive development of one side or one half of the body or an organ

C. Frequently associated with sectional areas of the gastrointestinal tract; the muscle is hyperechoic, and the inner core is hypoechoic

D. Congenital cystic malformation of the common bile duct

E. Photographing the scintillations emitted by radioactive substances injected into the body; this test is used to determine the outline and function of organs and tissues in which the radioactive substance collects or is secreted

F. Occurs when bowel prolapses into distal bowel and is propelled in an antegrade fashion

G. An autosomal recessive condition characterized by macroglossia, gigantism, hemihypertrophy, and exophthalmos; individuals may also manifest organomegaly and are at increased risk for development of certain abdominal neoplasms

H. Infant in the first 28 days of life

I. Located between the stomach and duodenum

J. Thickened muscle in the pylorus that prevents food from entering the duodenum; occurs more frequently in males

K. Closure or absence of some or all of the major bile ducts

L. A rapidly developing tumor of the kidney that usually occurs in children

M. A malignant hemorrhagic tumor composed principally of cells resembling neuroblasts that give rise to cells of the sympathetic system (especially the adrenal medulla)

N. Condition in pyloric stenosis in the neonatal period; after drinking, the infant experiences projectile vomiting secondary to the obstruction in the pylorus

Exercise 2

Label the following illustrations.

1. Diagram of hypertrophic pyloric stenosis (Fig. 22-14).

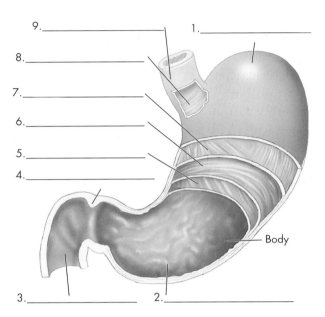

9._____   1._____

8._____

7._____

6._____

5._____

4._____

                                        ——— Body

3._____   2._____

THE PEDIATRIC ABDOMEN

Exercise 3

Fill in the blank(s) with the word(s) that best completes the statements or provide a short answer about the pediatric abdomen.

1. The right hepatic lobe should not extend more than _____ cm below the costal margin in the young infant.

2. The common bile duct should measure less than _____ mm in neonates, less than _____ mm in infants up to 1 year old, less than _____ mm in older children, and less than _____ mm in adolescents and adults.

3. The length of the gallbladder should not exceed the length of the _____.

4. The three most common causes for jaundice in the neonate are: _____, _____, and

   _____.

5. Identify the clinical features of biliary atresia in the neonate.

   _____

   _____

   _____

6. An abnormal cystic dilation of the biliary tree that most frequently affects the common bile duct is a(n)

_____.

7. When a choledochal cyst is present there is usually _____ of the common bile duct with associated

_____ ductal dilation.

8. The most common benign vascular liver tumor of early childhood is infantile hepatic _____.

9. The most common sonographic appearance of hemangioendothelioma is that of multiple _____

lesions and _____.

10. The most common primary malignant disease of the liver is _____ and occurs most frequently in children under 5 years of age.

11. The _____ is located between the stomach and duodenum.

12. _____ occurs most commonly in male infants between 2 and 6 weeks of age.

13. As the pyloric muscle thickens and elongates, the stomach outlet obstruction increases and vomiting is more

constant and _____.

14. A muscle thickness of _____ mm or greater on the long-axis view, a channel length of

_____ mm or greater, and pyloric muscle length of _____ or greater are reliable indicators of HPS.

15. In infants and young children, the progression of acute appendicitis to _____ is more rapid than in older children.

16. With ultrasound the acutely inflamed appendix is _____.

17. _____ produced by overlying transducer pressure is an additional finding consistent with appendicitis.

18. The most common acute abdominal disorder in early childhood is _____.

19. Alternating hypoechoic and hyperechoic rings surrounding an echogenic center as seen in a short-axis view of the

involved area is known as the _____ sign.

20. Intussusception may be reduced with _____ pressure or by air reduction.

Exercise 4

Provide a short answer for each question after evaluating the images.

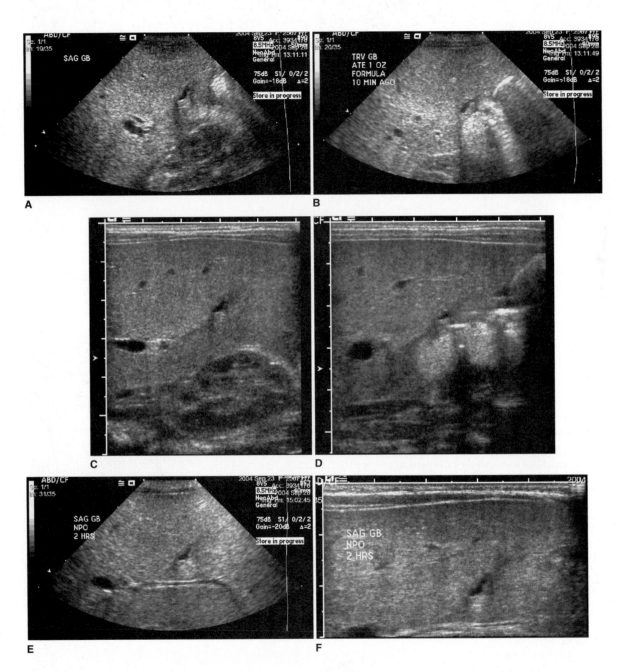

1. A 5-day-old infant presents with direct hyperbilirubinemia with unknown causes. Compare images **A** through **D** taken after eating to images **E** and **F** taken 2 hours later and identify the differences.

_____

_____

_____

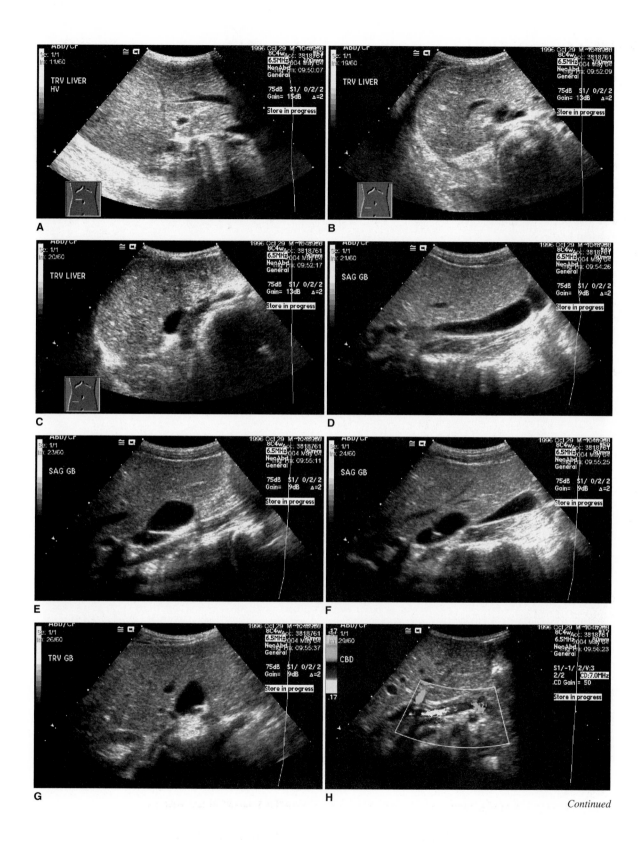

Continued

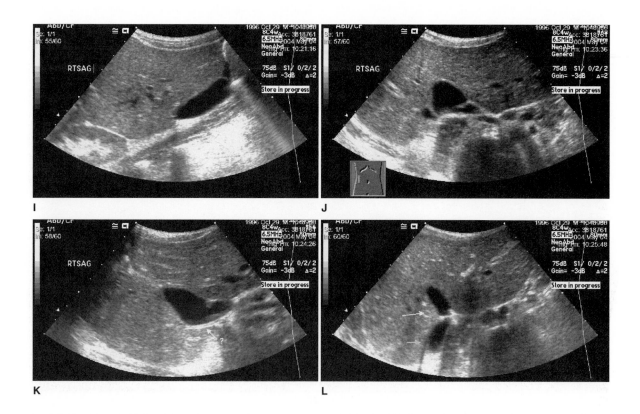

I

J

K

L

2. Look at images **E** and **F**. The cystic structure cephalic to the gallbladder in these sagittal images is:

_____

_____

_____

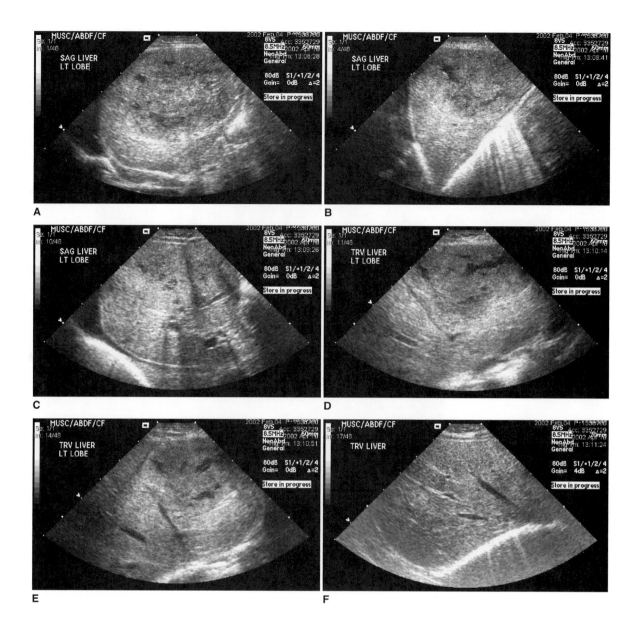

A

B

C

D

E

F

3. A 2-month-old infant with a history of a palpable abdominal mass and decrease in appetite was examined. The sonographic findings are:

_____

_____

_____

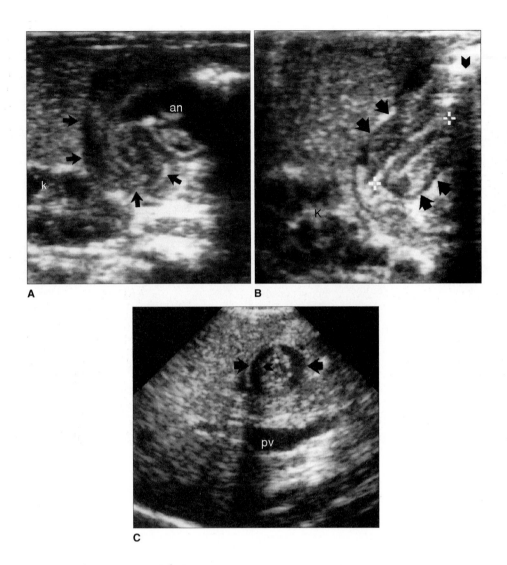

A

B

C

4. A neonate presented with projectile vomiting. The sonographic findings are:

_____

_____

_____

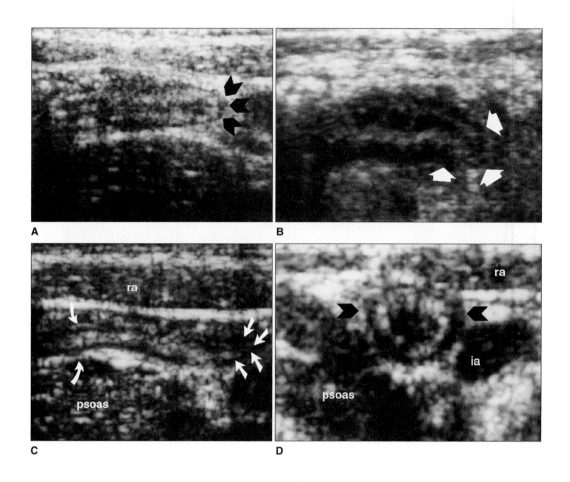

A

B

C

D

5. A child presented with nausea and vomiting, fever, and intense left lower quadrant pain. The sonographic finding is:

_____

_____

_____

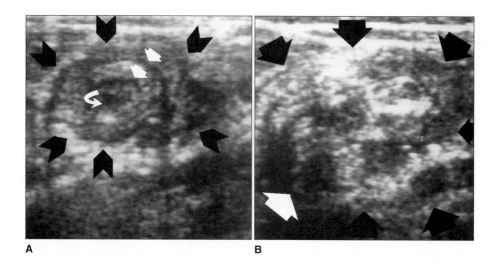

A   B

6. An infant presented with fever and peritoneal signs. The sonographic finding is:

_____

_____

_____

23 The Neonatal and Pediatric Kidneys and Adrenal Glands

KEY TERMS

Exercise 1

Match the following terms related to neonatal and pediatric kidneys with their definitions.

1. _____ adrenal hemorrhage

2. _____ arcuate arteries

3. _____ autosomal dominant polycystic kidney disease (ADPKD)

4. _____ autosomal recessive polycystic kidney disease (ARPKD)

5. _____ congenital mesoblastic nephroma

6. _____ cortex

7. _____ ectasia

8. _____ ectopic ureterocele

9. _____ hydronephrosis

10. _____ medullary pyramids

11. _____ multicystic dysplastic kidney (MCDK)

12. _____ neuroblastoma

13. _____ nephroblastomatosis

14. _____ polycystic renal disease

15. _____ posterior urethral valves

16. _____ Potter facies

17. _____ prune-belly syndrome

18. _____ pulmonary hypoplasia

19. _____ renal vein thrombosis

20. _____ ureteropelvic junction obstruction

A. Malignant tumor usually found in the adrenal glands

B. Dilation of the renal collecting system

C. Large and hypoechoic in the neonate

D. Poorly functioning enlarged kidneys

E. Most common benign renal tumor of the neonate and infant

F. Underdevelopment of the lung tissue that occurs in utero (secondary to oligohydramnios)

G. Classification of cystic renal disease

H. Abnormal persistence of fetal renal blastema (potential to develop into Wilms' tumor)

I. Most common neonatal obstruction of the urinary tract; results from intrinsic narrowing or extrinsic vascular compression

J. Lie at the base of the medullary pyramids and appear as echogenic structures

K. Congenital polycystic kidney disease that usually presents during middle age. Sometimes asymptomatic, the severity of the disease varies widely. Presents with hypertension, hematuria, and enlarged kidneys. Cysts can also form in the liver, spleen, and pancreas.

L. Adds cardiac and limb anomalies to the VATER syndrome

M. Most frequent malignant tumor in the neonate and infant

N. Dilation of any tubular vessel

O. Kidney becomes enlarged and edematous as a result of obstruction of the renal vein

P. Occurs more commonly in females (on left side); ectopic insertion and cystic dilation of distal ureter of duplicated renal collecting system

Q. Most common cause of bladder outlet obstruction in the male neonate

R. Occurs when the fetus is stressed during a difficult delivery or a hypoxic insult

S. Vertebral, anal, tracheoesophageal fistula and renal anomalies

T. Most common cause of renal cystic disease in the neonate; multiple cystic masses within the kidney; may have contralateral ureteral pelvic junction obstruction

21. _____ VACTER*L*

22. _____ VATER

23. _____ Wilms' tumor (nephroblastoma)

U. Triad of hypoplasia or deficiency of the abdominal musculature, cryptorchidism, and urinary tract anomalies

V. The outer rim of the kidney; the cortex is thin in the neonate, with an echogenicity similar to or slightly greater than that of the normal liver parenchyma

W. Rare, congenital polycystic renal disease also known as infantile polycystic disease; typically occurs with diffuse enlargement, sacculations, and cystic diverticula of the medullary portions of the kidneys

NEONATAL AND PEDIATRIC KIDNEYS AND ADRENAL GLANDS

Exercise 2
Fill in the blank(s) with the word(s) that best completes the statements about the neonatal and pediatric kidneys and adrenal glands.

1. In the second trimester, the kidney develops from small _____ composed of a central large pyramid with a thin peripheral rim of cortex.

2. As the renunculi fuse progressively, their adjoining cortices form a _____.

3. The former renunculi are at that point called "_____."

4. The _____ continue to grow throughout childhood, whereas the _____ become smaller in size.

5. The amount of cortical _____ is not present in the neonate and pediatric patient, thus allowing for clear distinction of the corticomedullary junction.

6. The _____ are large and hypoechoic and should not be mistaken for dilated calyces or cysts.

7. The surrounding cortex is quite thin, with echogenicity essentially similar to or slightly greater than that of normal _____ parenchyma.

8. The _____ vessels are seen as intense specular echoes at the corticomedullary junction.

9. At the site of the fetal lobulation, a parenchymal triangular defect may be identified in the anterosuperior or inferoposterior aspect of the kidney, known as a _____ defect.

10. Each adrenal gland lies immediately _____ to the upper pole of the kidney.

11. The normal urinary bladder is thin walled in the distended state and should measure less than _____ mm.

Exercise 3

Fill in the blank(s) with the word(s) that best completes the statements about the pathology of the neonatal and pediatric kidney and adrenal gland.

1. The dilatation of the urinary collecting system is known as _____.

2. The most common type of obstruction of the upper urinary tract is _____; it most often results from intrinsic narrowing or extrinsic vascular compression at the level of the ureteropelvic junction.

3. The obstruction produces _____ (proximal and/or distal) dilatation of the collecting system; however, the ureter is normal in caliber.

4. The most common cause of bladder outlet obstruction in the male neonate is _____ valves.

5. Urinary _____ or a perirenal _____ can result from high-pressure vesicoureteral reflux rupturing a calyceal fornix or tearing the renal parenchyma.

6. The ectopic _____ is seen as a fluid mass within the urinary bladder and is located inferomedially to the ureteral insertion of the lower pole ureter.

7. The triad of hypoplasia or deficiency of the abdominal musculature, cryptorchidism, and urinary tract anomalies is known as the _____ syndrome.

8. The most common cause of renal cystic disease presenting in the neonate is _____, and when hydronephrosis is excluded, it is the most common cause of an abdominal mass in the newborn.

9. Sonographically, the classic appearance of MCDK is of a unilateral mass resembling a bunch of grapes, which represents a cluster of discrete _____ cysts, the largest of which are peripheral.

10. The kidneys are hyperechoic and greatly enlarged with a hypoechogenic outer rim, which represents the cortex compressed by the expanded pyramids in _____. Pulmonary hypoplasia with respiratory distress and Potter facies may also be associated findings.

11. The most common intraabdominal malignant renal tumor is _____ in young children.

12. A _____ is a malignant tumor that arises in sympathetic chain ganglia and adrenal medulla; it may be detected on antenatal sonography or at birth.

13. About half of the neuroblastoma tumors arise in the medulla of the _____, although tumors have also been found in the neck, mediastinum, retroperitoneum, and pelvis.

14. Sonographically, adrenal _____ results in ovoid enlargement of the gland or a portion of the gland.

Exercise 4

Provide a short answer for each question after evaluating the images.

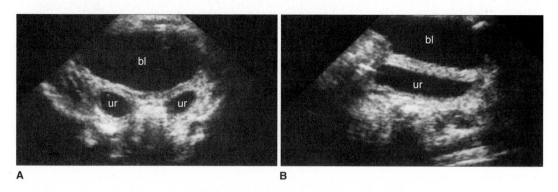

A   B

1. Identify whether this patient has obstructive or nonobstructive renal disease.

_____

_____

_____

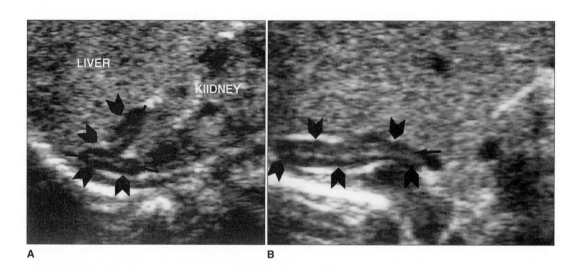

A   B

2. Identify the anatomic structure that the arrows are pointing to.

_____

_____

_____

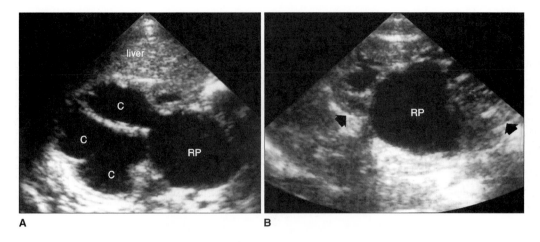

A   **B**

3. Identify whether this obstruction to the kidney is minor or major.

_____

_____

_____

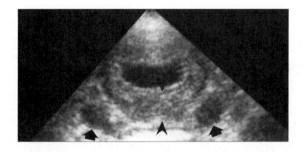

4. Identify the abnormality demonstrated in the transverse view of the neonatal bladder in image **A**.

_____

_____

_____

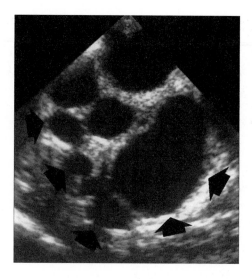

5. Does this neonate show sonographic evidence of hydronephrosis or multicystic dysplastic kidney disease?

_____

_____

_____

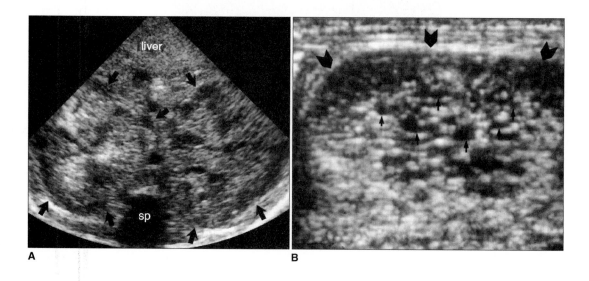

A   B

6. This neonate had abdominal distention at 1 day after birth. Describe the appearance of the kidneys.

_____

_____

_____

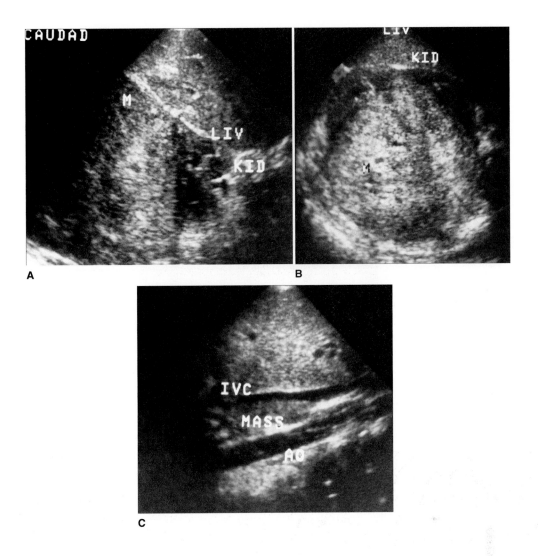

7. A 2-year-old with a palpable abdominal mass, nausea and vomiting, and appetite loss was imaged with ultrasound. Describe the findings.

_____

_____

_____

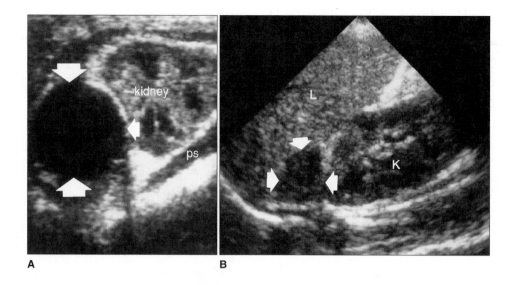

A   B

8. A 2-week-old male neonate with a history of neonatal infections, increased bilirubin, and an abdominal mass had an ultrasound. Describe the findings.

_____

_____

_____

24 Pediatric Congenital Anomalies of the Female Pelvis

KEY TERMS

Exercise 1
Match the following embryology and pathology terms with their definitions.

1. _____ bicornuate uterus

2. _____ hematometrocolpos

3. _____ hydrocolpos

4. _____ hydrometrocolpos

5. _____ isosexual

6. _____ oocytes

7. _____ oogonium

8. _____ paramesonephric ducts

9. _____ unicornuate uterus

10. _____ uterus didelphys

A. Fluid-filled vagina and uterus
B. (Müllerian ducts) Either of the paired ducts that form adjacent to the mesonephric ducts in the embryo
C. Duplication of the uterus and uterine horn or branches
D. Fluid-filled vagina
E. Anomaly of the uterus in which only one horn develops
F. A cell produced at an early stage in the formation of an ovum
G. Complete duplication of the uterus, cervix, and vagina
H. Blood-filled vagina and uterus
I. Concerning or characteristic of the same sex
J. The early or primitive ovum before it has developed completely

CONGENITAL ANOMALIES OF THE NEONATE

Exercise 2
Fill in the blank(s) with the word(s) that best completes the statements about the congenital anomalies of the neonate.

1. The first parts of the genital system to develop are the _____.

2. At about 16 weeks of gestation, the cortical cords break up into isolated cell clusters called primordial follicles,

   each of which contains an _____ derived from the primordial germ cell.

3. Before birth, all oogonia enlarge to form primary _____, and most of them have entered the first meiotic prophase, but this process remains in an arrested state until puberty.

4. All embryos have identical pairs of _____ ducts that develop into the female reproductive system.

5. Even though the genetic sex of an embryo is determined at fertilization by the kind of sperm that fertilizes

   the ovum, there are no morphologic indications of maleness or femaleness until the _____ gestational week.

6. External organs are fully developed by the _____ week.

7. The sonographic evaluation of the neonatal and pediatric pelvic cavity requires a distended _____ because only the transabdominal ultrasound technique is used.

8. In the newborn female, the uterus is prominent and thickened with a brightly _____ endometrial lining caused by the hormonal stimulation received in utero.

9. The uterus is pear shaped in configuration with the length approximately 3.5 cm with a fundus _____ than the cervix.

10. The maternal hormones stimulate the initial size of the uterine cavity after birth; as these hormones

    _____, so does the uterine size.

11. The uterus increases in size after the age of 7, with the greatest increase in size occurring after the onset of

    puberty, when the fundus becomes much _____ than the cervix.

12. It is not until _____ that the uterine shape and size dramatically changes. The uterine length increases to 5 to 7 cm and the fundus-to-cervix ratio becomes 3:1 (fundus is now greater than the cervix). The echogenicity and thickness of the endometrial lining vary according to the phase of the menstrual cycle.

13. The uterus is supplied by the bilateral _____ arteries, which are branches of the internal iliac arteries.

14. Color flow Doppler may demonstrate flow in the _____ tissue with little or no flow in the endometrium.

15. The appearance of the ovary in the neonatal period is _____ secondary to tiny cysts.

16. The blood supply to the ovary is from the _____ artery (originates directly from the aorta) and from the uterine artery, which supplies an adnexal branch to each ovary.

17. If müllerian anomalies are encountered, the _____ should be examined for ipsilateral renal agenesis or morphologic abnormalities.

18. Vaginal _____ is diagnosed by the development of hydrocolpos (fluid-filled vagina), hydrometrocolpos (fluid-filled vagina and uterus), or hematometrocolpos (blood-filled vagina and uterus).

19. Sonography demonstrates a uterus that is long and slender ("_____" shaped) and deviated to one side.

20. A complete duplication of the uterus, cervix, and vagina is _____.

21. A duplication of the uterus with a common cervix is _____.

22. The uterus is normal in size and shape externally; however, the cavity is T shaped with an irregular contour. This

    is associated with _____ exposure.

23. In _____ the embryo has the potential to develop as a male or female.

24. True _____ have both ovarian and testicular tissues.

25. True precocious puberty is always _____ and involves the development of secondary sexual characteristics and an increase in the size and activity of the gonads.

26. Precocious pseudopuberty involves the maturation of secondary sexual characteristics, but not the

_____ because there is no activation of the hypothalamic-pituitary-gonadal axis.

27. Excessive exogenous synthesis of gonadal _____ (by the adrenal gland, tumors, or cysts) is the most common cause of precocious pseudopuberty; prolonged exposure to exogenous gonadal hormones may mature the central nervous system and cause true precocious puberty in some children.

PATHOLOGY

Exercise 3
Fill in the blank(s) with the word(s) that best completes the statements about the pathology of the female pelvis.

1. Ovarian cysts develop from ovarian _____.

2. The _____ is secreted by the pituitary gland and causes an increase in both the number and size of the small follicles.

3. The most common primary complications are _____ and _____.

4. Torsion of the ovary may occur at any age, from the neonate to the adult; however, most torsion problems occur within the first _____ decades of life.

5. Torsion of the ovary and fallopian tube results from partial or complete rotation of the ovary on its

_____.

6. This results in compromise of arterial and venous flow, congestion of the ovarian parenchyma, and ultimately,

_____.

7. The most common pediatric germ cell tumor is the benign mature _____ or dermoid cyst.

8. Mural nodules and echogenic foci with acoustic shadowing are typical findings of _____ on ultrasound.

Exercise 4

Label the congenital uterine abnormalities present in the following illustrations.

1. Congenital uterine abnormalities (Fig. 24-5).

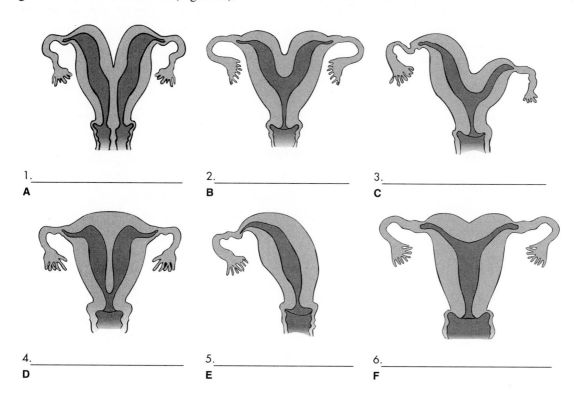

1. _____
A

2. _____
B

3. _____
C

4. _____
D

5. _____
E

6. _____
F

25 The Neonatal Hip

KEY TERMS

Exercise 1
Match the following anatomic terms with their definitions.

1. _____ abduction

2. _____ adduction

3. _____ fascia lata

4. _____ femoral triangle

5. _____ hip joint

6. _____ pelvic girdle

7. _____ saphenous opening

8. _____ sciatic nerve

A. Formed by the articulation of the head of the femur with the acetabulum of the hip bone

B. Deep fascia of the thigh

C. Movement away from the body

D. Largest nerve in the upper thigh.

E. Formation of the hip bones by the ilium, ischium, and pubis.

F. Movement toward the body

G. Description of a region at the front of the upper thigh, just below the inguinal ligament

H. Gap in the fascia lata, which is found 4 cm inferior and lateral to the pubic tubercle

Exercise 2
Match the following sonographic evaluation and pathology terms with their definitions.

1. _____ Barlow maneuver

2. _____ developmental displacement of the hip (DDH)

3. _____ frank dislocation

4. _____ Galeazzi sign

5. _____ Ortolani maneuver

6. _____ subluxated

A. The hip is laterally and posteriorly displaced to the extent that the femoral head has no contact with the acetabulum and the normal "U" configuration cannot be obtained on ultrasound.

B. Patient lies in the supine position. The examiner's hand is placed around the hip to be examined with the fingers over the femoral head. The hip is flexed 90 degrees, and the thigh is abducted.

C. The knee is lower in position on the affected side when the patient is supine and the knees are flexed. On physical exam the knee is lower in position on the affected side of the neonate with DDH when the patient is supine and the knees are flexed.

D. The patient lies in the supine position with the hip flexed 90 degrees and adducted. Downward and outward pressure is applied. If the hip is dislocated, the examiner will feel the femoral head move out of the acetabulum.

E. This occurs when the femoral head moves posteriorly and remains in contact with the posterior aspect of the acetabulum.

F. This is an abnormal condition of the hip that results in congenital hip dysplasia; includes dysplastic, subluxated, dislocatable, and dislocated hips.

Exercise 3

Label the following illustrations.
1. Coronal section of the right hip joint and articular surfaces of the right hip joint (Fig. 25-3, *A*).

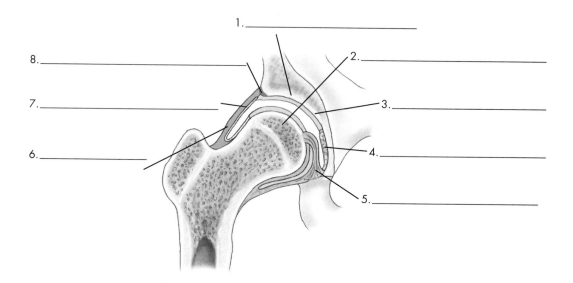

2. Coronal section of the right hip joint and arterial supply of the head of the femur.

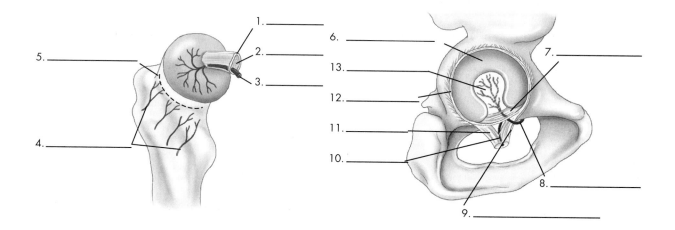

Exercise 4

Fill in the blank(s) with the word(s) that best completes the statements about the anatomy of the neonatal hip.

1. The _____ joints unite the two hip bones with the sacral part of the vertebral column.

2. The hip bones are the fusion of three separate bones: _____, _____, and

    _____; all together these form the pelvic girdle.

3. The bone of the upper thigh is the _____.

4. The femoral artery branches into the _____ artery, which is the main artery supply for the thigh muscles.

5. The largest nerve in the upper thigh is the _____ nerve.

6. The deep fascia of the thigh, the _____, forms a tough connective tissue surrounding the muscles.

7. The _____ is formed by the inguinal ligament, whereas the other two sides are formed by adductor longus (medially) and sartorius (laterally).

8. The contents of the femoral triangle include: the *femoral* _____, the *femoral* _____ and

_____, and the *femoral* _____.

9. The femoral vein and artery and the femoral canal are enclosed in a connective tissue sleeve, the femoral

_____.

10. The contents of the femoral triangle are separated from the more deeply lying hip joint by muscles; the

_____ is medial, and the _____ is lateral.

11. The articulation of the head of the femur with the acetabulum of the hip bone forms the _____.

12. The gluteus _____ muscle is the immediate cover for the upper part of the hip joint, whereas the obturator externus is found winding below it from front to back.

13. The _____ muscle is immediately posterior to the joint, whereas the obturator internus and the gemelli and quadratus femoris is lower down.

14. The rounded shape of the femur and the cup shape of the _____ form the "ball and socket" hip joint.

15. One of the strongest ligaments in the body is the _____; it is very important in standing and maintaining correct upright balance.

MOVEMENTS OF THE HIP

Exercise 5
Match the following terms regarding movements of the hip with their definitions.

1. _____ flexion

2. _____ extension

3. _____ abduction

4. _____ adduction

5. _____ medial rotation

6. _____ lateral rotation

A. Moving sideways outward
B. Turning inward
C. Bending forward
D. Turning outward
E. Bending backward
F. Moving sideways inward

Exercise 6

Fill in the blank(s) with the word(s) that best completes the statements about the movement of the hip.

1. The primary flexors of the hip are the _____ major, _____, and _____ femoris.

2. When the trochanter moves forward, the femur rotates _____, and when the trochanter moves backward, the femur rotates _____.

3. The medial rotators are the anterior fibers of gluteus _____ and _____.

4. The lateral rotators are the small muscles at the back of the joint: _____, _____, and _____ femoris, with assistance of the gluteus _____.

SONOGRAPHIC EVALUATION

Exercise 7

Fill in the blank(s) with the word(s) that best completes the statements or provide a short answer about the sonographic techniques of the neonatal hip.

1. Ossification of the femoral head begins between _____ and _____ months of age, occurs earlier in girls than boys, and is often complete by 1 year.

2. Sonography of the neonatal hip is performed with a _____ transducer.

3. Sonographically, the femoral head is _____ because it is cartilaginous and contains a focal echogenic ossification nucleus.

4. The femoral head sits within the acetabulum, which is _____ and has a deep concave configuration.

5. Two thirds of the head should be covered by the _____.

6. The basic hip anatomy is imaged in four different views:

   _____

   _____

   _____

7. The angle between the baseline and the acetabular roof line that represents the osseous acetabulum is the _____ angle.

8. The angle between the baseline and the inclination line is the _____ angle.

9. The _____ angle reflects changes in the cartilaginous acetabulum, which occur more quickly than do changes in the osseous acetabulum and may therefore be more sensitive than the _____ angle.

10. The _____ is performed with the infant in the supine position from the lateral aspect of the hip joint with the plane of the transducer oriented coronally with respect to the hip joint.

11. The transducer is maintained in the lateral position while the hip is moved into a 90-degree angle of flexion in the _____ view. During this assessment, the transducer is moved in an anteroposterior direction with respect to the body to visualize the entire hip.

12. A normal hip gives the appearance of a "ball on a spoon" in the midacetabulum. The _____ is the

    ball, the _____ forms the spoon, and the iliac line is the handle.

13. The transverse plane is rotated 90 degrees and moved posteriorly into a posterolateral position over the hip joint in

    the _____ view.

14. From the transverse and/or flexion view the leg is brought down into a neutral position to the _____ view.

PATHOLOGY

Exercise 8

Fill in the blank(s) with the word(s) that best completes the statements or provide a short answer about the pathology of the neonatal hip.

1. _____ causes of hip dislocation include traumatic and nontraumatic causes (i.e., neuromuscular diseases).

2. _____ dislocations occur in utero and are associated with neuromuscular disorders.

3. _____ of the hip includes dysplastic, subluxated, dislocatable, and dislocated hips.

4. Describe the multiple risk factors that may contribute to the developmental displacement of the hip.

   _____

   _____

   _____

5. Name the two basic maneuvers that are helpful in the diagnosis of DDH.

   _____

   _____

   _____

6. Sonographic signs of developmental displacement of the hip include:

   _____

   _____

   _____

7. A _____ hip is one in which the proximal femur moves (more than 6 mm on the left and 4 mm on the right) within the acetabulum, but cannot be displaced out of it.

8. A _____ hip is one in which the proximal femur can be displaced out of the acetabulum, but can be reduced.

9. A _____ hip is one in which the femoral head is displaced out of the acetabulum and cannot be reduced.

Exercise 9

Provide a short answer for each question after evaluating the images.

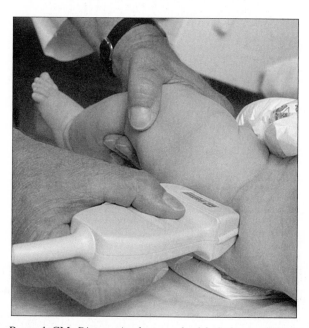

From Rumack CM: *Diagnostic ultrasound,* ed 2, St Louis, 1998, Mosby.

1. Name the view that the transducer is positioned to image.

_____

_____

_____

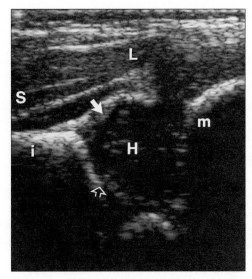

From Rumack CM: *Diagnostic ultrasound,* ed 2, St Louis, 1998, Mosby.

2. Identify the structure that the closed arrow is pointing to.

_____

_____

_____

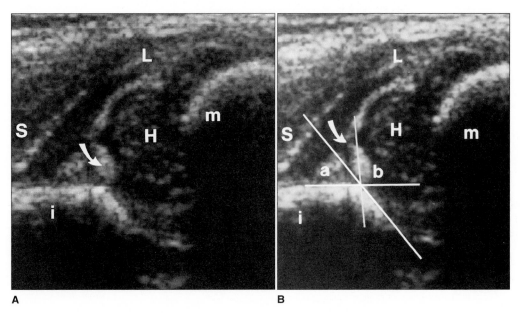

A   B

From Rumack CM: *Diagnostic ultrasound,* ed 2, St Louis, 1998, Mosby.

3. This coronal and/or neutral view of the hip demonstrates this abnormality.

_____

_____

_____

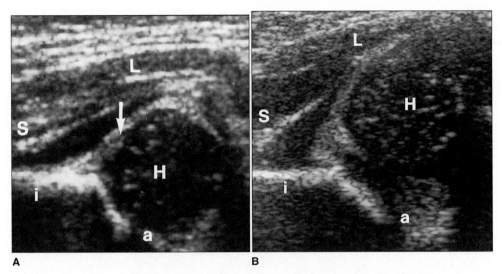

From Henningsen: *Clinical guide to ultrasonography,* St Louis, 2004, Mosby.

4. Describe the difference between image **A** and **B** in this coronal flexion view.

_____

_____

_____

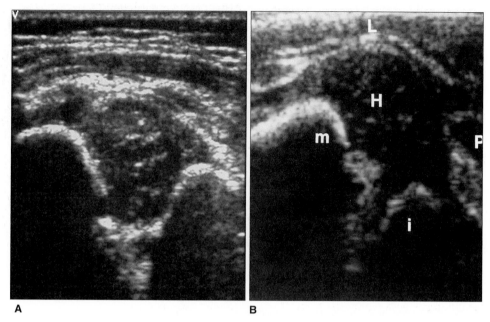

A   B

From Henningsen: *Clinical guide to ultrasonography,* St Louis, 2004, Mosby.

5. Describe the anatomy change in this transverse and/or flexion view between **A** and **B**.

_____

_____

_____

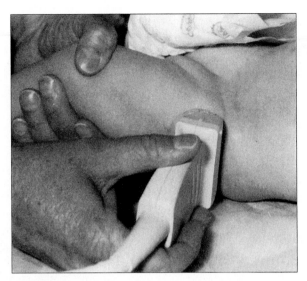

From Rumack CM: *Diagnostic ultrasound,* ed 2, St Louis, 1998, Mosby.

6. Identify the view that is demonstrated with the transducer.

_____

_____

_____

26 The Neonatal Spine

KEY TERMS

Exercise 1
Match the following neonatal spine terms with their definitions.

1. _____ cauda equina

2. _____ conus medullaris

3. _____ diastematomyelia

4. _____ filum terminale

5. _____ meningocele

6. _____ myelomeningocele

A. Protrusion of the meninges through the gap in the spine, the skin covering being vestigial

B. Bundle of nerve roots from the lumbar, sacral, and coccygeal spinal nerves that descend nearly vertically from the spinal cord until they reach their respective openings in the vertebral column

C. Slender tapering terminal section of the spinal cord

D. The caudal end of the spinal cord

E. The spinal cord and nerve roots are exposed, often adhering to the fine membrane that overlies them

F. A congenital fissure of the spinal cord, frequently associated with spina bifida cystica

Exercise 2
Match the following pathology terms with their definitions.

1. _____ dysraphism

2. _____ hydromyelia

3. _____ lipoma

4. _____ myeloschisis

5. _____ spina bifida aperta

6. _____ spina bifida occulta

7. _____ tethered spinal cord

A. Common benign tumor composed of fat cells

B. Open (non–skin-covered lesions) neural tube defects, such as myelomeningocele and meningocele

C. Dilation of the central canal of the spinal cord

D. Closed (skin-covered lesions) neural tube defects, such as spinal lipoma and tethered cord

E. Cleft spinal cord resulting from failure of the neural tube to close

F. Refers to the anomalies associated with incomplete embryologic development

G. Fixed spinal cord that is in an abnormal position

Exercise 3

Label the following illustrations.

1. Basic features of the vertebrae.

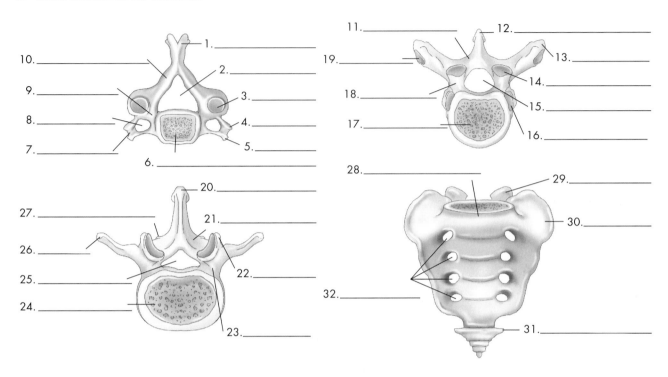

2. Longitudinal section of the sacrum.

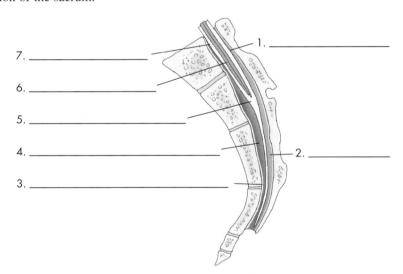

3. Joints in the cervical, thoracic, and lumbar regions of the vertebral column.

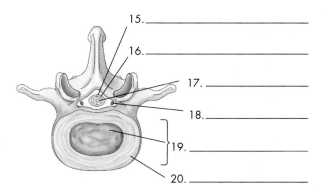

15. _____

16. _____

17. _____

18. _____

19. _____

20. _____

4. Section through the thoracic part of the spinal cord.

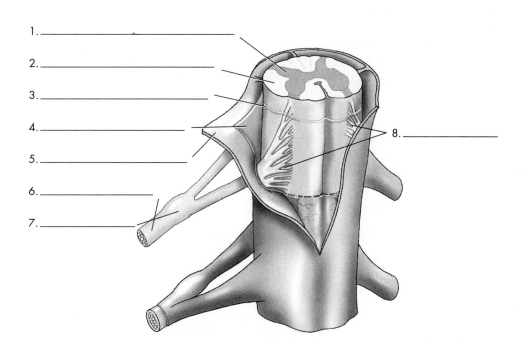

1. _____

2. _____

3. _____

4. _____

5. _____

6. _____

7. _____

8. _____

ANATOMY AND PATHOLOGY

Exercise 4

Fill in the blank(s) with the word(s) that best completes the statements about the anatomy of the neonatal spine.

1. Clinically, one of the signs that may lead to problems in the spine is when the infant presents with a

    _____ on the posterior surface of the body along the spinal canal.

2. Other suspicious findings that an abnormality may be present include a _____ or a raised midline

    area, a _____ patch, or even a tail-like projection from the lower spine.

3. The dimple may also be suspicious if it is of greater than _____ from the anus.

4. Spinal _____ includes disorders of the spine involving absent or incomplete closure of the neural tube.

5. The defects of the spinal canal occur in the first _____ weeks of life as the fetal nervous system develops.

6. The bony spine, meninges, and muscle form the _____.

7. Incomplete separation of the neural tube from the ectoderm may result in cord tethering, _____, or a dermal sinus.

8. If the neural tube fails to fold and fuse in the midline, defects, such as _____, occur.

9. Within the vertebral cavity lie the spinal cord, the roots of the spinal nerves, and the covering _____, which provide protection for the vertebral column.

Exercise 5

Fill in the blank(s) with the word(s) that best completes the statements about the anatomy of the vertebral column and spinal cord.

1. Each vertebra consists of a rounded body _____ and a vertebral arch _____.

2. These enclose a space called the vertebral _____, through which run the spinal cord and its coverings.

3. The vertebral arch consists of a pair of cylindrical pedicles, which form the sides of the arch, and a pair of

   flattened _____, which complete the arch posteriorly.

4. Laterally the sacrum articulates with the two iliac bones to form the _____ joints.

5. The laminae of the fifth sacral vertebra, and sometimes those of the fourth also, fail to meet in the midline,

   forming the sacral _____.

6. The _____ disks are responsible for one fourth of the length of the vertebral column.

7. Each disk consists of a peripheral part, the *annulus* _____, and a central part, the *nucleus*

   _____.

8. The spinal cord begins above at the foramen magnum, where it is continuous with the medulla oblongata of the

   brain. In the younger child, it is relatively longer and ends at the upper border of the _____ lumbar vertebra.

9. Inferiorly the cord tapers off into the conus _____, from the apex of which a prolongation of the pia

   mater, the filum _____, descends to be attached to the back of the coccyx.

10. The cord has a deep longitudinal fissure in the midline anteriorly, the *anterior* _____ *fissure*, and on the posterior surface a shallow furrow, the *posterior median sulcus*.

11. The lower nerve roots together are called the _____.

12. The spinal cord is surrounded by three meninges: the _____ mater, the _____ mater, and

the _____ mater.

13. The most external membrane is the _____ mater and is a dense, strong, fibrous sheet that encloses the
spinal cord and cauda equina.

14. The _____ mater is a delicate impermeable membrane covering the spinal cord and lying between
the pia mater internally and the dura mater externally.

15. The vascular membrane that closely covers the spinal cord is the _____ mater; below it fuses
with the filum terminale.

Exercise 6
Fill in the blank(s) with the word(s) that best completes the statements about the anatomy and pathology of the spinal cord.

1. The spinal cord is _____ with slightly echogenic borders and an echogenic line extending
longitudinally along its midline.

2. This central echo complex represents or is close to the cord's central _____.

3. The spinal cord and roots of the cauda equina are normally observed to _____ with the frequency of
the heartbeat, and there is also a superimposed motion that occurs with respirations.

4. The _____ spinal cord is a pathologic fixation of the spinal cord in an abnormal caudal location so that
the cord suffers mechanical stretching, distortion, and ischemia with daily activities, growth, and development.

5. The tethered spinal cord, in addition to being in a more caudal location, is often fixed _____ within
the canal.

6. Lipomas are usually _____ and may present as a small or large mass.

7. _____ shows a flat nontubulated cord (neural placode) with nerve roots extending into the defect.

8. In contrast, a _____ shows nothing but fluid within the sac.

9. _____ seem to have a high association with tethered spinal cord.

Exercise 7

Provide a short answer for each question after evaluating the images.

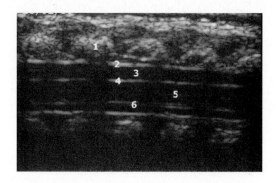

1. Identify the structures numbered 1 through 6 on this image.

_____

_____

_____

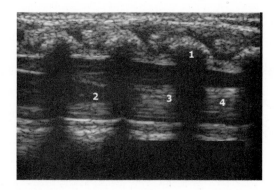

2. Identify the structures numbered 1 through 4 on this sagittal image.

_____

_____

_____

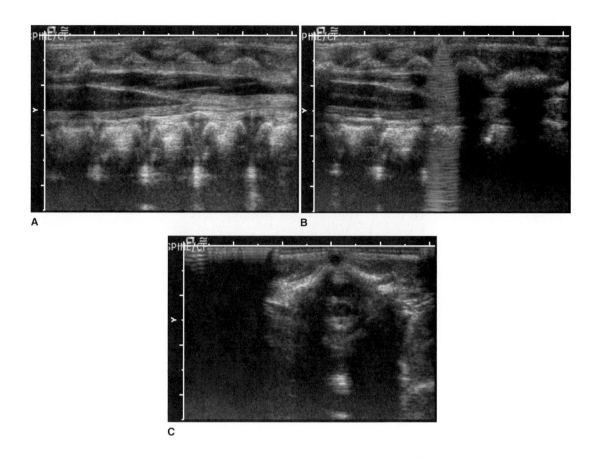

A

B

C

3. A neonate presented with fatty mass near the lower back with increased areas of pigmentation. Describe the sonographic finding.

_____

_____

_____

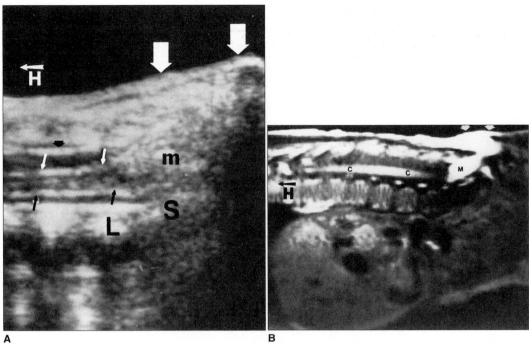

From Rumack CM: *Diagnostic ultrasound,* ed 2, St Louis, 1998, Mosby.

4.   Would this mass be considered more likely to be a leptomyelolipoma or a myelomeningocele?

_____

_____

_____

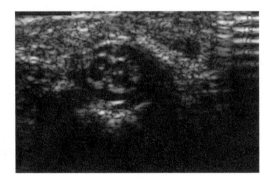

5.   This image is representative of this abnormality of the neonatal spine.

_____

_____

_____

27 Anatomic and Physiologic Relationships within the Thoracic Cavity

KEY TERMS

Exercise 1
Match the following heart and cardiac cycle terms with their definitions.

1. _____ atrioventricular valves

2. _____ endocardium

3. _____ epicardium

4. _____ myocardium

5. _____ pericardium

6. _____ semilunar valves

A. Outer layer of the heart wall

B. Inner layer of the heart wall

C. Sac surrounding the heart, reflecting off the great arteries

D. Valves located between the atria and ventricle

E. Thickest muscle in the heart wall

F. Valves located in the aortic or pulmonic artery

Exercise 2
Match the following electrical conduction system and auscultation terms with their definitions.

1. _____ continuous murmur

2. _____ depolarization

3. _____ diastolic murmur

4. _____ electrocardiography

5. _____ frequency

6. _____ intensity

7. _____ murmur

8. _____ repolarization

9. _____ systolic murmur

A. The predominant frequency band of the murmur varies from high to low as determined by auscultation.

B. The method of recording the electrical activity generated by the heart muscle.

C. The systolic murmur begins with or after the time of the first heart sound and ends at or before the time of the second heart sound.

D. This describes the electrical activity that triggers contraction of the heart muscle.

E. A murmur is a relatively prolonged series of auditory vibrations of varying intensity (loudness), frequency (pitch), quality, configuration, and duration. The murmur is produced by structural changes and/or hemodynamic events in the heart or blood vessels.

F. The diastolic murmur begins with or after the time of the second heart sound and ends at or before the time of the first heart sound.

G. This begins just before the relaxation phase of cardiac muscle activity.

H. The murmur begins in systole and continues without interruption through the time of the second heart sound into all or part of diastole.

I. Murmurs, both systolic and diastolic, vary from grade 1 to grade 6. A grade 1 murmur is very faint with progression to a grade 6 murmur that is exceptionally loud and heard with the stethoscope.

Exercise 3

Label the following illustrations.

1. Anterior view of the right ventricle (Fig. 27-4).

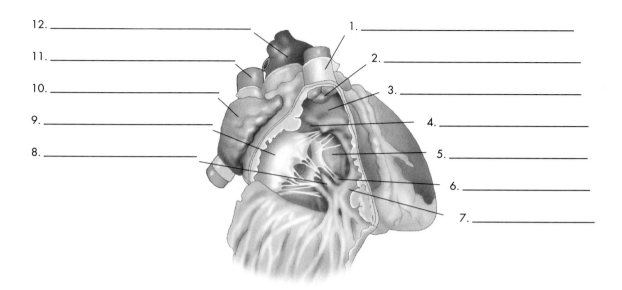

2. Posterolateral view of the left atrium and ventricle.

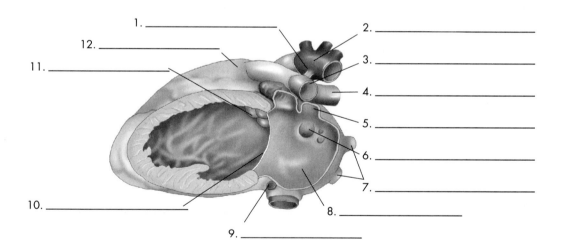

3. Right atrium viewed from the right side.

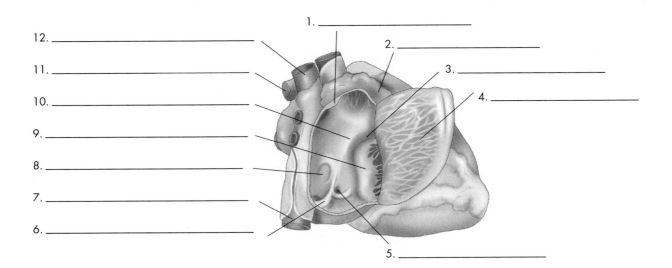

12. _____

11. _____

10. _____

9. _____

8. _____

7. _____

6. _____

1. _____

2. _____

3. _____

4. _____

5. _____

4. Tricuspid valve.

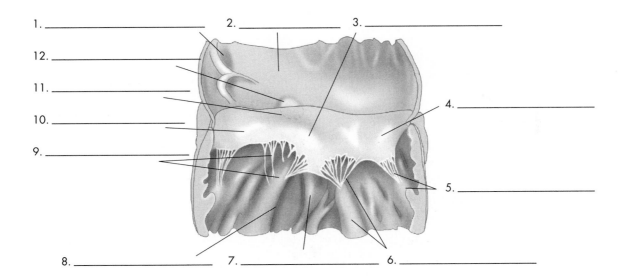

1. _____

12. _____

11. _____

10. _____

9. _____

8. _____

2. _____

3. _____

4. _____

5. _____

7. _____

6. _____

5. Mitral valve.

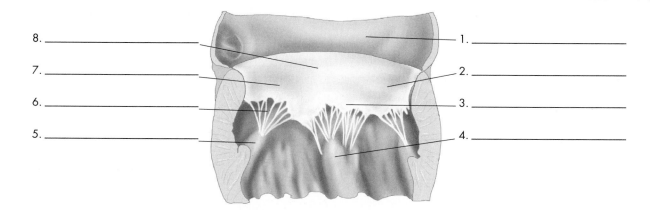

8. _____   1. _____
7. _____   2. _____
6. _____   3. _____
5. _____   4. _____

6. Posterolateral view of the left ventricle.

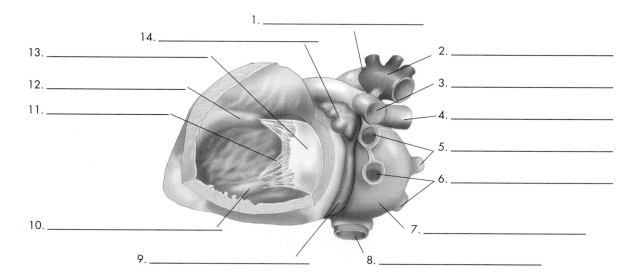

1. _____
14. _____
13. _____   2. _____
12. _____   3. _____
11. _____   4. _____
                              5. _____
                              6. _____
10. _____   7. _____
9. _____   8. _____

7. Long-axis view of the heart.

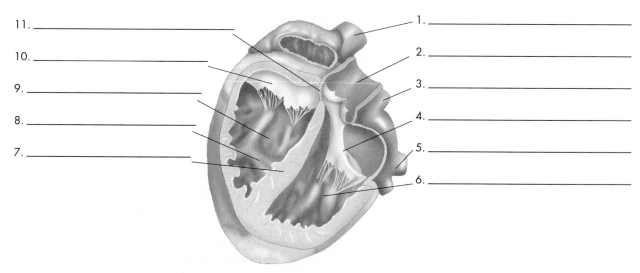

11. _____   1. _____
10. _____   2. _____
9. _____   3. _____
8. _____   4. _____
7. _____   5. _____
                              6. _____

Chapter **27** **Anatomic and Physiologic Relationships within the Thoracic Cavity**

8. Aortic valve.

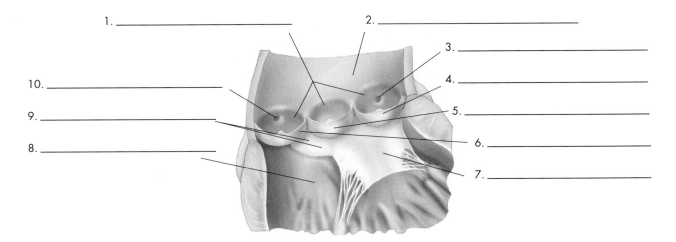

9. Aortic arch and branches.

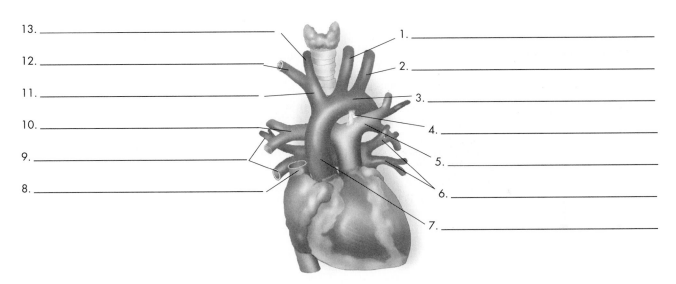

Exercise 4

Match the following landmarks of the thorax with their locations.

1. _____ midaxillary line

2. _____ sternal angle

3. _____ costal margin

4. _____ midsternal line

5. _____ xiphoid

6. _____ suprasternal notch

7. _____ midclavicular line

A. Lies in the median plane over the sternum

B. Superior margin of the manubrium sterni; lies opposite the lower border of the body of the second thoracic vertebra

C. Angle between the manubrium and the body of the sternum; also known as the angle of Louis

D. Lowest point of the sternum

E. Runs vertically from a point midway between the anterior and posterior axillary folds

F. Vertical line from the midpoint of the clavicle

G. Lower boundary of the thorax, formed by the cartilages of the seventh through tenth ribs and the ends of the eleventh and twelfth cartilages

Exercise 5

Fill in the blank(s) with the word(s) that best completes the statements about the anatomy of the cardiovascular system.

1. The cardiovascular system delivers _____ blood to tissues in the body and removes _____ products from these tissues.

2. The thoracic cavity lies within the thorax and is separated from the abdominal cavity by the _____.

3. The junction between the manubrium and the body of the sternum is a prominent ridge called the

   _____.

4. The greater part of the thoracic cavity is occupied by two lungs that are enclosed by the _____.

5. The pleural reflection between the costal and diaphragmatic portions of the parietal pleura is known as the

   _____.

6. The heart lies obliquely in the chest, posterior to the sternum, with the greater portion of its muscular mass lying

   slightly to the _____ of midline.

7. The right heart is located more _____ than its left side chambers.

8. The right atrium is _____ to the left atrium and lies to the _____ of the sternum.

9. The left atrium becomes the most _____ chamber to the left of the sternum.

10. The _____ layer lines the fibrous pericardium and is reflected around the roots of the great vessels to become continuous with the visceral layer of serous pericardium.

11. The slit between the parietal and visceral layers is the _____.

12. The intimal lining of the heart is the _____ and is continuous with the intima of the vessels connecting to it.

13. The muscular part of the heart is the _____.

14. The primary purpose of the atrium is to act as a _____ chamber that drives the blood into the relaxed ventricular cavity.

15. The left ventricle has the greatest muscle mass because it must pump blood to _____, whereas the

    right ventricle needs only enough pressure to pump the blood to the _____.

16. The _____ enters the upper posterior border and the _____ enters the lower posterolateral border of the right atrium.

17. The medial wall of the right atrium is formed by the _____ septum.

18. The _____ part of the membranous septum separates the right atrium and left ventricle.

19. The inferior vena cava is guarded by a fold of tissue called the _____ valve, and the coronary sinus is

    guarded by the _____ valve.

20. The _____ drains the blood supply from the heart wall.

21. The valve that separates the right atrium from the right ventricle is the _____ valve.

22. The base of the right ventricle lies on the diaphragm, and the roof is occupied by the crista _____, which lies between the tricuspid and pulmonary orifices.

23. The outflow portion of the right ventricle, or _____, is smooth walled and contains few trabeculae.

24. The valve that separates the left atrium from the left ventricle is the _____ valve.

25. The functions of the _____ are to prevent the opposing borders of the leaflets from inverting into the atrial cavity, to act as mainstays of the valves, and to form bands or foldlike structures that may contain muscle.

26. The smaller end of the ventricle represents the _____ of the heart, and the larger end, near the orifice

of the mitral valve, is near the _____ of the heart.

27. The ventricular septum is formed of _____, _____, _____, and

_____ parts.

28. The _____ septum is located just inferior to the aortic root in the area of the left ventricular outflow tract.

29. The _____ arise from the right and left coronary cusps.

Exercise 6
Fill in the blank(s) with the word(s) that best completes the statements about the cardiac cycle and conduction system of the heart.

1. The heart beats in sinus rhythm at _____ beats per minute.

2. The forceful contraction of the cardiac chambers is _____, and the relaxed phase of the cycle

is _____.

3. During diastole the venous blood enters the _____ from the superior and inferior venae cavae.

4. Oxygenated blood returns from the lungs through the _____ to enter the left atrium.

5. The _____ pressure in the ventricular cavity closes the atrioventricular valves.

6. The blood fills the sinuses of _____ and forces the cusps to close.

7. The conducting system of the heart consists of specialized cardiac muscle in the _____ node,

_____ node, _____ bundle, and _____ fibers.

8. The _____ node initiates the normal cardiac impulse and is often called the pacemaker of the heart.

9. The _____ node is located in the right posterior portion of the interatrial septum.

10. Atrial contraction follows the _____ wave on ECG and generates the atrial systolic activity.

11. The impulse spreads via the Purkinje fibers to activate the ventricles, generating the _____ waves of the ECG.

12. The _____ interval is measured from the beginning of the P wave to the beginning of the QRS complex.

13. The _____ wave represents ventricular repolarization.

14. The _____ Law of the heart states that the output of the heart increases in proportion to the degree of diastolic stretch of the muscle fibers.

15. The longer the initial resting length of the cardiac muscle, called _____, the greater the strength of contraction of the following beat.

16. The shortening velocity of cardiac muscle is inversely related to the _____.

Exercise 7

Fill in the blank(s) with the word(s) that best completes the statements about cardiac physiology.

1. When the blood moves in smooth layers, which slide against each other, this is known as _____ flow.

2. When the blood cells move in different directions with varying velocities, it is known as _____ flow.

3. The flow dynamics depend on the fluid _____ and the _____ of molecules in the fluid.

4. The _____ profile is such that as fluid moves through a tube, fluid layers in the center have a higher velocity than those on outer surfaces.

5. The _____ profile states that as flow accelerates and converges, more fluid travels at velocities closer to peak velocity than layers in the center.

6. In _____ the ventricles eject blood into the aorta and pulmonary artery.

7. In _____ the ventricles fill with blood from the atria and flow to the body organs.

8. The blood flow through a constriction creates a _____ pressure upstream from constriction.

9. The high fluid pressure forces blood through the constriction in the form of laminar _____ velocity jet.

10. The normal left ventricular ejection fraction is _____%.

11. Myocardial ischemia may occur in situations in which blood pressure is acutely _____.

28 Introduction to Echocardiographic Evaluation and Techniques

KEY TERMS

Exercise 1

Match the following echocardiographic terms with their definitions.

1. _____ color flow mapping (CFM)

2. _____ continuous wave probe

3. _____ diastole

4. _____ Doppler frequency

5. _____ pulsed wave transducer

6. _____ spectral analysis waveform

7. _____ systole

A. Red blood cells move from a lower-frequency sound source at rest toward a higher-frequency sound source; change in frequency is called the Doppler shift in frequency.

B. Part of the cardiac cycle in which the ventricles are filling with blood; the tricuspid and mitral valves are open during this time.

C. Sound is continuously emitted from one transducer and continuously received by a second transducer.

D. Graphic display of the flow velocity over time

E. Ability to display blood flow in multiple colors, depending on the velocity, direction of flow, and extent of turbulence

F. Part of the cardiac cycle in which the ventricles are pumping blood through the outflow tract into the pulmonary artery or the aorta

G. Single crystal that sends and receives sound intermittently; a pulse of sound is emitted from the transducer, which also receives the returning signal.

ECHOCARDIOGRAPHIC EXAMINATION

Exercise 2

Match the following nomenclature and image orientation terms with their definitions.

1. _____ apical

2. _____ four chamber

3. _____ long axis

4. _____ parasternal

5. _____ short axis

6. _____ subcostal

7. _____ suprasternal

A. Transducer placed over the area bounded superiorly by the left clavicle, medially by the sternum, and inferiorly by the apical region

B. Transects the heart perpendicular to the dorsal and ventral surfaces of the body and parallel with the long axis of the heart

C. Transducer placed in the suprasternal notch

D. Transects the heart approximately parallel with the dorsal and ventral surfaces of the body

E. Transducer located near the body midline and beneath the costal margin

F. Transects the heart perpendicular to the dorsal and ventral surfaces of the body and perpendicular to the long axis of the heart

G. Transducer located over the cardiac apex (at the point of maximal impulse)

Exercise 3

Fill in the blank(s) with the word(s) that best completes the statements about the echocardiographic examination.

1. The cardiac window is found between the _____ and _____ intercostal spaces, slightly to the left of the sternal border. The cardiac window may be considered that area on the anterior chest where the heart is just beneath the skin surface, free of lung interference.

2. Doppler echocardiography has emerged as a valuable noninvasive tool in clinical cardiology to provide

   _____ information about the function of the cardiac valves and chambers of the heart.

3. The best quality Doppler signals are obtained when the sample volume is _____ to the direction of flow.

4. Blood flow toward the transducer is displayed by a time velocity waveform _____ the baseline at

   point zero, or a _____ deflection.

5. The maximum frequency shift that can be measured by a pulsed Doppler system is called the _____ limit and is one half of the pulsed repetition frequency.

6. The _____ waveform allows the operator to print a graphic display of what the audio signal is recording as it provides a representation of blood flow velocities over time.

7. The Doppler equation is based on the principle that the velocity of blood flow is _____ proportional to the Doppler frequency shift and the speed of sound in tissue and is inversely related to twice the frequency of transmitted ultrasound and the cosine of the angle of incidence between the ultrasound beam and the direction of blood flow.

Exercise 4

Identify the proper echocardiographic view demonstrated in each image.

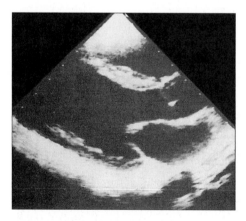

1. _____

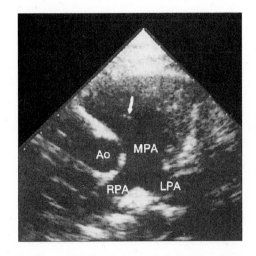

2. _____

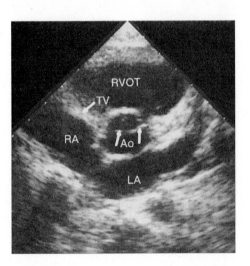

3. _____

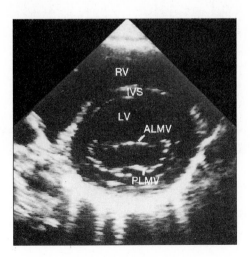

4. _____

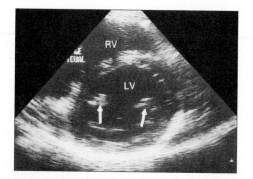

5. _____

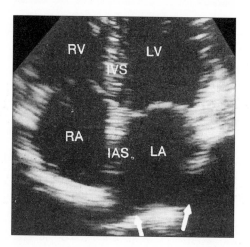

6. _____

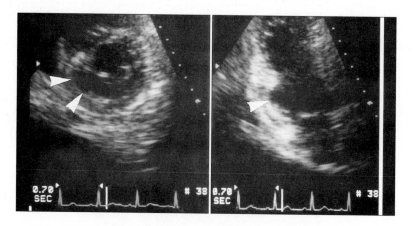

7. _____

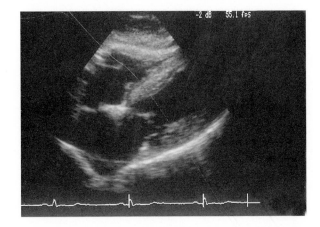

8. _____

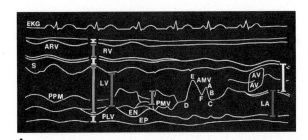

A

B

9. _____

29 Introduction to Fetal Echocardiography

KEY TERMS

Exercise 1
Match the following embryology of the cardiovascular system terms with their definitions.

1. _____ atrioventricular node

2. _____ bulbus cordis

3. _____ foramen ovale

4. _____ left and right atrium

5. _____ left and right ventricle

6. _____ septum primum

7. _____ septum secundum

8. _____ sinoatrial node

A. Filling chamber of the heart

B. First part of the atrial septum to grow from the dorsal wall of the primitive atrium; fuses with the endocardial cushions

C. Primitive chamber that forms the right ventricle

D. Pumping chamber of the heart

E. Area of cardiac muscle that receives and conducts the cardiac impulse

F. Forms in the wall of the sinus venosus near its opening into the right atrium

G. Also termed fossa ovale; opening between the free edge of the septum secundum and the dorsal wall of the atrium

H. Grows into the atrium to the right of the septum primum

Exercise 2
Match the following fetal circulation and echocardiographic terms with their definitions.

1. _____ bicuspid aortic valve

2. _____ ductus arteriosus

3. _____ fossa ovale

4. _____ inferior vena cava

5. _____ main pulmonary artery

6. _____ mitral valve

7. _____ patent ductus arteriosus

8. _____ pulmonary veins

9. _____ right ventricle

A. Venous return from the head and upper extremities into the upper posterior medial wall of the right atrium

B. Four pulmonary veins bring blood from the lungs back into the posterior wall of the left atrium; there are two upper (right and left) and two lower (right and left) pulmonary veins.

C. Pumping chamber of the heart

D. Also termed foramen ovale; opening between the free edge of the septum secundum and the dorsal wall of the atrium

E. Atrioventricular valve between the left atrium and left ventricle

F. Two leaflets instead of the normal three leaflets with asymmetric cusps

G. Atrioventricular valve found between the right atrium and right ventricle

H. Venous return into the right atrium of the heart along the posterior lateral wall

10. _____ superior vena cava

11. _____ tricuspid valve

I. Open communication between the pulmonary artery and descending aorta that does not constrict after birth

J. Communication between the pulmonary artery and descending aorta that closes after birth

K. Main artery that carries blood from the right ventricle to the lungs

ANATOMY

Exercise 3

Label the following illustrations.

1. The heart during the fourth week of development.

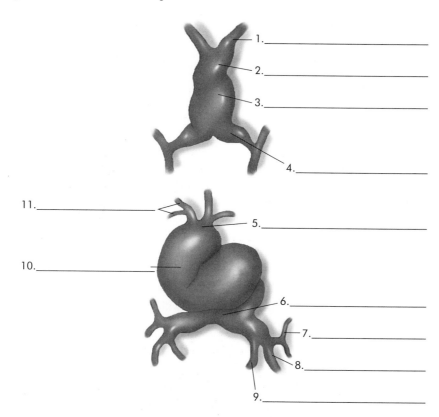

1. _____

2. _____

3. _____

4. _____

11. _____

5. _____

10. _____

6. _____

7. _____

8. _____

9. _____

2.   The partitioning of the primitive atrioventricular canal, atrium, and ventricle in the developing heart.

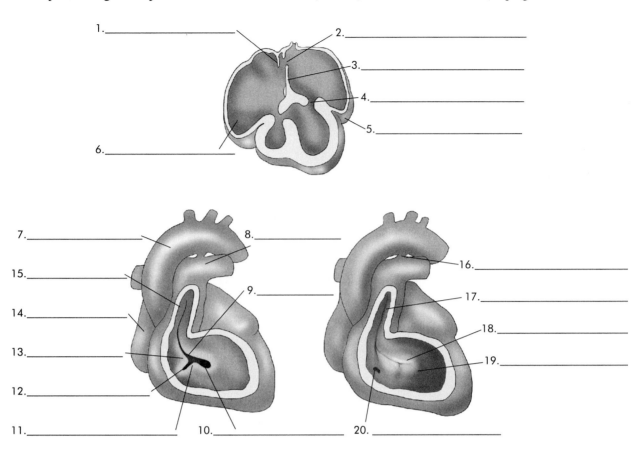

1._____
2._____
3._____
4._____
5._____
6._____
7._____
8._____
9._____
10._____
11._____
12._____
13._____
14._____
15._____
16._____
17._____
18._____
19._____
20._____

3.   Fetal circulation.

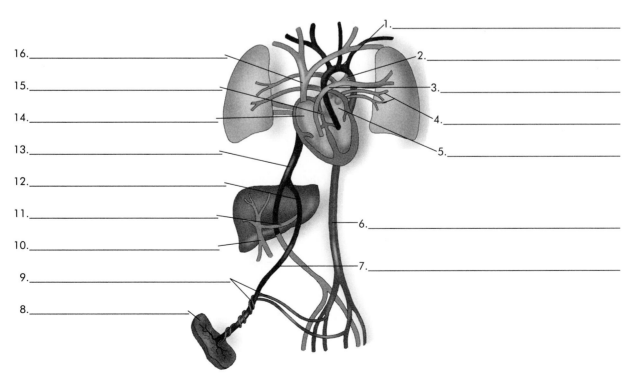

1._____
2._____
3._____
4._____
5._____
6._____
7._____
8._____
9._____
10._____
11._____
12._____
13._____
14._____
15._____
16._____

Exercise 4

Fill in the blank(s) with the word(s) that best completes the statements about the embryology and physiology of the fetal heart.

1. The cardiovascular system is the first organ system to reach a functional state; by the end of the _____

   week, circulation of blood has begun, and the heart begins to beat in the _____ week.

2. The vascular system begins during the third week in the wall of the _____, the connecting stalk, and the chorion.

3. The _____ veins return blood from the embryo, and the _____ veins return blood from the yolk sac.

4. The _____ veins return oxygenated blood from the placenta (only one umbilical vein persists).

5. _____ develop in the atrioventricular region of the heart.

6. The _____ grows from the dorsal wall of the primitive atrium and fuses with the endocardial cushions.

7. As the *foramen secundum* develops, another membranous fold, the _____, grows into the atrium to the right of the septum primum.

8. There is also an opening between the free edge of the septum secundum and the dorsal wall of the atrium, the

   _____.

9. The right ventricle is formed from the _____.

10. Communication is open between the right and left sides of the heart through the _____ and between

    the aorta and the pulmonary artery via the _____.

11. A small amount of oxygenated blood from the inferior vena cava is diverted by the _____ and remains in the right atrium to mix with deoxygenated blood from the superior vena cava and *coronary sinus.*

12. Some of the blood from the inferior vena cava is directed by the lower border of the _____ (the crista dividens) through the *foramen ovale* into the *left atrium.*

13. The blood in the right atrium flows through the three-leaflet _____ into the _____ and

    leaves the right ventricle through the _____.

14. Most of this blood from the right heart passes through the connection of the _____ into the *descending aorta;* only a very small amount goes to the lungs.

15. The pulmonary veins enter the _____ of the left atrium.

16. The blood then flows from the left atrium into the _____ through the bicuspid _____ and

    leaves the heart through the _____.

17. The septum primum forms the _____ of the fossa ovalis.

18. The _____ usually constricts shortly after birth (usually within 24 to 48 hours), once the left-sided pressures exceed the right-sided pressures.

19. The normal fetal heart rate is between _____ beats per minute.

20. If the heart rate is too slow (less than 60 beats per minute), it is called _____; a heart rate more than 200 beats per minute is termed _____.

Exercise 5

Fill in the blank(s) with the word(s) that best completes the statements about the anatomy and sonographic technique of the fetal heart.

1. The fetal heart lies in a _____ position within the thorax, and the apex of the heart (the left ventricle) is directed toward the left hip.

2. The right heart is slightly _____ in utero than the left heart.

3. The right and left sides may be identified by the opening flap of the patent foramen ovale; in utero the foramen opens _____ the left atrium.

4. The _____ stretches horizontally across the right ventricle near the apex.

5. Normally the tricuspid valve is located just slightly _____ to the mitral valve.

6. The right and left ventricular width measurements are performed in the four-chamber view at the level of the _____ annulus.

7. The pulmonary artery normally is _____ and to the _____ of the aorta.

8. The _____ membranous septum is best seen on the apical four-chamber view at the level of the atrioventricular valves, whereas the _____ may be seen on the long-axis view.

9. On the long-axis view, the continuity of the right side of the _____ with the _____ wall of the aortic root is important to rule out the presence of a membranous ventricular septal defect (VSD), conal truncal abnormality (such as truncus arteriosus), endocardial cushion defect, or tetralogy of Fallot.

10. Normally the three cusps open in _____ to the full extent of the aortic root and close in a midposition in _____.

11. On the short-axis view, normally the right ventricular outflow tract and pulmonary artery "drape" _____ to the circular aorta.

12. The sonographer may find the fetal spine in the sagittal plane and angle slightly inward toward the left chest to search for the _____.

13. The three head and neck branch arteries (_____, _____, and _____) may be seen to arise from the perfect curve of the aortic arch as they ascend into the fetal head.

14. A second "arch-type" pattern (which appears as large as the aorta) is shown as the transducer is angled inferior from

the aortic arch. This represents the _____, a communication between the pulmonary artery and the aorta.

Exercise 6
Provide a short answer for each question after evaluating the images.

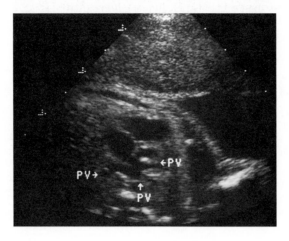

1. The pulmonary vein not shown is:

_____

_____

_____

_____

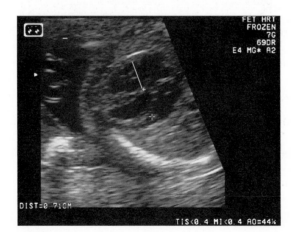

2. The left ventricle should be measured at the level of this structure.

_____

_____

_____

_____

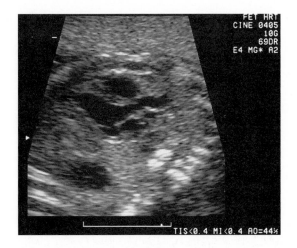

3. This image shows the mitral valve in this stage of the cardiac cycle.

_____

_____

_____

_____

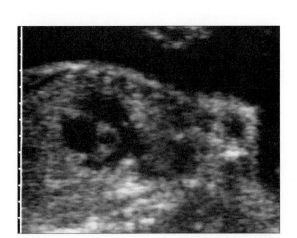

4. This image shows this important relationship.

_____

_____

_____

_____

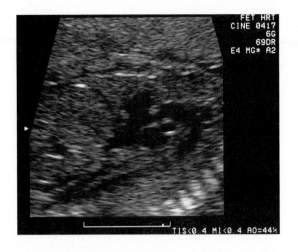

5. Is this image showing the ductus arteriosus or the aortic arch?

_____

_____

_____

_____

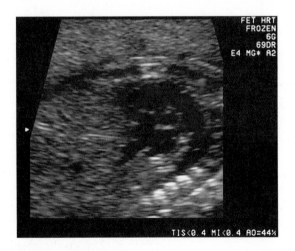

6. This image represents this anatomic structure.

_____

_____

_____

_____

30 Fetal Echocardiography: Congenital Heart Disease

KEY TERMS

Exercise 1

Match the following congenital heart disease terms with their definitions.

1. _____ atrial septal defects

2. _____ atrioventricular septal defect (AVSD)

3. _____ bicuspid aortic valve

4. _____ cardiomyopathy

5. _____ coarctation of the aorta

6. _____ dextrocardia

7. _____ dextroposition

8. _____ levocardia

9. _____ levoposition

10. _____ mesocardia

11. _____ myocarditis

12. _____ partial anomalous pulmonary venous return

13. _____ pericardial effusion

14. _____ ventricular septal defect

A. Disease of the myocardial tissue in the heart. This disease process is caused by several problems, including exposure to a virus, such as Coxsackie or mumps, or a bacterial infection.

B. The heart is in the right chest with the apex pointed to the right of the thorax.

C. This is an atypical location of the heart in the middle of the chest with the cardiac apex pointing toward the midline of the chest.

D. This is a condition in which the pulmonary veins do not all enter the left atrial cavity.

E. This is the normal position of the heart in the left chest with the cardiac apex pointed to the left.

F. Congenital abnormality that causes two of the three aortic leaflets to fuse together, resulting in a two-leaflet valve, instead of the normal three-leaflet valve. Usually the cusps are asymmetric in size and position. May be the cause of adult aortic stenosis and/or insufficiency.

G. Narrowing of the aortic arch (discrete, long segment, or tubular). Most commonly occurs as a shelflike protrusion in the isthmus of the arch or at the site of the ductal insertion near the left subclavian artery.

H. This is a cardiac disease process of necrosis and destruction of myocardial cells and also an inflammatory infiltrate.

I. This is a condition in which the heart is located in the right side of the chest, and the cardiac apex points medially or to the left.

J. This is a condition in which the heart is displaced farther toward the left chest, usually in association with a space-occupying lesion.

K. Defects that provide communication between the left atrium and the right atrium. The three most common forms of atrial septal defects are ostium secundum, ostium primum, and sinus venosus.

L. Defect in the ventricular septum that provides communication between the right and left chambers of the heart. Most common congenital lesion in the heart.

M. This is an abnormal collection of fluid surrounding the epicardial layer of the heart.

N. Failure of the endocardial cushion to fuse. This defect of the central heart provides communication between the ventricles, between the atria, or between the atria and ventricles. AVSD is subdivided into the complete, incomplete, and partial forms.

Exercise 2

Match the following right and left ventricular terms with their definitions.

1. _____ aortic stenosis

2. _____ Ebstein's anomaly of the tricuspid valve

3. _____ hypoplastic left heart syndrome

4. _____ hypoplastic right heart syndrome

5. _____ tetralogy of Fallot

6. _____ mitral atresia

7. _____ mitral regurgitation

8. _____ pulmonary stenosis

9. _____ subpulmonic stenosis

10. _____ supravalvular pulmonic stenosis

11. _____ tricuspid atresia

A. This is the most common form of cyanotic heart disease characterized by a high, membranous ventricular septal defect; large, anteriorly placed aorta; pulmonary stenosis; and right ventricular hypertrophy.

B. This is an abnormal pulmonary valve characterized by thickened, domed leaflets, which restrict the amount of blood flowing from the right ventricle to the pulmonary artery to the lungs.

C. Also called congenital mitral stenosis. Abnormal development of the mitral leaflet (valve between the left atrium and left ventricle). May lead to development of hypoplastic left ventricle.

D. This is an abnormal narrowing in the main pulmonary artery superior to the valve opening.

E. Abnormal displacement of the septal leaflet of the tricuspid valve toward the apex of the right ventricle. The right ventricle above this leaflet becomes the "atrialized" chamber.

F. This is an interruption of the growth of the tricuspid leaflet that begins early in cardiac embryology.

G. Underdevelopment of the right ventricular outflow tract secondary to pulmonary stenosis. Tricuspid atresia is also often found.

H. This is an abnormal development of the cusps of the aortic valve, which results in thickened and domed leaflets.

I. Underdevelopment of the left ventricle with aortic and/or mitral atresia. Left ventricle is extremely thickened compared with the right ventricle.

J. This occurs when the mitral leaflet is deformed and unable to close properly, allowing blood to leak from the left ventricle into the left atrium during systole.

K. This occurs when a membrane or muscle bundle obstructs the outflow tract into the pulmonary artery.

Exercise 3

Match the following abnormality and dysrhythmia terms with their definitions.

1. _____ atrioventricular block

2. _____ corrected transposition of the great arteries

3. _____ cor triatriatum

4. _____ ductal constriction

5. _____ premature atrial contractions (PACs) and premature ventricular contractions (PVCs)

6. _____ single ventricle

7. _____ supraventricular tachyarrhythmias

8. _____ total anomalous pulmonary venous return

9. _____ transposition of the great arteries

10. _____ truncus arteriosus

A. Benign condition that arises from the electrical impulses generated outside the cardiac pacemaker (sinus node). Immature development of the electrical pacing system causes irregular heartbeats scattered throughout the cardiac cycle.

B. Right atrium and left atrium are connected to the morphologic left and right ventricle, respectively, and the great arteries are transposed.

C. Congenital heart lesion in which only one great artery arises from the base of the heart. The pulmonary trunk, systemic arteries, and coronary arteries arise from this single great artery.

D. This is a congenital anomaly in which there are two atria but only one ventricular chamber, which receives both the mitral and tricuspid valves.

E. This occurs when the transmission of the electrical impulse from the atria to the ventricles is blocked.

F. This is a condition in which the pulmonary veins do not return at all into the left atrial cavity; the veins may return into the right atrial cavity or into a chamber posterior to the left atrial cavity.

G. This occurs when flow is diverted from the ductus secondary to tricuspid or pulmonary atresia or secondary to maternal medications given to stop early contractions.

H. This occurs when the left atrial cavity is partitioned into two compartments; pulmonary veins drain into an accessory left atrial chamber proximal to the true left atrium.

I. Abnormal condition that exists when the aorta is connected to the right ventricle and the pulmonary artery is connected to the left ventricle. The atrioventricular valves are normally attached and related.

J. This is an abnormal cardiac rhythm above 200 beats per minute with a conduction rate of 1:1.

CONGENITAL HEART DISEASE

Exercise 4

Fill in the blank(s) with the word(s) that best completes the statements about congenital heart disease.

1. The most common type of congenital heart disease is the _____, followed by atrial septal defects and then pulmonary stenosis.

2. _____ is usually found when extrinsic factors, such as a space-occupying large diaphragmatic hernia or hypoplasia of the right lung are present.

3. In the four-chamber view, a hypoechoic area in the peripheral part of the epicardial and/or pericardial interface

   of _____ or less is considered within normal limits and does not represent a pericardial effusion.

4. The _____ defect is the defect in the central atrial septum near the foramen ovale and is the most difficult to see in utero because the flap of the foramen ovale is mobile at this period of development.

5. The _____ defect is usually associated with the chromosome abnormality of trisomy 21 and often will have a cleft mitral valve and abnormalities of the atrioventricular septum.

6. The flap of the foramen ovale should not be so large as to touch the lateral wall of the atrium; when this redundancy of the foramen occurs, the sinoatrial node may become agitated in the right atrium and cause fetal

   _____.

7. The (perimembranous) ventricular septal defect may be classified as _____, _____, or

   _____.

8. Ventricular septal defects may close with the formation of _____ tissue that is commonly found along the right side of the septal defect.

9. The failure of the endocardial cushion to fuse is termed an _____ atrioventricular septal defect.

10. The most primitive form of endocardial cushion defect is called _____ atrioventricular septal defect. This defect has a single, undivided, free-floating leaflet stretching across both ventricles.

11. The findings in tricuspid atresia are a large dilated _____ ventricular cavity with a small,

    underdeveloped _____ ventricular cavity.

12. The portion of the right ventricle underlying the adherent tricuspid valvular tissue is quite thin and functions as a

    receiving chamber analogous to the right atrium. This is referred to as the _____ *chamber*.

13. The right heart is underdeveloped because of obstruction of the right ventricular outflow tract secondary to

    _____.

14. A large septal defect with mild-to-moderate pulmonary stenosis is classified as _____ disease, and a

    large septal defect with severe pulmonary stenosis is considered _____ disease ("blue baby" at birth).

15. If the override is greater than 50%, the condition is called a _____ ventricle. (Both great vessels arise from the right heart.)

16. In pulmonic stenosis, the abnormal pulmonic cusps become thickened and _____ during diastole.

17. In a _____, the raphe between the cusp tissue has not separated; thus the leaflet opens asymmetrically and may show "doming" on the parasternal long-axis view.

18. _____ occurs when a membrane covers the left ventricular outflow tract.

19. _____ is characterized by a small, hypertrophied left ventricle with aortic and/or mitral dysplasia or atresia.

20. _____ is an abnormal condition that exists when the aorta is connected to the right ventricle and the pulmonary artery is connected to the left ventricle. The atrioventricular valves are normally attached and related.

21. _____ shows an abnormal, large, single great vessel arising from the ventricles. Usually an infundibular ventricular septal defect is present. Significant septal override is present.

22. In the normal fetus, the ductus arteriosus transmits about 55% to 60% of combined ventricular output from the

    _____ to the aorta.

23. _____ tumors tend to be multiple and involve the septum. This tumor is associated with tuberous sclerosis (50% to 86%).

24. _____ occurs when the left atrial cavity is partitioned into two compartments. This anomaly is characterized by drainage of the pulmonary veins into an accessory left atrial chamber that lies proximal to the true left atrium.

25. An enlarged _____ system can serve an important function as a conveyor of inferior vena caval blood to the right atrium even though the inferior vena cava itself communicates with the left atrium.

26. In _____ the venous return may be totally into the right atrium or into a "common chamber" posterior to the left atrium, into the superior or inferior vena cava, or into the left subclavian vein, azygos vein, or portal vein.

FETAL CARDIAC RHYTHM

Exercise 5

Fill in the blank(s) with the word(s) that best completes the statements about the fetal cardiac rhythm.

1. _____ contractions arise from the electrical impulses generated outside the cardiac pacemaker (sinus node).

2. To adequately assess the fetal rhythm, the ventricular and atrial rates must be analyzed _____.

3. The aortic leaflets may signify the ventricular _____ event, whereas the atrial wall signifies the

   _____ event.

4. _____ include abnormal rhythms above 200 beats per minute with a conduction rate of 1:1.

5. In atrial flutter, the _____ rate is recorded at 300 to 460 beats per minute with a normal ventricular rate.

6. _____ shows the atria to have a rate of more than 400 beats per minute with a ventricular rate of 120 to 200 beats per minute.

7. With supraventricular tachycardia the fetus develops _____ filling of the ventricles, decreased cardiac output, and right ventricular volume overload leading to subsequent congestive heart failure.

8. When the transmission of the electrical impulse from the atria to the ventricles is blocked, the condition is called an

   _____ .

9. In _____ heart block, atrial and ventricular rates are independent of each other, with the atrial rate slower.

Exercise 6

Provide a short answer for each question after evaluating the images.

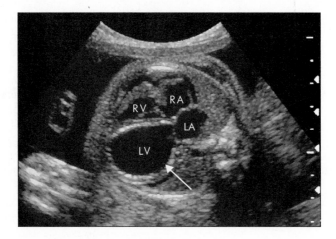

1. From this image identify and answer the following questions:
   a. Where is the fetal spine? (Use a clock identification.)
   b. Describe the left ventricle.
   c. What is the ratio of the cardiac circumference to the thoracic circumference?
   d. What would you expect the contractility to be?

_____

_____

_____

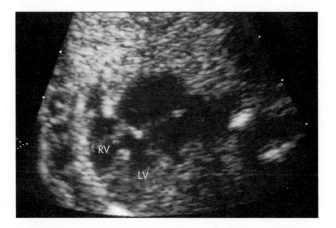

2. This 4CV demonstrates this fetal defect.

_____

_____

_____

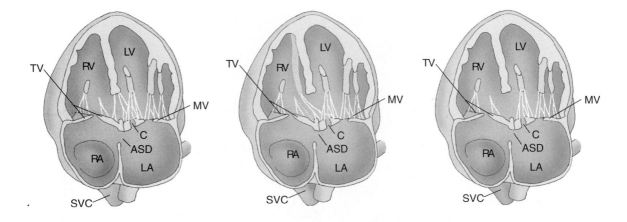

3. Describe the difference between the illustrations.

_____

_____

_____

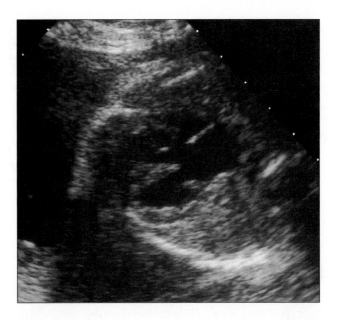

4. Describe the fetal cardiac defect in this image.

_____

_____

_____

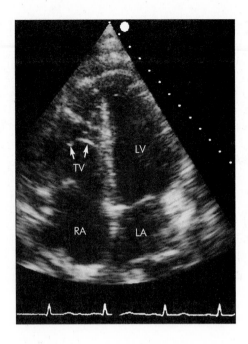

5. Describe the fetal cardiac anomaly in this fetus with tricuspid regurgitation.

_____

_____

_____

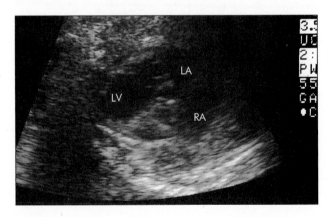

6. Describe the fetal cardiac anomaly.

_____

_____

_____

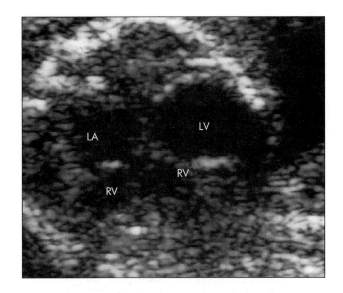

7. Describe the fetal cardiac anomaly.

_____

_____

_____

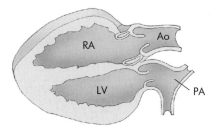

8. Describe the illustration and the cardiac anomaly.

_____

_____

_____

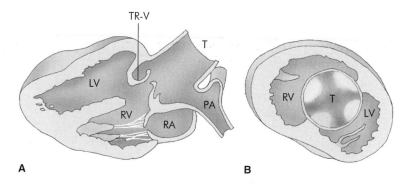

9. Describe the illustration and the cardiac anomaly.

_____

_____

_____

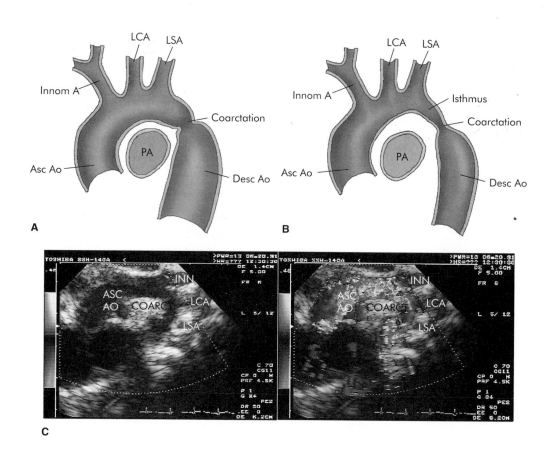

10. Identify the illustration that shows a long segment coarctation.

_____

_____

_____

31 Extracranial Cerebrovascular Evaluation

KEY TERMS

Exercise 1

Match the following extracranial terms with their definitions.

1. __I__ amaurosis fugax
2. __M__ aphasia
3. __E__ ataxia
4. __C__ bruit
5. __L__ collateral pathway
6. __B__ common carotid artery (CCA)
7. __N__ CVA
8. __Q__ diplopia
9. __A__ dysarthria
10. __D__ dysphagia
11. __O__ external carotid artery (ECA)
12. __K__ hemiparesis
13. __G__ internal carotid artery (ICA)
14. __J__ RIND
15. __P__ TIA
16. __H__ vertebral artery
17. __F__ vertigo

A. Difficulty with speech because of impairment of the tongue or muscles essential to speech
B. Arises from the aortic arch on the left side and from the innominate artery on the right side
C. Noise caused by tissue vibration produced by turbulence that causes flow disturbance
D. Inability to swallow or difficulty in swallowing
E. Gait disturbances
F. Sensation of having objects move about the person or sensation of moving around in space
G. Larger of the two terminal branches of the CCA
H. Large branch of the subclavian arteries
I. Transient partial or complete loss of vision in one eye
J. Reversible ischemic neurologic deficit
K. Unilateral partial or complete paralysis
L. Occurs when one vessel becomes obstructed; smaller side branches of the vessel provide alternative flow pathways
M. Inability to communicate by speech or writing
N. Cerebrovascular accident
O. Smaller of the two terminal branches of the CCA
P. Transient ischemic attack
Q. Double vision

Exercise 2

Label the following illustrations.

1. Anatomy of the extracranial carotid system.

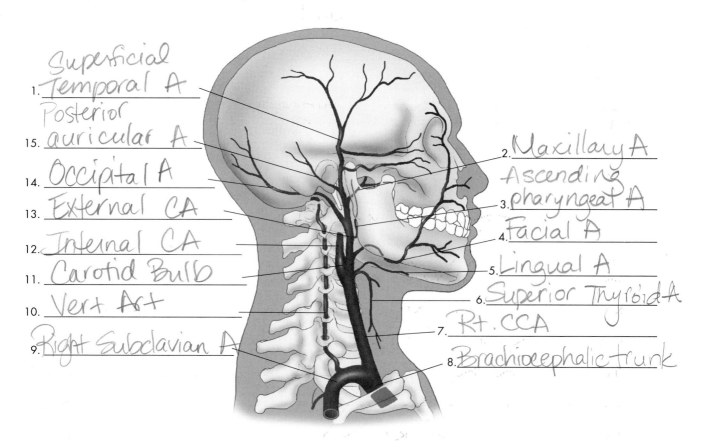

1. Superficial Temporal A
15. Posterior auricular A
14. Occipital A
13. External CA
12. Internal CA
11. Carotid Bulb
10. Vert Art
9. Right Subclavian A

2. Maxillary A
3. Ascending pharyngeal A
4. Facial A
5. Lingual A
6. Superior Thyroid A
7. Rt. CCA
8. Brachiocephalic trunk

Exercise 3

Fill in the blank(s) with the word(s) that best completes the statements or provide a short answer about the anatomy of extracranial cerebrovascular imaging.

1. The ascending aorta originates from the ___left___ ventricle of the heart.

2. The first branch is the ___brachiocephalic___ trunk (innominate artery), the ___left___ CCA the second, and the ___left___ subclavian artery the third branch in approximately 70% of cases.

3. The right CCA and the right subclavian artery are divided by the ___innominate___ artery, which gives rise to the right vertebral artery.

4. Each CCA ascends through the superior mediastinum anterolaterally in the neck and lies ___medial___ to the jugular vein.

5. The left common carotid is usually ___longer___ than the right, because it originates from the aortic arch.

6. The termination of the CCA is the carotid ___bifurcation___, which is the origin of the ICA and the ECA.

7. The ECA originates at the midcervical level and is usually the ___smaller___ of the two terminal branches of the CCA.

8. The larger of the CCA terminal branches is usually the _ICA_.

9. Identify the four main segments into which the ICA can be divided: _cervical_, _petrous_, _cavernous_ and _cerebral_.

10. In the majority of individuals, the ICA lies _posterolateral_ to the ECA and courses medially as it ascends in the neck.

11. The vertebral arteries are large branches of the _subclavian_ arteries.

12. The _extravertebral_ segment of the vertebral artery courses superiorly and medially from its subclavicular origin to enter the transverse foramen of the sixth cervical vertebra.

STROKE

Exercise 4

Fill in the blank(s) with the word(s) that best completes the statements or provide a short answer about stroke risk factors, warning signs, and symptoms.

1. A stroke or "brain attack" is caused by an _interruption_ of blood flow to the brain (ischemic stroke) or by a ruptured intracranial blood vessel (intracranial hemorrhage).

2. Approximately 80% of all known strokes are _ischemic_, and the remaining 20% are hemorrhagic.

3. The nonmodifiable risk factors are: _age_, _sex_, and _race_.

4. List the modifiable or controllable risk factors of stroke. _HTN, atrial fibrillation, cardiac disease, diabetes mellitus, elevated cholesterol, smoking, sedentary lifestyle_

5. Symptoms of weakness or numbness of a leg or arm on one side of the body indicate disease in the _contralateral_ carotid system.

6. Ocular symptoms, however, suggest disease in the carotid system on the _ipsilateral_.

7. Other cerebrovascular (carotid and vertebral territory) symptoms are: _amaurosis fugax_ (transient partial or complete loss of vision in one eye, often described as a shade or curtain being lowered over the eye), _hemiparesis_ (unilateral partial or complete paralysis), _dysarthria_ (difficulty with speech because of impairment of the tongue or muscles essential to speech), _aphasia_ (inability to communicate by speech or writing), _dysphagia_ (inability or difficulty in swallowing), _ataxia_ (gait disturbances), _diplopia_ (double vision), and _vertigo_ (sensation of having objects move about the person or sensation of moving around in space).

Exercise 5

Fill in the blank(s) with the word(s) that best completes the statements about the technical aspects of carotid duplex imaging.

1. Arm pressures are recorded, and a difference of _≥ 20_____ mm Hg pressure between arms suggests a proximal stenosis and/or occlusion of the subclavian or innominate artery on the side of the lower pressure.

2. In the normal setting, the CCA spectral waveform will demonstrate a ___low_____ resistance pattern (end diastole above the zero baseline) because blood travels from the CCA to the brain via the ICA.

3. The CCA Doppler signal will display a _positive_____ Doppler shift throughout the cardiac cycle.

4. The ICA demonstrates blood flow velocity that is _continuous___ and _above_____ the zero baseline throughout the cardiac cycle.

5. The normal color pattern of the ICA will have _continuous___ color throughout the cardiac cycle because the ICA has diastolic blood flow caused by the low peripheral resistance of the brain.

6. The ECA demonstrates a more _pulsatile____ Doppler signal (minimum diastolic flow) because it supplies blood to the skin and muscular bed of the scalp and face.

7. The ECA usually has a _faster_____ slope to peak systole and blood flow velocity at or very close to zero in late diastole.

8. The vertebral arteries are located by angling the transducer slightly _laterally___ from a longitudinal view of the middle or proximal CCA.

Exercise 6

Fill in the blank(s) with the word(s) that best completes the statements or provide a short answer about the interpretation of carotid duplex imaging.

1. The _highest_____ velocity obtained from an ICA stenosis is used to classify the degree of narrowing.

2. If there is reversal of vertebral artery blood flow direction secondary to a significant obstruction proximal to the origin of the vertebral artery in the ipsilateral subclavian or innominate artery, a _subclavian steal__ is present.

3. The evaluation of normal subclavian arteries produces _multiphasic__ high-resistance Doppler signals.

4. Identify the important information that should be included in the interpretation of a carotid duplex imaging examination. 1) loc. of stenosis / 2) extent of plaque + patency of distal ICA 3) presence of tortuosity/kinking of vessels / 4) plaque characteristics (smooth vs. irregular surface, calcification)

5. Carotid duplex imaging performed after carotid endarterectomy may reveal _residual__ or _recurrent__ stenosis in the ipsilateral ICA and disease progression in the contralateral ICA.

Exercise 7

Fill in the blank(s) with the word(s) that best completes the statements or provide a short answer about the pathology of the extracranial vessels.

1. The echogenicity of plaque is usually described as _homo_ if it demonstrates a uniform level of echogenicity and texture throughout the plaque and _hetero_ if the plaque has mixed areas of echogenicity and textures.

2. A _calcified_ plaque is usually visualized with an accompanying acoustic shadow that obscures imaging information deep to it.

3. When describing if the ICA is occluded, the color PRF should be _decreased_ to document the presence of any slow-moving blood flow, and the color gain should be increased to enhance any blood flow that may be present.

4. The ICA should be sampled at _multiple_ sites with Doppler.

5. A nonatherosclerotic disease that usually affects the media of the arterial wall is _fibromuscular dysplasia_

Exercise 8

Provide a short answer for each question after evaluating the images.

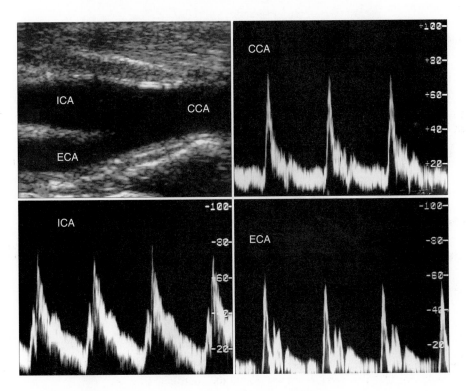

1. Name the vessel(s) that demonstrate(s) a higher resistance flow pattern.

    ECA

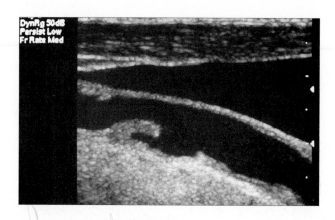

2. This image of the carotid artery demonstrates:

irregular plaque post surf

_____

_____

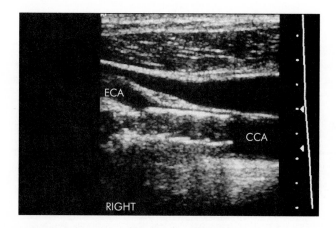

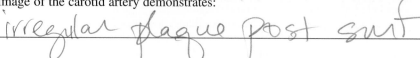

3. The image of the carotid artery shown in this postoperative patient is:

bright echoes from lumen of stent

_____

_____

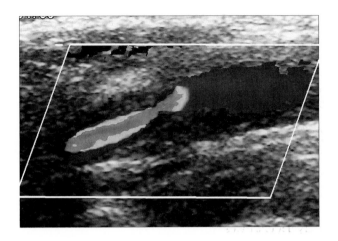

4. This image demonstrates:

doppler aliasing from the narrowed
lumen—carotid stenosis

32 Intracranial Cerebrovascular Evaluation

KEY TERMS

Exercise 1
Match the following intracranial anatomic terms with their definitions.

1. _____ anterior cerebral artery (ACA)

2. _____ anterior communicating artery (AcoA)

3. _____ basilar artery (BA)

4. _____ circle of Willis

5. _____ internal carotid artery (ICA)

6. _____ middle cerebral artery (MCA)

7. _____ posterior cerebral artery (PCA)

8. _____ posterior communicating artery (PcoA)

9. _____ vertebral artery

A. A polygon vascular ring at the base of the brain

B. A short vessel that connects the anterior cerebral arteries at the interhemispheric fissure

C. Courses posteriorly and medially from the ICA to join the posterior cerebral artery

D. Branch of the subclavian artery

E. Smaller of the two terminal branches of the ICA

F. Originates from the terminal basilar artery and courses anteriorly and laterally

G. Formed by the union of the two vertebral arteries

H. Arises from the common carotid artery to supply the anterior brain and meninges

I. Large terminal branch of the ICA

Exercise 2
Match the following intracranial terms with their definitions.

1. _____ cerebral vasospasm

2. _____ mean velocity

3. _____ ophthalmic artery

4. _____ subclavian steal syndrome

5. _____ submandibular window

6. _____ suboccipital window

7. _____ transorbital window

8. _____ transtemporal window

A. Characterized by symptoms of brain stem ischemia associated with a stenosis or occlusion of the left subclavian, innominate, or right subclavian artery proximal to the origin of the vertebral artery

B. Transducer is placed on the posterior aspect of the neck inferior to the nuchal crest

C. First branch of the ICA

D. Transducer is placed on the temporal bone cephalad to the zygomatic arch anterior to the ear

E. Vasoconstriction of the arteries

F. Transducer is placed at the angle of the mandible and angled slightly medially and cephalad toward the carotid canal

G. Transducer is placed on the closed eyelid

H. Based on the time average of the outline velocity (maximum velocity envelope)

Exercise 3

Label the following illustrations.
1. The arteries of the circle of Willis.

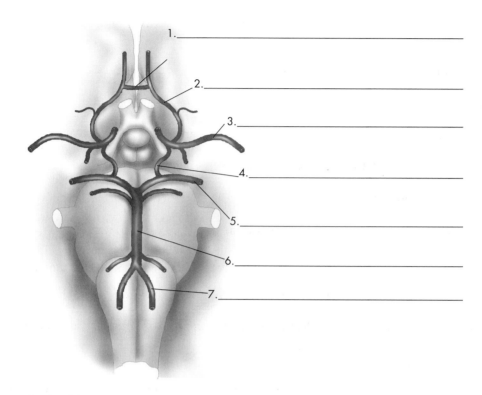

1. _____

2. _____

3. _____

4. _____

5. _____

6. _____

7. _____

2. Identify the pathway of blood in the subclavian steal.

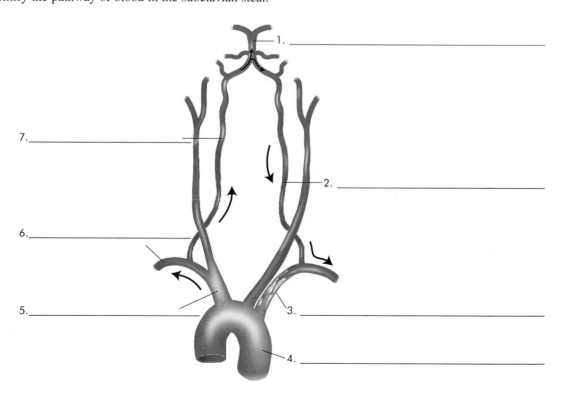

1. _____

7. _____

2. _____

6. _____

5. _____

3. _____

4. _____

Exercise 4

Fill in the blank(s) with the word(s) that best completes the statements about the anatomy of the intracranial cerebrovascular system.

1. Blood supply to the brain is provided by the _____ (anterior) and _____ (posterior) arteries.

2. The first branch of the ICA is the _____ artery that courses anterior laterally and slightly downward through the optic foramen to supply the globe, orbit, and adjacent structures.

3. The artery that courses posteriorly and medially from the ICA to join the posterior cerebral artery is the

   _____ artery.

4. The larger terminal branch of the ICA is the _____ artery.

5. The terminal branches of the MCA anastomose with terminal branches of the _____ cerebral and

   _____ cerebral arteries.

6. The smaller of the two terminal branches of the ICA is the _____ artery.

7. A short vessel that connects the ACAs at the interhemispheric fissure is the _____ artery.

8. The large branches of the subclavian arteries are the _____ arteries.

9. The artery that is formed by the union of the two vertebral arteries and is evaluated during TCD imaging is the

   _____ artery.

10. The arteries that originate from the terminal basilar artery and course anteriorly and laterally are the

    _____ arteries.

11. A polygon vascular ring at the base of the brain that permits communication between the right and left cerebral

    hemispheres (via the ACoA) and between the anterior and posterior systems (via the PCoAs) is the

    _____.

Exercise 5

Fill in the blank(s) with the word(s) that best completes the statements about the hemodynamics of the intracranial cerebrovascular system.

1. The percentage of red blood cells by volume in whole blood and a major determinant of blood viscosity is

   _____.

2. Blood viscosity is an important factor influencing intracranial arterial blood _____ velocity.

3. A deficiency of CO_2 in the blood is known as hypocapnia or _____ and causes a decrease in the MCA mean velocity and an increase in the PI.

4. An excess of CO_2 in the blood is referred to as hypercapnia or _____ and causes an increase in MCA mean velocity and a decrease in the PI.

Exercise 6

Fill in the blank(s) with the word(s) that best completes the statements about the sonographic technique of intracranial evaluation.

1. The approach that is performed with the patient in the supine position with the head aligned straight with the body

   is the _____ window.

2. When evaluating the vertebrobasilar system, the best results are obtained with the patient lying on his or her side

   with the head bowed slightly toward the chest. This is called the _____ window.

3. The large, circular, anechoic area seen from the suboccipital window is the _____, and the bright,

   echogenic reflection is from the _____ bone.

4. The _____ window evaluation provides information about the ophthalmic artery and the carotid siphon.

5. To evaluate the extracranial distal ICA, the transducer is placed at the angle of the mandible and angled slightly

   medially and cephalad toward the carotid canal with the _____ window.

PATHOLOGY

Exercise 7

Fill in the blank(s) with the word(s) that best completes the statements about the pathology of the intracranial cerebrovascular system.

1. The most common cause of SAH is leakage of blood from intracranial cerebral aneurysms into the

   _____ space.

2. The hemodynamic effect of vasospasm produces an _____ in blood flow velocity coupled with a
   pressure drop distal to the narrowed segment.

3. When there is increased intracranial pressure or the vasomotor reserve has been exhausted, cerebral blood flow

   can be reduced to critical levels resulting in _____ or _____.

4. Intracranial arterial _____ cause characteristic alterations in the Doppler signal (audio and spectral
   waveform), including focal increases in velocity, local turbulence, and a poststenotic drop in velocity.

5. An artery providing collateral circulation usually demonstrates an _____ blood flow velocity.

6. Brain stem ischemia associated with a stenosis or occlusion of the left subclavian, innominate, or right subclavian

   artery proximal to the origin of the vertebral artery is a symptom of _____ syndrome.

7. The "stealing" of blood from the _____ artery, via retrograde vertebral artery flow, causes the patient

   to experience neurologic symptoms of brain stem ischemia.

8. Blood flow is normally _____ from the transducer (suboccipital approach) in the vertebrobasilar

system. If flow is _____ the transducer in a vertebral artery and the basilar artery, there is evidence of a steal.

Exercise 8

Provide a short answer for each question after evaluating the images.

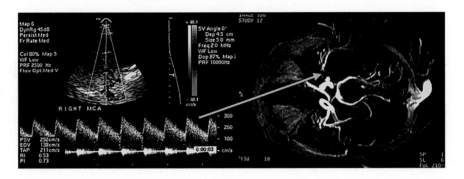

1. Describe the abnormality demonstrated on this transcranial image.

_____

_____

_____

33 Peripheral Arterial Evaluation

KEY TERMS

Exercise 1

Match the following peripheral arterial terms with their definitions.

1. _____ anterior tibial artery

2. _____ arteritis

3. _____ axillary artery

4. _____ brachial artery

5. _____ claudication

6. _____ dorsalis pedis artery

7. _____ innominate artery

8. _____ ischemic rest pain

9. _____ necrosis

10. _____ popliteal artery

11. _____ profunda femoris artery

12. _____ pseudoaneurysm

13. _____ radial artery

14. _____ reactive hyperemia

15. _____ subclavian artery

16. _____ superficial femoral artery

17. _____ thoracic outlet syndrome

18. _____ tibial-peroneal trunk

19. _____ ulnar artery

A. Continuation of the anterior tibial artery on the top of the foot

B. Perivascular collection (hematoma) that communicates with an artery or a graft and has the presence of pulsating blood entering the collection

C. Continuation of the axillary artery

D. Posterior and lateral to the superficial femoral artery

E. Changes in arterial blood flow to the arms may be related to intermittent compression of the proximal arteries (or neural and venous structures)

F. Takes off after the anterior tibial artery and bifurcates into the posterior tibial artery and the peroneal artery

G. Inflammation of an artery

H. Begins at the opening of the adductor magnus muscle and travels behind the knee in the popliteal fossa

I. Originates at the inner border of the scalenus anterior and travels beneath the clavicle to the outer border of the first rib to become the axillary artery

J. Branch of the brachial artery that runs parallel to the radial artery in the forearm

K. Walking-induced muscular discomfort of the calf, thigh, hip, or buttock

L. First branch artery from the aortic arch

M. Branch of the brachial artery that runs parallel to the ulnar artery in the forearm

N. Begins at the popliteal artery and travels down the lateral calf in the anterior compartment to the level of the ankle

O. Courses the length of the thigh through Hunter's canal and terminates at the opening of the adductor magnus muscle

P. The death of areas of tissue

Q. Alternative method to stress the peripheral arterial circulation

R. Continuation of the subclavian artery

S. Implies critical ischemia (lack of blood) of the distal limb when the patient is at rest

Exercise 2

Label the following illustrations.
1. The arteries of the lower extremity.

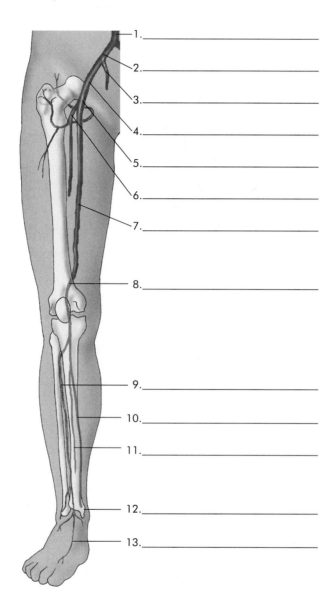

1. _____

2. _____

3. _____

4. _____

5. _____

6. _____

7. _____

8. _____

9. _____

10. _____

11. _____

12. _____

13. _____

2. The arteries of the upper extremity.

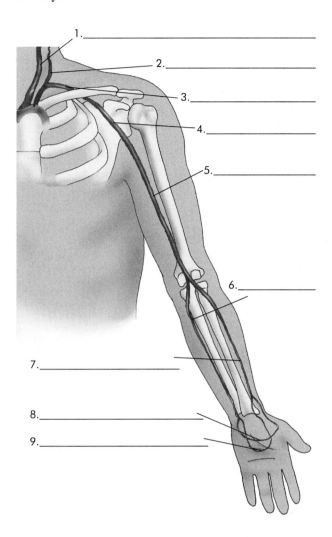

1._____

2._____

3._____

4._____

5._____

6._____

7._____

8._____

9._____

Exercise 3

Fill in the blank(s) with the word(s) that best completes the statements about the anatomy of peripheral arterial testing.

1. The descending aorta is divided into a(n) _____ section and a(n) _____ section.

2. The abdominal aorta terminates in the _____ of the right and left common iliac arteries (approximately at the level of the fourth lumbar vertebra).

3. Each of the common iliac arteries bifurcates into an internal iliac artery (_____ artery) that supplies the pelvis and an external iliac artery that continues distally to supply the lower extremity.

4. The external iliac artery terminates at the inguinal ligament, where it becomes the _____ artery.

5. The common femoral artery originates beneath the inguinal ligament and terminates by dividing into the

   superficial femoral and _____ arteries.

6. The popliteal artery begins at the opening of the adductor magnus muscle and travels behind the knee in the

   _____ fossa.

7. The popliteal artery terminates distally into the _____ tibial artery and the tibial _____ trunk.

8. A continuation of the anterior tibial artery on the top of the foot is the _____ artery.

9. The artery that is located deep within the calf and travels near the medial aspect of the fibula is the

   _____ artery.

10. The artery that originates at the inner border of the scalenus anterior and travels beneath the clavicle to the outer

    border of the first rib is the _____ artery.

11. The brachial artery is a continuation of the _____ artery.

12. The radial artery begins at the _____ artery bifurcation.

Exercise 4

Fill in the blank(s) with the word(s) that best completes the statements or provide a short answer about the risk factors and symptoms of peripheral arterial disease.

1. List the several risk factors that are associated with peripheral occlusive arterial disease.

   _____

   _____

   _____

2. Symptoms of lower extremity occlusive arterial disease are _____ and _____ pain.

3. Ischemic rest pain implies critical ischemia of the _____ limb when the patient is at rest.

INDIRECT ARTERIAL TESTING

Exercise 5

Fill in the blank(s) with the word(s) that best completes the statements about indirect arterial testing.

1. Before beginning the examination, there should be a _____ minute rest period to allow the patient's blood pressure to stabilize and legs to recover from walking to the examination room.

2. Segmental pressures are obtained with the patient in the _____ position; the legs should be at the same

   level as the _____ because this position prevents hydrostatic pressure artifact.

3. To obtain pressures comparable with direct intraarterial measurements, the blood pressure cuff must have a width

   _____ greater than the diameter of the limb.

4. Pressures may be falsely _____ in obese patients, and a proximal thigh pressure may be

   _____ in extremely thin patients.

5. Pulse volume recordings measure changes in _____ limb volume with each cardiac cycle.

Exercise 6

Fill in the blank(s) with the word(s) that best completes the statements or provide a short answer about arterial stress testing.

1. In a normal individual without occlusive arterial disease, blood flow will _____ with exercise because

   of a _____ in peripheral vascular resistance.

2. Identify the contraindications to lower-extremity arterial stress testing.

   _____

   _____

   _____

3. Indirect arterial testing is helpful in predicting the likelihood of the _____ of skin lesions.

ARTERIAL DUPLEX IMAGING

Exercise 7

Fill in the blank(s) with the word(s) that best completes the statements or provide a short answer about arterial duplex imaging.

1. Arterial duplex imaging provides direct anatomic and physiologic information, but it does not provide information

   regarding overall limb _____.

2. Duplex imaging distinguishes between a stenosis and an _____, determines the length of the disease

   segment and _____ of the distal vessels, evaluates the results of intervention (angioplasty, stent

   placement), aids in diagnoses of aneurysms and _____, and monitors patients' postoperative course
   with continuing bypass graft surveillance.

3. If a _____ degree angle cannot be maintained, documentation of the angle used during the examination
   is important, especially in following the patient over time.

4. In normal vessels, the arterial Doppler signal is _____ from the abdominal aorta to the tibial arteries at
   the ankle.

5. The aortic characteristic waveform has a high-velocity _____ flow component during systole (ventricular contraction), followed by a brief _____ of flow in early diastole (because of peripheral resistance), and a final low-velocity forward flow phase in late diastole (elastic recoil of the vessel wall).

6. Peak systolic velocity gradually _____ from the proximal to the distal arteries.

7. List the three major changes in the spectral Doppler arterial waveform that occur because of a significant stenosis.

_____

_____

_____

8. A pseudoaneurysm may be unilocular or multilocular and may partially contain _____.

9. Identification of the _____ of the pseudoaneurysm is important when ultrasound-guided compression therapy is attempted and color Doppler imaging permits identification of the vessel of origin, which is important when planning surgical interventions.

10. During _____, blood flows from the native artery into the pseudoaneurysm and during _____ blood flow returns to the native artery.

Exercise 8
Provide a short answer for each question after evaluating the images.

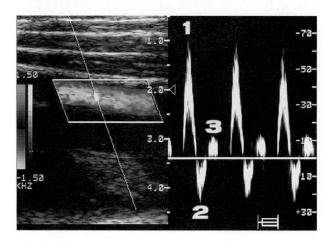

1. Describe the flow pattern in the femoral artery tracing.

_____

_____

_____

_____

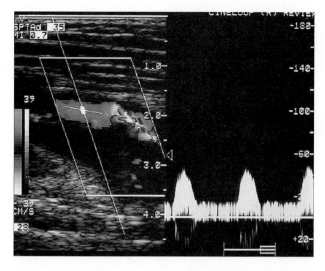

2. This patient presented with claudication. There was a 40-mm Hg drop in pressure from the upper to the lower thigh. This Doppler signal is proximal to the narrowed segment. It shows:

_____

_____

_____

_____

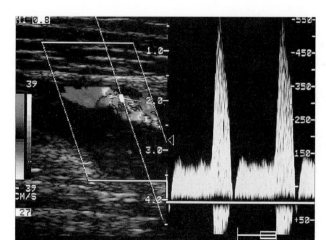

3. Describe what this waveform tells about flow in the distal superficial femoral artery.

_____

_____

_____

_____

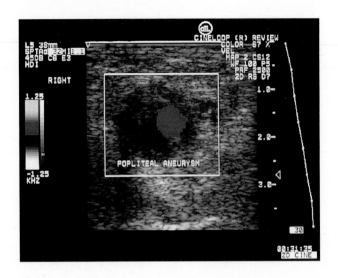

4. This image is taken along the posterior distal femoral area. It demonstrates this vascular abnormality.

_____

_____

_____

_____

34 Peripheral Venous Evaluation

KEY TERMS

Exercise 1

Match the following anatomic terms with their definitions.

1. _J_ anterior tibial veins

2. _D_ axillary vein

3. _F_ cephalic vein

4. _L_ common iliac vein

5. _A_ gastrocnemius veins

6. _H_ innominate veins

7. _C_ perforating veins

8. _K_ popliteal vein

9. _E_ posterior tibial veins

10. _B_ respiratory phasicity

11. _I_ subclavian vein

12. _G_ valves

A. Paired veins that lie in the medial and lateral gastrocnemius muscles; terminate into the popliteal vein

B. Blood flow velocity changes with respiration

C. Connect the superficial and deep venous systems

D. Begins where the basilic vein joins the brachial vein in the upper arm and terminates beneath the clavicle at the outer border of the first rib

E. Originate from the plantar veins of the foot and drain blood from the posterior compartment of the lower leg

F. Begins on the thumb side of the dorsum of the hand and joins the axillary vein just below the clavicle

G. Folds of the intima that temporarily close to permit blood flow in one direction only

H. Right vein: courses vertically downward to join the left innominate vein below the first rib to form the superior vena cava; left vein: longer than right, courses from left chest to the right beneath the sternum to join the right innominate vein

I. Continuation of the axillary vein joins the internal jugular vein to form the innominate vein

J. Drain blood from the dorsum of the foot and anterior compartment of the calf

K. Originates from the confluence of the anterior tibial vein with the posterior and peroneal veins

L. Formed by the confluence of the internal and external iliac veins

Exercise 2

Match the following peripheral venous terms with their definitions.

1. __F__ augmentation

2. __K__ basilic vein

3. __A__ common femoral vein

4. __D__ deep femoral vein

5. __J__ greater saphenous vein

6. __H__ lesser saphenous vein

7. __L__ peroneal veins

8. __C__ posterior arch vein

9. __E__ pulmonary embolism

10. __I__ soleal sinuses

11. __B__ superficial femoral vein

12. __G__ varicose veins

A. Formed by the confluence of the profunda femoris and the superficial femoral vein; also receives the greater saphenous vein

B. Originates at the hiatus of the adductor magnus muscle in the distal thigh and ascends through the adductor (Hunter's) canal

C. Main tributary of the greater saphenous vein

D. Travels with the profunda femoris artery to unite with the superficial femoral vein to form the common femoral vein

E. Blockage of the pulmonary circulation by foreign matter

F. Blood flow velocity increases with distal limb compression or with the release of proximal limb compression

G. Dilated, elongated, tortuous superficial veins

H. Originates on the dorsum of the foot and ascends posterior to the lateral malleolus and runs along the midline of the posterior calf. Vein terminates as it joins the popliteal vein.

I. Large venous reservoirs that lie in the soleus muscle and empty into the posterior tibial or peroneal veins

J. Originates on the dorsum of the foot and ascends anterior to the medial malleolus and along the anteromedial side of the calf and thigh; joins the common femoral vein in the proximal thigh

K. Originates on the small finger side of the dorsum of the hand and enters the brachial veins in the upper arm

L. Drain blood from lateral compartment of the lower leg

ANATOMY

Exercise 3

Label the following illustrations.

1. The deep veins of the lower extremity.

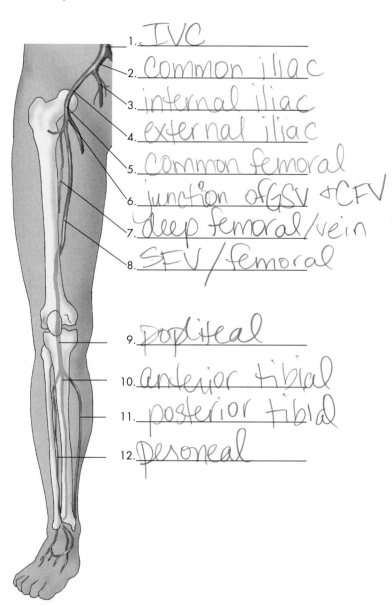

1. IVC
2. Common iliac
3. internal iliac
4. external iliac
5. Common femoral
6. junction of GSV & CFV
7. deep femoral/vein
8. SFV/femoral

9. popliteal
10. anterior tibial
11. posterior tibial
12. peroneal

2. The greater saphenous vein.

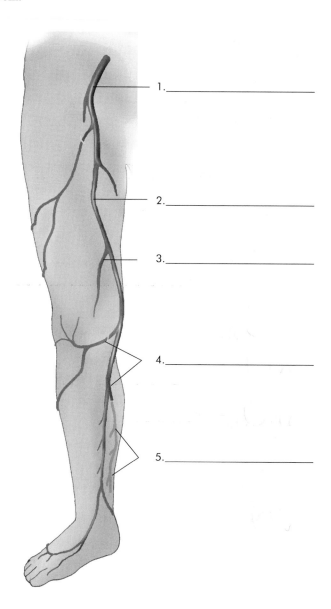

1._____

2._____

3._____

4._____

5._____

3. The lesser saphenous vein.

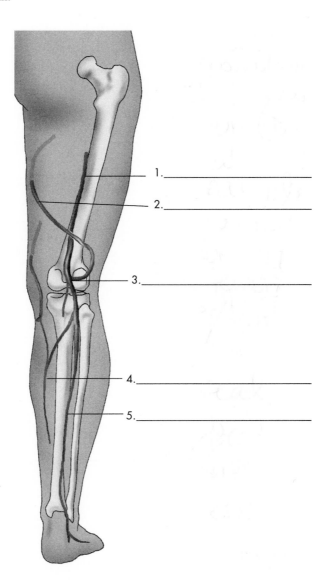

1._____

2._____

3._____

4._____

5._____

4. The deep veins of the upper extremity.

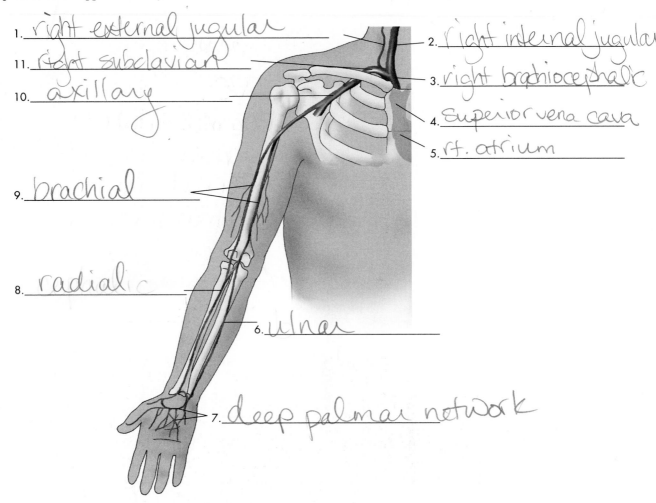

1. right external jugular

11. right subclavian

10. axillary

9. brachial

8. radial

6. ulnar

7. deep palmar network

2. right internal jugular

3. right brachiocephalic

4. Superior vena cava

5. rt. atrium

5. The superficial veins of the upper extremity.

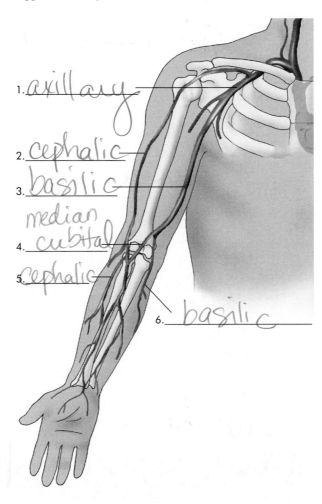

1. *axillary*
2. *cephalic*
3. *basilic*
   median
4. *cubital*
5. *cephalic*
6. *basilic*

PERIPHERAL VENOUS EVALUATION

Exercise 4

Fill in the blank(s) with the word(s) that best completes the statements about the risk factors and symptoms of vascular disease.

1. A potentially lethal complication of acute DVT is __*PE*__.

2. The chronic process, __*Post thrombotic*__ syndrome, is a complication following DVT.

3. Identify the three factors associated with thrombus formation, Virchow's triad.

   hypercoagulable state

   venous stasis

   vein wall injury

4. Varicose veins are dilated, elongated, tortuous __*superficial*__ veins.

5. The venous systems of the lower and upper extremities consist of __*ant tib*__ / *superf*, __*post tib*__ / *deep*, and

   perforating (__*communicating*__) veins.

6. Perforating veins provide a channel between the _deep_ and _superficial_ veins.

7. Venous blood flow is normally from the _superficial_ veins to the _deep_ veins.

8. Venous valves are important in maintaining _unidirectional_ blood flow from the peripheral veins to the central veins.

Exercise 5

Fill in the blank(s) with the word(s) that best completes the statements about the technical aspects of venous duplex imaging.

1. If the patient is symptomatic, it helps to locate the _area_ of pain and to measure any limb swelling at the _calf_ level.

2. The bed or table should be placed in reverse Trendelenburg (head elevated) position, which promotes venous _distention_ and optimizes visualization of the veins.

3. The leg being evaluated is _externally_ rotated and the knee slightly _flexed_.

4. In general compared with the common femoral artery, the common femoral vein will _collapse_ with light-to-moderate transducer pressure on the skin and usually will _change_ in size with respiration.

5. If superficial thrombophlebitis is suspected, the _GSV_ vein should be followed along its entire length.

6. If the saphenous vein is not visualized, _reduce_ the pressure on the transducer to make sure that the vein is not inadvertently being compressed.

7. The popliteal vein is evaluated from a _posterior_ approach with the patient's knee rotated externally, with the patient in the _decubitus_ position, or with the patient in the _prone_ position with the foot elevated on a pillow to eliminate extrinsic compression of the vein.

8. The popliteal vein usually lies _superficial_ to the popliteal artery.

Exercise 6

Fill in the blank(s) with the word(s) that best completes the statements or provide a short answer about the peripheral venous examination.

1. Identify the three components that the interpretation criteria for venous duplex imaging are based on.

free of echoes

compresses fully

normal venous Doppler signal

2. The most significant diagnostic criteria during venous imaging is how the vein responds to transducer _pressure_.

3. If the vein still does not _compress_, remember that visualization of the thrombus is quite variable.

4. At times the thrombus is very _echogenic_ and may blend into the surrounding tissue, and at other times the clot is _anechoic_.

5. The purpose of superficial vein mapping is to determine the vein's suitability for use as a _bypass conduit_ and to identify its anatomic route.

6. The purpose of venous reflux testing is to identify the presence and the location of _incompetent_ venous valves.

7. The term _superficial_ femoral vein is often used to describe the deep venous system in the thigh in venous duplex imaging reports. It may be advisable to use the term *femoral vein* in venous duplex imaging reports when describing the deep venous system in the thigh.

Exercise 7
Provide a short answer for each question after evaluating the images.

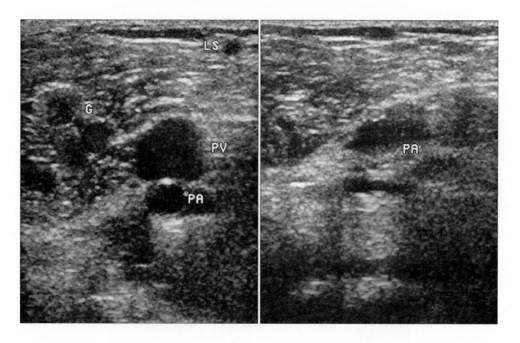

1. Identify which image was made with transducer pressure.

_____

_____

_____

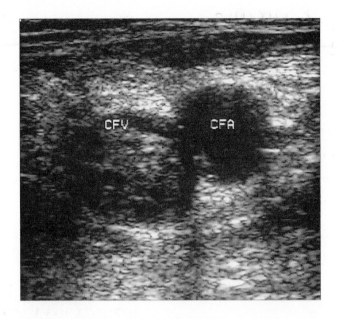

2. This image over the common femoral artery is made with transducer pressure. Describe the sonographic findings.

thrombos

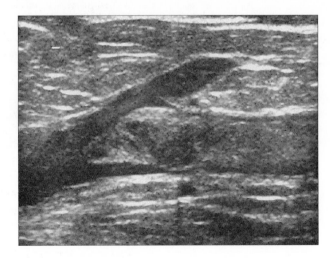

3. The patient presented with tenderness and swelling of the upper thigh. Describe the sonographic findings.

floating clot in femoral vein

35 Normal Anatomy and Physiology of the Female Pelvis

KEY TERMS

Exercise 1

Match the following pelvic anatomic terms with their definitions.

1. ___E___ coccygeus muscles

2. ___J___ false pelvis

3. ___B___ iliacus muscle

4. ___H___ iliopectineal line

5. ___D___ levator ani

6. ___K___ obturator internus muscle

7. ___F___ piriformis muscle

8. ___A___ polymenorrhea

9. ___I___ psoas major muscle

10. ___G___ striations

11. ___C___ true pelvis

A. An abnormally frequent recurrence of the menstrual cycle; a menstrual cycle of less than 21 days

B. Paired triangular, flat muscle that covers the inner curved surface of the iliac fossae; arises from the iliac fossae and joins the psoas major muscles to form the lateral walls of the pelvis

C. Pelvic cavity found below the brim of the pelvis

D. One of two muscles of the pelvic diaphragm that stretch across the floor of the pelvic cavity like a hammock, supporting the pelvic organs and surrounding the urethra, vagina, and rectum; a broad thin muscle that consists of the pubococcygeus, iliococcygeus, and puborectalis

E. One of two muscles in the pelvic diaphragm; located on the posterior pelvic floor where it supports the coccyx

F. A flat, pyramidal muscle arising from the anterior sacrum, passing through the greater sciatic notch to insert into the superior aspect of the greater trochanter of the femur; serves to rotate and abduct the thigh

G. Parallel longitudinal lines commonly seen in muscle tissue when imaged sonographically; appear as hyperechoic parallel lines running in the long axis of the hypoechoic muscle tissue

H. A bony ridge on the inner surface of the ilium and pubic bones that divides the true and false pelves

I. Paired muscle that originates at the transverse process of the lumbar vertebrae and extends inferiorly through the false pelvis on the pelvic sidewall, where it unites with the iliacus muscle to form the iliopsoas muscle before inserting into the lesser trochanter of the femur; serves to flex the thigh toward the pelvis

J. Portion of the pelvis found above the brim; that portion of the abdominal cavity cradled by the iliac fossae

K. A triangular sheet of muscle that arises from the anterolateral pelvic wall and surrounds the obturator foramen; passes through the lesser sciatic foramen and inserts into the medial aspect of the greater trochanter of the femur; serves to rotate and abduct the thigh

319

Exercise 2

Match the following female pelvic terms with their definitions.

1. _S_ anteverted

2. _I_ anteflexed

3. _M_ broad ligament

4. _G_ cardinal ligament

5. _Q_ corpus albicans

6. _L_ corpus luteum

7. _C_ estrogen

8. _N_ mesosalpinx

9. _H_ mesovarium

10. _I_ mesometrium

11. _A_ oocyte

12. _X_ ovarian ligament

13. _F_ ovum

14. _P_ perimetrium

15. _D_ postmenopause

16. _W_ progesterone

17. _K_ rectouterine recess (pouch)

18. _U_ retroflexed

19. _B_ retroverted

20. _V_ round ligament

21. _R_ space of Retzius

22. _J_ suspensory ligament

23. _E_ uterosacral ligament

24. _O_ vesicouterine recess (pouch)

A. An incompletely developed or immature ovum

B. Refers to the position of the uterus when the entire uterus is tipped posteriorly so that the angle formed between the cervix and vaginal canal is greater than 90 degrees

C. A steroidal hormone secreted by the theca interna and granulosa cells of the ovarian follicle that stimulates the development of the female reproductive structures and secondary sexual characteristics; promotes the growth of the endometrial tissue during the proliferative phase of the menstrual cycle

D. Time period of life after menopause

E. Posterior portion of the cardinal ligament that extends from the cervix to the sacrum

F. The female egg; a secondary oocyte released from the ovary at ovulation

G. Wide bands of fibromuscular tissue arising from the lateral aspects of the cervix and inserting along the lateral pelvic floor; a continuation of the broad ligament that provides rigid support for the cervix

H. The posterior portion of the broad ligament that is drawn out to enclose and hold the ovary in place

I. Refers to the position of the uterus when the uterine fundus bends forward toward the cervix

J. Paired ligaments that extend from the infundibulum of the fallopian tube and the lateral aspect of the ovary to the lateral pelvic wall

K. Area in the pelvic cavity between the rectum and the uterus that is likely to accumulate free fluid

L. An anatomic structure on the surface of the ovary, consisting of a spheroid of yellowish tissue that grows within the ruptured ovarian follicle after ovulation; acts as a short-lived endocrine organ that secretes progesterone to maintain the decidual layer of the endometrium should conception occur

M. A broad fold of peritoneum draped over the fallopian tubes, uterus, and the ovaries; extends from the sides of the uterus to the side walls of the pelvis, dividing the pelvis from side to side and creating the vesicouterine pouch anterior to the uterus and the rectouterine pouch posteriorly; it is divided into mesometrium, mesosalpinx, and mesovarium

N. The upper portion of the broad ligament that encloses the fallopian tubes

O. Area in the pelvic cavity between the urinary bladder and the uterus

P. A serous membrane enveloping the uterus

Q. A pale white spot on the surface of the ovary that results from the degeneration of the corpus luteum

R. Located between the anterior bladder wall and the pubic symphysis; contains extraperitoneal fat

S. Refers to the position of the uterus when the uterus is tipped slightly forward so that the cervix forms a 90-degree angle or less with the vaginal canal; most common uterine position

T. The portion of the broad ligament below the mesovarium, composed of the layers of peritoneum that separate to enclose the uterus

U. Refers to the position of the uterus when the uterine fundus bends posteriorly upon the cervix

V. Paired ligaments that originate at the uterine cornua, anterior to the fallopian tubes and course anterolaterally within the broad ligament to insert into the fascia of the labia majora; holds the uterus forward in its anteverted position

W. A steroidal hormone produced by the corpus luteum that helps prepare and maintain the endometrium for the arrival and implantation of an embryo

X. A paired ligament that extends from the inferior and/or medial pole of the ovary to the uterine cornua

Exercise 3

Match the following physiologic terms with their definitions.

1. ___D___ amenorrhea

2. ___G___ dysmenorrhea

3. ___B___ follicle-stimulating hormone

4. ___I___ gonadotropin

5. ___A___ gonadotropin-releasing hormone

6. ___L___ luteinizing hormone

7. ___H___ menarche

8. ___E___ menopause

9. ___J___ menses

10. ___C___ menorrhagia

11. ___F___ oligomenorrhea

12. ___K___ premenarche

A. A hormone secreted by the hypothalamus that stimulates the release of the follicle-stimulating hormone and luteinizing hormone by the anterior pituitary gland

B. A hormone secreted by the anterior pituitary gland that stimulates the growth and maturation of graafian follicles in the ovary

C. Abnormally heavy or long menstrual periods

D. An absence of menstruation

E. Refers to the cessation of menstruation

F. Abnormally light menstrual periods

G. Pain associated with menstruation

H. Refers to the onset of menstruation and the commencement of cyclic menstrual function; usually occurs between 9 and 17 years of age

I. A hormonal substance that stimulates the function of the testes and the ovaries

J. The periodic flow of blood and cellular debris that occurs during menstruation

K. Time period in young girls before the onset of menstruation

L. A hormone secreted by the anterior pituitary gland that stimulates ovulation and then induces luteinization of the ruptured follicle to form the corpus luteum

Exercise 4

Label the following illustrations.
1.   Pelvic cavity viewed from above.

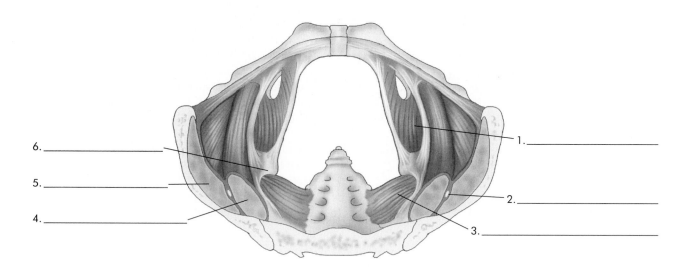

6. _____

5. _____

4. _____

1. _____

2. _____

3. _____

2.   The floor of the pelvis.

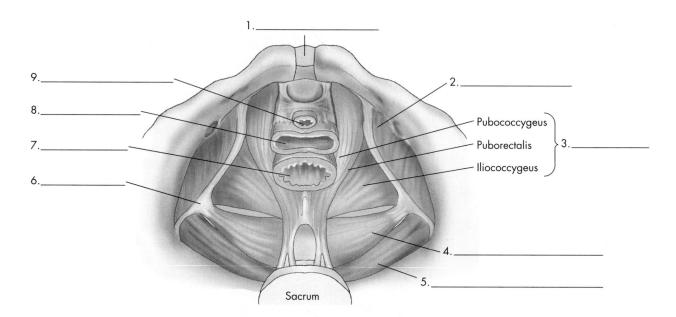

1. _____

9. _____

8. _____

7. _____

6. _____

2. _____

{ Pubococcygeus

Puborectalis } 3. _____

Iliococcygeus

4. _____

5. _____

Sacrum

3. Lateral view of the pelvis.

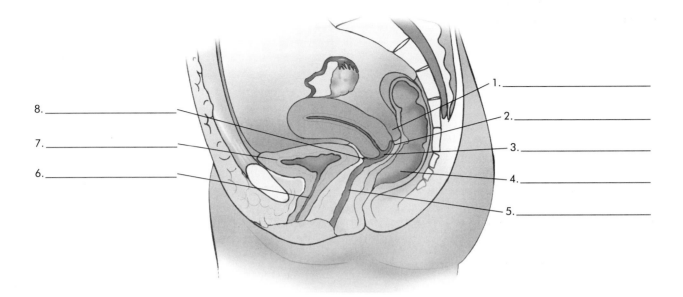

8. _____
7. _____
6. _____

1. _____
2. _____
3. _____
4. _____
5. _____

4. Coronal view of the vagina, cervix, and uterus.

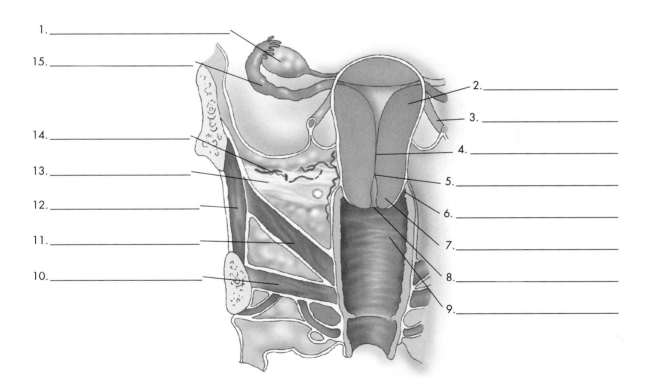

1. _____
15. _____
14. _____
13. _____
12. _____
11. _____
10. _____

2. _____
3. _____
4. _____
5. _____
6. _____
7. _____
8. _____
9. _____

5. Normal female pelvic anatomy.

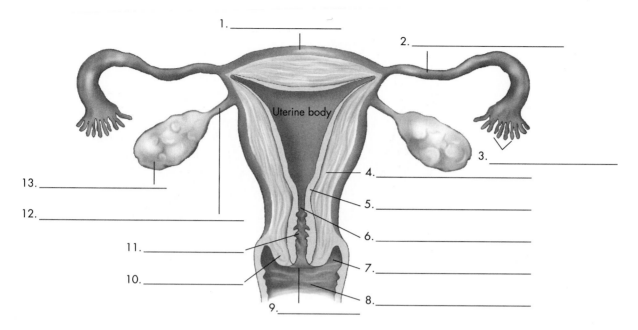

1._____

2._____

3._____

13._____

12._____

11._____

10._____

9._____

4._____

5._____

6._____

7._____

8._____

Uterine body

6. Identify the uterine positions.

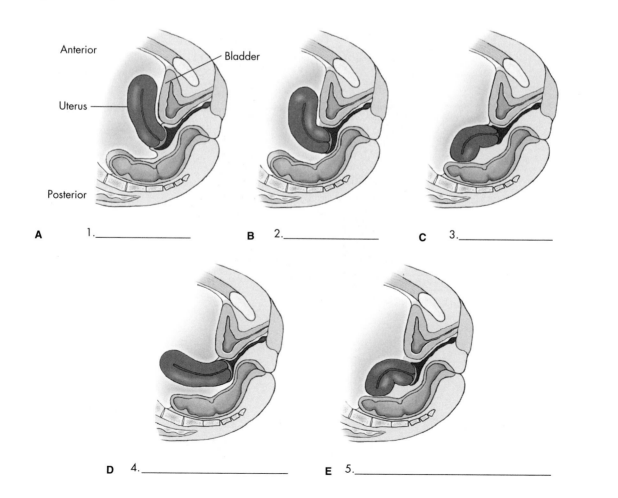

Anterior

Bladder

Uterus

Posterior

A 1._____ B 2._____ C 3._____

D 4._____ E 5._____

7. Diagram of the fallopian tube.

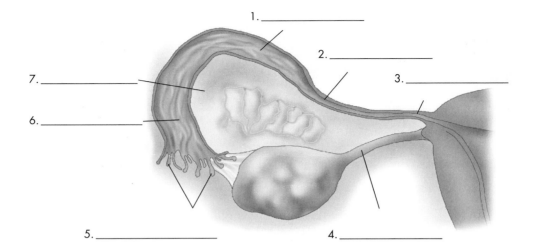

1. _____

2. _____

3. _____

7. _____

6. _____

5. _____

4. _____

8. Blood is supplied to the uterus and vagina by the uterine and vaginal arteries.

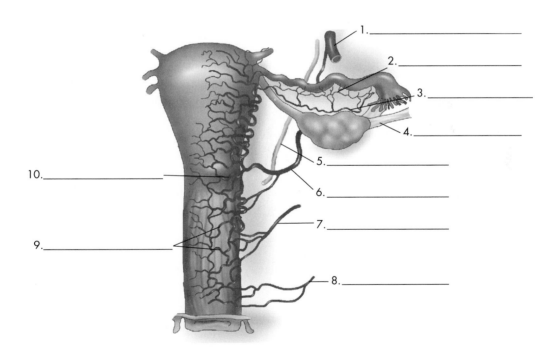

1. _____

2. _____

3. _____

4. _____

5. _____

6. _____

7. _____

8. _____

10. _____

9. _____

Exercise 5

Fill in the blank(s) with the word(s) that best completes the statements about the rectouterine space.

1. The anterior cul-de-sac, or _____ pouch, is located anterior to the fundus of the uterus between the urinary bladder and the uterus.

2. The posterior cul-de-sac, or _____ pouch, is located posterior to the uterus between the uterus and the rectum.

3. The rectouterine pouch is often referred to as the pouch of _____ and is normally the most inferior and most posterior region of the peritoneal cavity.

4. One additional area that is sonographically significant is the retropubic space, which is also called the space of

   _____.

5. The retropubic space normally can be identified between the _____ bladder wall and the pubic symphysis.

6. The retropubic space normally contains subcutaneous fat, but a hematoma or abscess in this location may displace

   the urinary bladder _____.

7. The greatest quantity of free fluid in the cul-de-sac normally occurs immediately following _____ when the mature follicle ruptures.

Exercise 6

Fill in the blank(s) with the word(s) that best completes the statements about the physiology of the menstrual cycle.

1. The average menstrual cycle is approximately _____ days in length, beginning with the first day of menstrual bleeding.

2. The menstrual cycle is regulated by the _____ and is dependent upon the cyclic release of estrogen and progesterone from the ovaries.

3. During the menarchal years, an _____ is released once a month by one of the two ovaries. This process is known as ovulation.

4. Ovulation normally occurs midcycle on about day _____ of a 28-day cycle.

5. The secretion of the _____ by the anterior pituitary gland causes the ovarian follicles to develop during the first half of the menstrual cycle.

6. This phase of the ovulatory cycle, known as the _____ phase, begins with the first day of menstrual bleeding and continues until ovulation on day 14.

7. The _____ hormone level will typically increase rapidly 24 to 36 hours before ovulation in a process known as the LH surge.

8. The cells in the lining of the ruptured ovarian follicle begin to multiply and create the corpus luteum, or yellow

   body, during the _____ phase.

9. The phase of endometrial regeneration is called the _____ phase and will last until luteinization of the graafian follicle around ovulation.

10. The endometrial phase after ovulation is referred to as the _____ phase and extends from approximately day 15 to the onset of menses (day 28). The secretory phase of the endometrial cycle corresponds to the luteal phase of the ovarian cycle.

SONOGRAPHIC EVALUATION

Exercise 7

Fill in the blank(s) with the word(s) that best completes the statements about the anatomy and sonographic technique of the female pelvis.

1. The approach that requires a full urinary bladder for use as an "acoustic window" and typically necessitates the use of a 3.5- to 5-MHz transducer for adequate penetration is the _____ approach.

2. An _____ examination is performed with an empty bladder and allows the use of a higher-frequency transducer, typically 7.5 to 10 MHz.

3. The transabdominal scan offers a _____ field of view for a general screening of the pelvic anatomy.

4. When using a transabdominal scanning technique, a _____ urinary bladder is essential.

5. The _____ are folds of skin at the opening of the vagina; the labia _____ being the thicker external folds and the _____ being the thin folds of skin between the labia majora.

6. The _____ bones make up the anterior and lateral margins of the bony pelvis, whereas the _____ and _____ form the posterior wall.

7. The margins of the posterolateral wall of the true pelvis are formed by the _____ and _____ muscles.

8. The anterolateral walls of the pelvic cavity are formed by the hip bones and the _____ muscles that rim the ischium and pubis.

9. The lower margin of the pelvic cavity, the pelvic floor, is formed by the _____ and _____ muscles and is known as the pelvic diaphragm.

10. The area below the pelvic floor is the _____.

11. The muscles of the false pelvis include the _____ major and _____ muscles.

12. The muscles that arise from the lower part of the pubic symphysis and surround the lower part of the rectum, forming a sling, are the _____ muscles.

13. A collapsed muscular tube that extends from the external genitalia to the cervix of the uterus is the _____.

14. The cervix lies _____ to the urinary bladder and urethra and _____ to the rectum and anus.

15. The largest organ in the normal female pelvis when the urinary bladder is empty is the _____.

16. At the lateral borders of the uterine fundus are the _____ where the fallopian tubes enter the uterine cavity.

17. The cervix is constricted at its upper end by the _____ os and at its lower end by the _____ os.

18. The point where the uterus bends either anteriorly (anteversion) or posteriorly (retroversion) with an empty

    bladder is the _____.

19. The uterine wall consists of three histologic layers: the_____, the _____, and

    the _____.

20. The endometrium consists primarily of two layers: the superficial functional layer (zona _____) and the

    deep basal layer (zona _____).

21. The uterus is supported in its midline position by paired _____ ligaments, _____

    ligaments, _____ ligaments, and _____ ligaments.

22. The average uterine position is considered to be _____ and _____.

23. The _____ are contained in the upper margin of the broad ligament and extend from the uterine cornua
    of the uterus laterally where they curve over the ovary.

24. The fallopian tubes are divided into four anatomic portions: the _____ (lateral

    segment), _____ (middle segment), _____ (medial segment), and _____ (segment
    that passes through the uterine cornua).

25. The _____ is often referred to as the fimbriated end of the fallopian tube because it contains fringelike
    extensions, called fimbriae, which move over the ovary directing the ovum into the fallopian tube after ovulation.

26. The ovaries are usually located _____ to the external iliac vessels and _____ to the internal
    iliac vessels and ureter.

27. The cortex of the ovary consists primarily of follicles in varying stages of development and is covered by a layer

    of dense connective tissue, the _____.

28. The central _____ is composed of connective tissue containing blood, nerves, lymphatic vessels, and
    some smooth muscle at the region of the hilum.

29. The ovaries produce the reproductive cell, the *ovum*, and two known hormones:_____, secreted by the

    follicles, and _____, secreted by the corpus luteum.

30. The common _____ arteries course anterior and medial to the psoas muscles, providing blood to the
    pelvic cavity and lower extremities.

31. The _____ iliac arteries extend into the pelvic cavity along the posterior wall and provide multiple
    branches that perfuse the pelvic structures to include the urinary bladder, uterus, vagina, and rectum.

32. The _____ arteries extend through the myometrium to the base of the endometrium, where straight and
    spiral arteries branch off of the radial arteries to supply the zona basalis of the endometrium.

33. The _____ arteries will lengthen during the regeneration of the endometrium after menses to traverse
    the endometrium and supply the zona functionalis.

36 The Sonographic and Doppler Evaluation of the Female Pelvis

KEY TERMS

Exercise 1
Match the following patient preparation and sonographic technique terms with their definitions.

1. __B__ adnexa
2. __H__ anteverted
3. __F__ coronal
4. __D__ endometrium
5. __L__ introitus
6. __A__ menarche
7. __N__ menopause
8. __J__ myometrium
9. __C__ parity
10. __M__ premenarche
11. __G__ retroverted
12. __K__ sagittal
13. __E__ translabial
14. __I__ transperineal

A. State after reaching puberty in which menses occurs normally every 21 to 28 days

B. Structure or tissue next to or near another related structure

C. Pregnancy

D. Inner lining of the uterine cavity, which appears echogenic to hypoechoic on ultrasound, depending on the menstrual cycle

E. Across or through the labia

F. Refers to a horizontal plane through the longitudinal axis of the body to image structures from anterior to posterior

G. Bending backwards

H. Tipped forward

I. Across or through the perineum

J. Middle layer of the uterine cavity that appears very homogeneous with sonography

K. Refers to a vertical plane through the longitudinal axis of the body that divides it into two portions

L. An opening or entrance into a canal or cavity, as the vagina

M. Time before the onset of menses

N. When menses have ceased permanently

Exercise 2
Match the following sonographic evaluation terms with their definitions.

1. __G__ arcuate vessels
2. __E__ internal os
3. __A__ menstruation
4. __H__ Pourcelot resistive index

A. Days 1 to 4 of the menstrual cycle; endometrial canal appears as a hypoechoic central line representing blood and tissue

B. Technique that uses a catheter inserted into the endometrial cavity, with the instillation of saline solution or contrast medium, to fill the endometrial cavity for the purpose of demonstrating abnormalities within the cavity or uterine tubes

5. _C_ proliferative phase

6. _F_ proliferative phase (late)

7. _I_ pulsatility index

8. _D_ secretory phase

9. _B_ sonohysterography

C. Days 5 to 9 of the menstrual cycle; endometrium appears as a single thin stripe with a hypoechoic halo encompassing it; creates the "three-line sign"

D. Days 15 to 28 of the menstrual cycle; the endometrium is at its greatest thickness and echogenicity with posterior enhancement

E. Inner surface of the cervical os

F. Days 10 to 14 of the menstrual cycle; ovulation occurs; the endometrium increases in thickness and echogenicity

G. Small vessels found along the periphery of the uterus

H. Doppler measurement that takes the highest systolic peak minus the highest diastolic peak divided by the highest systolic peak

I. Doppler measurement that uses peak systole minus peak diastole divided by the mean

SAGITTAL AND CORONAL LANDMARKS

Exercise 3

Label the following illustrations.

1. Endovaginal sagittal plane.

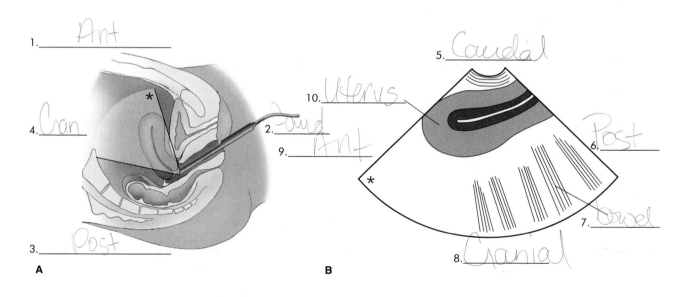

1. Ant
4. Cran
3. Post

A

5. Caudal
10. Uterus
2. Caud
9. Ant
6. Post
7. bowel
8. Cranial

B

SONOGRAPHIC EVALUATION

Exercise 4

Fill in the blank(s) with the word(s) that best completes the statements about the sonographic and Doppler evaluation of the female pelvis.

1. The full bladder _displaces_ the bowel and its contained gas from the field of view and _flattens_ the anteflexed uterus slightly so that it is more perpendicular to the transducer angle.

2. The bladder shape may be helpful because a well-distended bladder typically has a _△_ or elongated shape on midline scans.

3. The _____ vessels can be used as a landmark to identify the lateral adnexal borders.

4. If pathology is present, documentation of the _____ (Morison's pouch and subphrenic area) and

   bilateral _____ areas must be obtained.

5. In endovaginal scanning, it is necessary to advance the transducer slightly, angling _ant_____ to visualize
   the fundus, and withdraw

   slightly, away from the external os, while angling _post_____ to see the cervix and rectouterine recess.

6. These measurements of the uterus and ovaries should be documented: _length_____, _width_____,

   and _axial_____.

7. The thickness of the endometrium should be measured in the _sagittal_____ plane.

8. Pelvic muscles may be mistaken for ovaries, fluid collections, or masses. A _____ bilateral arrange-
   ment indicates that they are muscles.

9. Sonographically, sections of the _____ muscle are seen at the posterior lateral corners of the bladder at
   the level of the vagina and cervix.

10. The muscle that is best visualized sonographically in a transverse plane with caudal angulation at the most inferior

    aspect of the bladder is the _____ muscle.

11. The muscles that are located on either side of the midline posterior to the upper half of the uterine body and

    fundus are the _____ muscles.

12. To assess the uterine vessels, the sonographer interrogates just _____ to the cervix and lower uterine
    segment at the level of the internal os.

13. A _____, highly resistive flow pattern in the ovary is shown during the follicular phase of the
    menstrual cycle.

14. At ovulation the maximum velocity increases and the RI _____.

15. The middle uterine layer is the _____ of the uterus; this layer should have a homogeneous echotexture
    with smooth-walled borders.

16. The _____ of the uterus is hypoechoic and surrounds the relatively echogenic endometrial stripe,
    creating a subendometrial halo.

17. Calcifications may be seen in the _____ arteries in postmenopausal women and appear as peripheral
    linear echoes with shadowing.

18. The body of the uterus is separated from the cervix by the isthmus at the level of the _____ and is
    identified by the narrowing of the canal.

19. The axis of the uterine body relative to the cervix is referred to as the _____ , whereas _____
    refers to the axis of the cervix relative to the vagina.

20. The best way to measure the cervical-fundal dimension of the uterus in the longitudinal plane is the

_____ technique.

21. During menstruation (days 1 to 4) the _____ canal appears as a hypoechoic central line representing blood and tissue reaching 4 to 8 mm, including the basal layer in this measurement.

22. As menses progress (days 3 to 7), the hypoechoic echo that represented blood disappears, and the endometrial

stripe is a discrete thin _____ line that is usually only 2 to 3 mm.

23. In the early proliferative phase (days 5 to 9), the endometrial canal appears as a _____ stripe.

24. The layer that is seen as a hyperechoic halo encompassing the stripe is the _____ layer.

25. The layer of the endometrium that represents the thin surrounding hyperechoic outermost echo is the

_____ layer.

26. During the _____ (luteal) phase (days 15 to 28), the endometrium is at its greatest thickness and echogenicity with posterior enhancement.

27. Sonographically the postmenopausal endometrial complex is seen as a thin _____ line measuring less than 8 mm unless a hormone regimen is followed.

28. If the tubes are distended with or surrounded by a sufficient amount of _____, they can be easily outlined by the contrasting fluid.

29. Typically the ovary is located just _____ to the uterus and _____ to the internal iliac vessels, which can be used as a landmark to localize the ovary.

30. The best sonographic marker for the ovary is identification of a _____, which has the classic appearance of being thin walled and anechoic with through-transmission posteriorly.

31. The posterior cul-de-sac, or _____, is the most posterior and inferior reflection of the peritoneal cavity. It is located between the rectum and vagina and is also known as the pouch of Douglas.

32. _____ involves the instillation of sterile saline solution into the endometrial cavity.

Exercise 5

Provide a short answer for each question after evaluating the images.

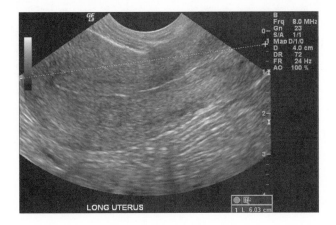

1. In this image, identify the location of the fundus of the uterus. Identify the location of the cervix.

_____

_____

_____

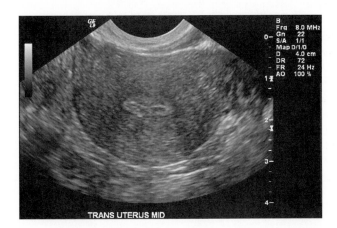

2. Identify the structure in the center of the uterine cavity.

_____

_____

_____

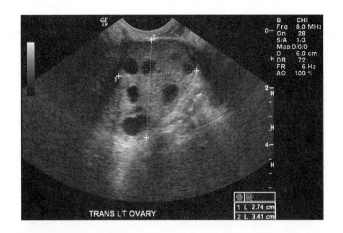

3. Describe the structures seen within the ovary.

_____

_____

_____

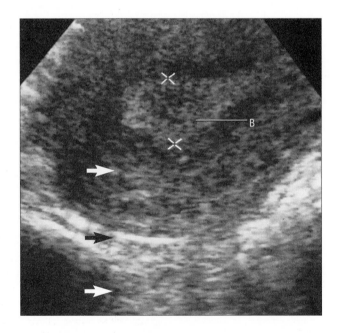

4. Identify the stage of the cycle that this image demonstrates.

_____

_____

_____

37 Pathology of the Uterus

KEY TERMS

Exercise 1
Match the following cervical and vaginal pathology terms with their definitions.

1. __C__ cervical polyp
2. __F__ cervical stenosis
3. __A__ dysmenorrhea
4. __D__ ectocervix
5. __I__ ectopic pregnancy
6. __B__ Gartner's duct cyst
7. __H__ leiomyoma
8. __E__ nabothian cyst
9. __G__ squamous cell carcinoma

A. Pain in association with menstruation
B. Small cyst within the vagina
C. Hyperplastic protrusion of the epithelium of the cervix; may be broad based or pedunculated
D. A portion of the canal of the uterine cervix that is lined with squamous epithelium
E. Benign tiny cyst within the cervix
F. Acquired condition with obstruction of the cervical canal
G. Most common type of cervical cancer
H. Most common benign gynecologic tumor in women during their reproductive years
I. Pregnancy occurring outside the uterine cavity

Exercise 2
Match the following uterine pathology terms with their definitions.

1. __B__ adenomyosis
2. __D__ curettage
3. __E__ intramural leiomyoma
4. __C__ metrorrhea
5. __A__ submucosal leiomyoma
6. __F__ subserosal leiomyoma

A. Type of leiomyoma found to deform the endometrial cavity and cause heavy or irregular menses
B. Benign invasive growth of the endometrium that may cause heavy, painful menstrual bleeding
C. Irregular, acyclic bleeding
D. Scraping with a curet to remove the contents of the uterus, as is done following inevitable or incomplete abortion; to obtain specimens for use in diagnosis; and to remove growths, such as polyps
E. Most common type of leiomyoma; deforms the myometrium intrauterine contraceptive device, a device inserted into the endometrial cavity to prevent pregnancy
F. Type of leiomyoma that may become pedunculated and appear as an extrauterine mass

Exercise 3

Match the following endometrial pathology terms with their definitions.

1. ___D___ endometrial carcinoma

2. ___I___ endometrial hyperplasia

3. ___B___ endometrial polyp

4. ___F___ endometritis

5. ___H___ hematometra

6. ___C___ hydrometra

7. ___E___ pyometra

8. ___G___ sonohysterography

9. ___A___ tamoxifen

A. An antiestrogen drug used in treating carcinoma of the breast

B. Pedunculated or sessile well-defined mass attached to the endometrial cavity

C. Obstruction of the uterus and/or the vagina characterized by an accumulation of fluid

D. Malignancy characterized by abnormal thickening of the endometrial cavity; usually associated with irregular bleeding in perimenopausal and in postmenopausal women

E. Obstruction of the uterus and/or the vagina characterized by an accumulation of pus

F. Infection within the endometrium of the uterus

G. Injection of sterile saline into the endometrial cavity under ultrasound guidance

H. Obstruction of the uterus and/or vagina characterized by an accumulation of blood

I. Condition that results from estrogen stimulation to the endometrium without the influence of progestin; frequent cause of bleeding

PATHOLOGY

Exercise 4

Fill in the blank(s) with the word(s) that best completes the statements about the pathology of the uterus.

1. The most common finding, seen frequently in middle-aged women, is the presence of __Nabothian cysts__.

2. Clinical findings of irregular bleeding may be the result of __cervical polyps__, a condition that arises from the hyperplastic protrusion of the epithelium of the endocervix or ectocervix.

3. An acquired condition with obstruction of the cervical canal at the internal or external os resulting from radiation therapy, previous cone biopsy, postmenopausal cervical atrophy, chronic infection, laser or cryosurgery, or cervical carcinoma is __cervical stenosis__.

4. A vaginal __cuff__ is seen in hysterectomy patients after surgery.

5. The most common cystic lesion of the vagina is the __Gartner's duct__ cyst; it usually is found incidentally during sonographic examination.

6. The most common congenital abnormality of the female genital tract is an __imperforate hymen__ resulting in obstruction.

7. This benign tumor is called a __leomyoma__ and is the most common gynecologic tumor, occurring in approximately 20% to 30% of women over the age of 30 with a higher incidence in African-American women.

8. Myomas are _estrogen_ dependent and may increase in size during pregnancy, although about one half of all myomas show little change during pregnancy.

9. Leiomyomas are characterized as _submucosal_ (displacing or distorting the endometrial cavity with subsequent irregular or heavy menstrual bleeding), _intramural_ (confined to the myometrium, the most common type), or _subserosal_ (projecting from the peritoneal surface of the uterus, sometimes becoming pedunculated and appearing as extrauterine masses).

10. _Submucosal_ myomas may erode into the endometrial cavity and cause irregular or heavy bleeding, which may lead to anemia.

11. The earliest sonographic finding of _myomas_ is demonstration of uterine enlargement with a heterogeneous texture and contour distortion along the interface between the uterus and the bladder.

12. The most common cause of uterine calcifications is _myomas_; a less common cause is _arcuate_ artery calcification in the periphery of the uterus.

13. The ectopic occurrence of nests of endometrial tissue within the myometrium is _adenomyosis_ and is more extensive in the posterior wall.

14. Uterine _arteriovenous_ malformations (AVMs) consist of a vascular plexus of arteries and veins without an intervening capillary network.

15. The most common cause of abnormal uterine bleeding in both premenopausal and postmenopausal women that develops from unopposed estrogen stimulation is _endometrial hyperplasia_.

16. Ideally a woman using _sequential_ hormones should be studied at the beginning or end of her hormone cycle when the endometrium is theoretically at its thinnest.

17. Sonographically, _polyps_ appear toward the end of the luteal phase and are represented by a hypoechoic region within the hyperechoic endometrium.

18. _Endometritis_ most often occurs in association with PID, in the postpartum state, or following instrumentation invasion.

19. Intrauterine _synechiae_ (endometrial adhesions, Asherman's syndrome) are found in women with posttraumatic or postsurgical histories. (This includes uterine curettage and may be a cause of infertility or recurrent pregnancy loss.)

20. The earliest change of a(n) _endometrial carcinoma_ tumor is a thickened endometrium and is also associated with endometrial hypertrophy and polyps.

21. Sonographically a thickened endometrium (studies have reported endometrial thickness greater than 4mm to 5mm is abnormal) must be considered _cancer_ until proved otherwise.

22. The _intrauterine contraceptive_ device appears as highly echogenic linear structures in the endometrial cavity within the uterine body that are separate from the normal, central endometrial echoes.

Provide a short answer for each question after evaluating the images.

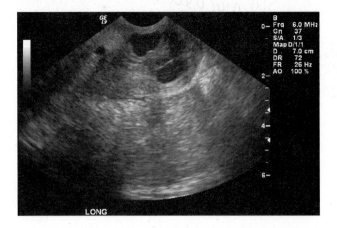

1. Identify the abnormality that is demonstrated in the endovaginal sagittal image of the cervical canal.

   Nabothian cysts

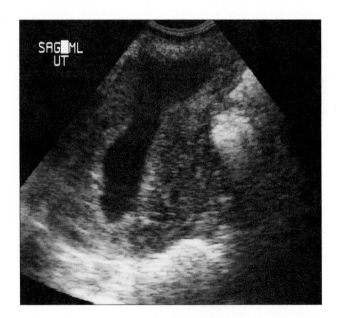

2. A 63-year-old asymptomatic woman on cyclic hormone replacement therapy demonstrates this abnormality of the lower uterine segment.

   Cervical stenosis

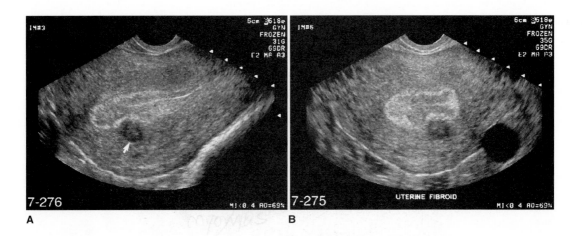

A   B

3. Sagittal and coronal images of the uterus demonstrate these findings on the sonogram.

A. submucosal liemyoma

B. cyst on exterior uterus

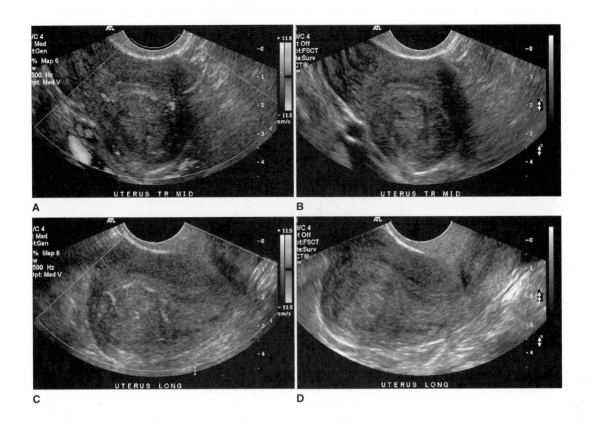

A

B

C

D

4. Sagittal endovaginal images of the uterus demonstrate this finding.

intramural lieomyoma (posterior to endometrium)

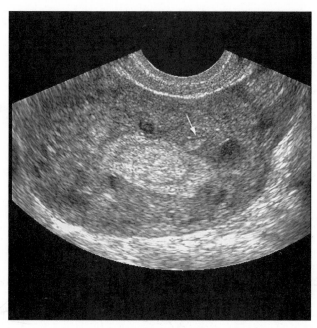

From Rumack C, Wilson S, Charboneau W: *Diagnostic ultrasound,* ed 3, St Louis, 2005, Mosby.

5. Sagittal endovaginal image of the uterine cavity demonstrates this finding.

adenomyosis (swiss cheese

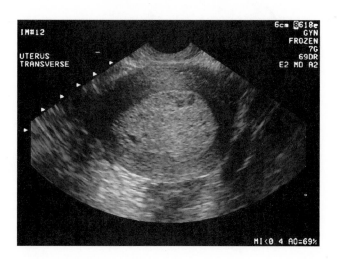

6. A patient presented with continuous vaginal bleeding for 3 weeks. Identify the sonographic findings.

endometrial hyperplasia

38 Pathology of the Ovaries

KEY TERMS

Exercise 1

Match the following sonographic evaluation terms with their definitions.

1. __C__ androgen

2. __F__ cystadenocarcinoma

3. __A__ cystadenoma

4. __E__ estrogen

5. __D__ pulsatility index

6. __G__ resistive index

7. __B__ simple ovarian cyst

A. A benign adenoma containing cysts

B. Smooth, well-defined cystic structure that is filled completely with fluid

C. Substance that stimulates the development of male characteristics, such as the hormones testosterone and androsterone

D. Peak-systolic velocity minus end-diastolic velocity divided by the mean velocity

E. The female hormone produced by the ovary

F. A malignant tumor that forms cysts

G. Peak-systolic velocity minus the end-diastolic velocity divided by the peak-systolic velocity

Exercise 2

Match the following ovarian pathology terms with their definitions.

1. __L__ corpus luteum cyst

2. __G__ dermoid tumor

3. __D__ endometriosis

4. __B__ follicular cyst

5. __I__ functional cyst

6. __E__ Meigs' syndrome (fibroma)

7. __N__ mucinous cystadenocarcinoma   multilocular

8. __K__ mucinous cystadenoma multilocular

9. __C__ ovarian carcinoma

10. __M__ ovarian torsion

11. __H__ paraovarian cyst

12. __O__ polycystic ovarian syndrome

A. Most common type of ovarian carcinoma; may be bilateral with multilocular cysts

B. Benign cyst within the ovary that may occur and disappear on a cyclic basis

C. Malignant tumor of the ovary that may spread beyond the ovary and metastasize to other organs via the peritoneal channels

D. Multilocular cysts that occur in patients with hyperstimulation

E. Benign tumor of the ovary associated with ascites and pleural effusion

F. Second most common benign tumor of the ovary; unilocular or multilocular

G. Benign tumor composed of hair, muscle, teeth, and fat

H. Cystic structure that lies adjacent to the ovary

I. Results from the normal function of the ovary

J. Gynecologic tumors that arise from the surface epithelium and cover the ovary and the underlying stroma

K. Benign tumor of the ovary that contains thin-walled multilocular cysts

13. ___A___ serous cystadenocarcinoma   *most common ov. carc*
blatter w/ multilocular cysts

14. ___F___ serous cystadenoma   *2nd most common benign*

15. ___J___ surface epithelial-stromal tumors

16. ___D___ theca-lutein cysts   *hyper stim*

L. A small endocrine structure that develops within a ruptured ovarian follicle and secretes progesterone and estrogen

M. Partial or complete rotation of the ovarian pedicle on its axis

N. Malignant tumor of the ovary with multilocular cysts

O. Endocrine disorder associated with chronic anovulation

P. Occurs when functioning endometrial tissue invades other sites outside the uterus

ANATOMY

Exercise 3

Label the following illustrations.

1. Normal anatomy of the female pelvis.

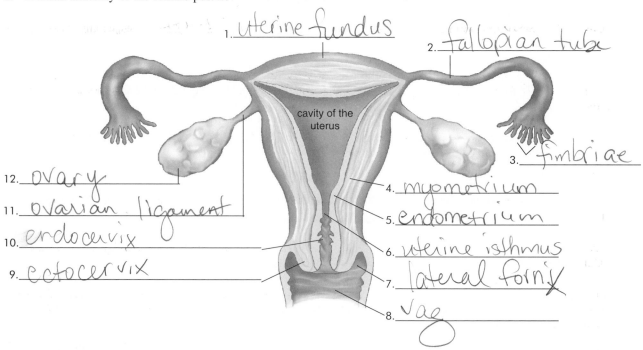

1. *uterine fundus*
2. *fallopian tube*
3. *fimbriae*
4. *myometrium*
5. *endometrium*
6. *uterine isthmus*
7. *lateral fornix*
8. *vag*
9. *ectocervix*
10. *endocervix*
11. *ovarian ligament*
12. *ovary*

cavity of the uterus

PATHOLOGY

Exercise 4

Fill in the blank(s) with the word(s) that best completes the statements about the pathology of the ovaries.

1. In the anteflexed midline uterus, the ovaries are usually identified *laterally* or *posterolaterally*

2. Following hysterectomy, the ovaries tend to be located more *medially* and directly superior to the vaginal cuff.

3. The normal ovary has a *homogenous* echotexture, which may exhibit a central, more echogenic medulla with small anechoic or cystic follicles seen in the cortex.

4. Small anechoic or cystic follicles may be seen _peripherally_ in the cortex.

5. During the early _proliferative_ phase, many follicles develop and increase in size until about day 8 or 9 of the menstrual cycle.

6. The _cumulus oophorus_ may occasionally be detected as an eccentrically located, cystlike, 1-mm internal mural protrusion.

7. If the fluid in the nondominant follicles is not reabsorbed, a(n) _follicular_ cyst develops.

8. The occurrence of fluid in the cul-de-sac is commonly seen after ovulation and peaks in the early _luteal_ phase.

9. Following ovulation in the luteal phase, a mature _corpus luteum_ develops and may be identified sonographically as a small hypoechoic or isoechoic structure peripherally within the ovary.

10. Any simple _cyst_ that hemorrhages may appear as a complex mass.

11. The more sonographically complex the tumor, the more likely it is to be _malignant_, especially if associated with ascites.

12. Patients with normal menstrual cycles are best scanned in the first _10_ days of the cycle; this prevents confusion with normal changes in intraovarian blood flow because high diastolic flow occurs in the luteal phase.

13. A mass showing a complete absence of or very little diastolic flow (very elevated RI and PI values) is usually _benign_.

14. Duplex Doppler reveals prominent _diastolic_ flow in corpus luteum cysts. This low-velocity waveform is present throughout the luteal phase of the cycle.

15. Echogenic, free intraperitoneal fluid in the cul-de-sac can help confirm the diagnosis of a _ruptured_ or leaking hemorrhagic cyst.

16. The largest of the functional cysts are _theca-lutein cysts_ and appear as very large, bilateral, multiloculated cystic masses. This mass is associated with high levels of human chorionic gonadotropin (hCG) and is seen most frequently in association with gestational trophoblastic disease.

17. A frequent iatrogenic complication of ovulation induction is _ovarian hyperstimulation syndrome_. The ovaries are enlarged, but measure less than 5 cm in diameter.

18. An endocrinologic disorder associated with chronic anovulation with an imbalance of LH and FSH resulting in abnormal estrogen and androgen production is _polycystic ovarian syndrome_.

19. Paraovarian cysts account for approximately 10% of adnexal masses; they arise from the _broad_ ligament and usually are of mesothelial or paramesonephric origin.

20. Endometriosis is a common condition in which functioning _endometrial_ tissue is present outside the uterus.

21. The localized form consists of a discrete mass called an endometrioma, or _chocolate cyst_.

22. Endometriosis may appear as bilateral or unilateral ovarian cysts with patterns ranging from anechoic to solid, depending on the amount of _blood_ and its organization.

23. Torsion of the ovary is caused by partial or __complete__ rotation of the ovarian pedicle on its axis.

24. Ovarian torsion produces an enlarged __edematous__ ovary, usually greater than 4 cm in diameter.

25. Unilocular or thinly septated cysts are more likely __benign__.

26. Multilocular thickly septated masses and masses with solid nodules are more likely __malignant__

27. Ovarian cancer can present as either a complex, cystic, or a solid mass, but is more likely preponderantly __cystic__.

28. The incidence of ovarian cancer is greatly __increased__ in women who have had breast and colon cancer.

29. Malignant tumor growth is dependent on __angiogenesis__ with the development of abnormal tumor vessels. This leads to decreased vascular resistance and higher diastolic flow velocity.

30. Ultrasonography demonstrates a completely cystic mass, a cystic mass with an echogenic mural nodule representing a "__dermoid plug__," a __fat-fluid__ level, high amplitude echoes with __shadowing__ (e.g., teeth or bone), or a complex mass with internal __internal echoes__.

31. The __ovaries__ are more involved with metastatic disease than any other pelvic organ.

Exercise 5

Provide a short answer for each question after evaluating the images.

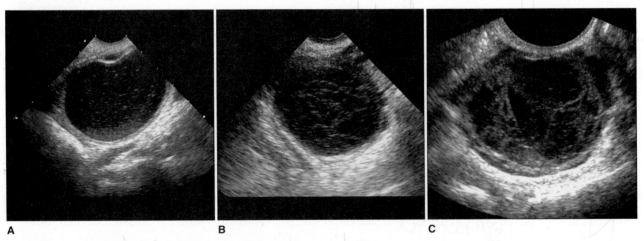

A   B   C

From Rumack C, Wilson S, Charboneau W: *Diagnostic ultrasound,* ed 3, St Louis, 2005, Mosby.

1. Identify the anomaly that is most likely represented in these images.

__hemorrhagic cyst__

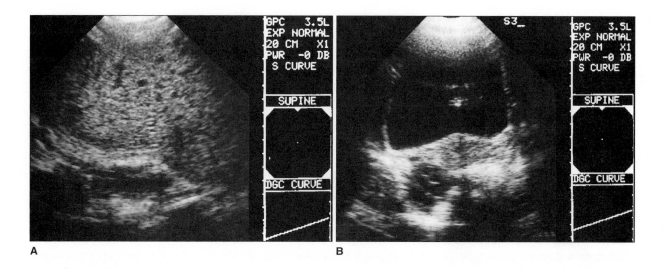

2. A patient in her 15th week of pregnancy presented with hyperemesis and uterine size larger than dates. The sonogram shows:

molar pregnancy w/ theca lutein cysts

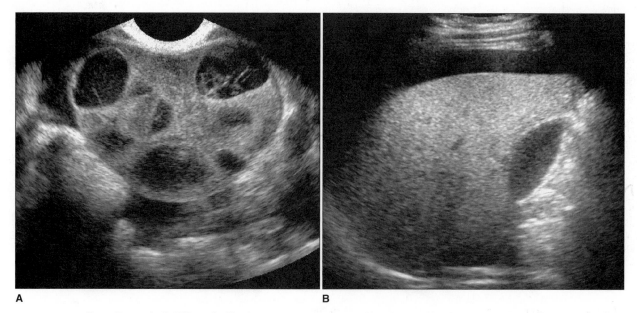

From Rumack C, Wilson S, Charboneau W: *Diagnostic ultrasound,* ed 3, St Louis, 2005, Mosby.

3. A patient on fertility drugs presented for an ultrasound. Describe your findings.

Ovarian hyperstimulation w/ an enlarged ovary w/ multiple complicated cysts

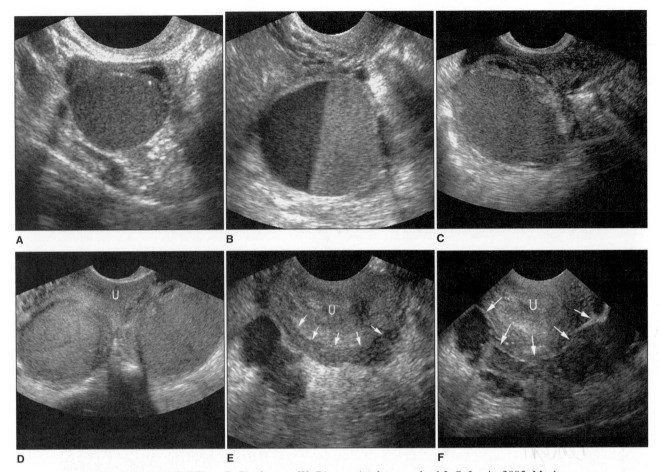

From Rumack C, Wilson S, Charboneau W: *Diagnostic ultrasound,* ed 3, St Louis, 2005, Mosby.

4. A patient with severe pelvic pain. Describe the ultrasound findings.

endometriosis

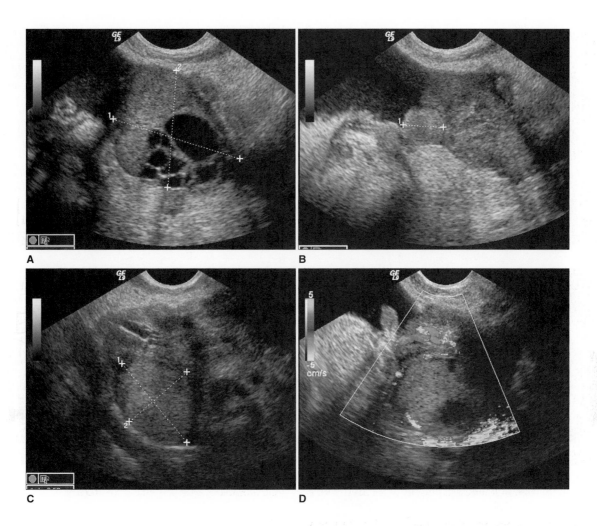

5. A 42-year-old female presented with mild abdominal distention and bloating for 1 month. Describe the findings.

ovarian carcinoma w/ bilateral metastases

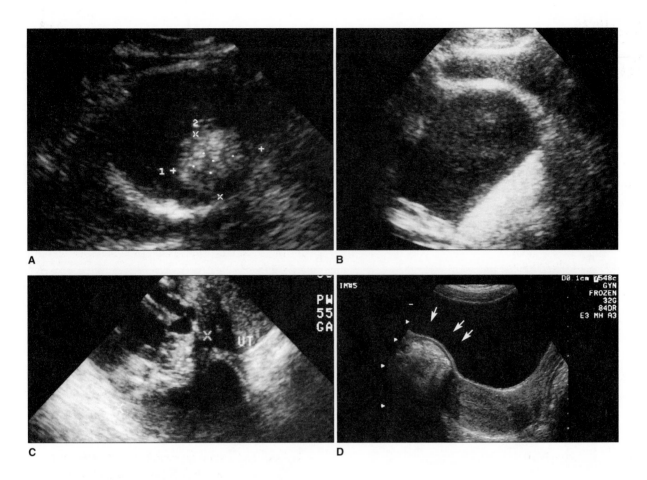

A   B

C   D

6. These images most likely represent this abnormality.

dermoid tumor

_____

_____

39 Pathology of the Adnexa

KEY TERMS

Exercise 1

Match the following adnexa pathology terms with their definitions.

1. _____ adenomyosis

2. _____ chlamydia

3. _____ endometrioma

4. _____ endometriosis

5. _____ endometritis

6. _____ hydrosalpinx

7. _____ myometritis

8. _____ oophoritis

9. _____ parametritis

10. _____ pelvic inflammatory disease

11. _____ periovarian inflammation

12. _____ pyosalpinx

13. _____ salpingitis

14. _____ tubo-ovarian abscess

15. _____ tubo-ovarian complex

A. Fluid within the fallopian tube

B. Infection that involves the fallopian tube and the ovary

C. Localized tumor of endometriosis most frequently found in the ovary, cul-de-sac, rectovaginal septum, and peritoneal surface of the posterior wall of the uterus

D. All-inclusive term that refers to all pelvic infections

E. Infection within the endometrium of the uterus

F. Infection within the fallopian tubes

G. A condition that occurs when functioning endometrial tissue invades sites outside the uterus

H. Infection within the ovary

I. Fusion of the inflamed dilated tube and ovary

J. Infection within the uterine serosa and broad ligaments

K. Enlarged ovaries with multiple cysts and indistinct margins

L. An organism that causes a great variety of diseases, including genital infections in men and women

M. Infection within the myometrium of the uterus

N. Benign invasive growth of the endometrium into the muscular layer of the uterus

O. Retained pus within the inflamed fallopian tube

PATHOLOGY

Exercise 2

Fill in the blank(s) with the word(s) that best completes the statements about the pathology of the adnexa.

1. Infrequently a pelvic infection may ascend the right flank, causing a perihepatic inflammation that may mimic

   liver, gallbladder, or right renal pain. This perihepatic inflammation is called the _____ syndrome.

2. Sexually transmitted PID is spread via the _____ of the pelvic organs through the cervix into the pelvic cavity.

3. Infection in the uterine endometrium is known as _____; inflammation in the fallopian tubes is called

   acute _____.

4. As the dilated tube becomes obstructed, it becomes filled with pus (_____).

5. Clinically, patients with pelvic inflammatory disease may present with intense pelvic _____ and

   tenderness described as dull, aching, with constant _____ discharge.

6. An obstructed tube filled with serous secretions is a _____; this can occur as a result of PID, endometriosis, or postoperative adhesions.

7. Severe and chronic pyosalpinx often contains _____, _____ mucoid pus, which does not transmit sound as well as serous fluid or blood.

8. The complex collection is called a _____ complex with the adhesive, edematous, and inflamed serosa that may further adhere to the ovary and/or other peritoneal surfaces, which distorts anatomy. As the infection worsens, periovarian adhesions may form.

9. The inflammation of the peritoneum, the serous membrane lining the abdominal cavity and covering the viscera, is

   _____ .

10. Endometriosis has two forms—internal and external. Internal endometriosis (_____) occurs within the

    uterus. The external form (_____) is outside the uterus and may be found in the pouch of Douglas, surface of the ovary and fallopian tube and uterus, broad ligaments, and rectovaginal septum.

11. Endometriomas may appear as bilateral or unilateral ovarian cysts with patterns ranging from

    _____ to _____, depending on the amount of blood and its organization.

12. Pain and the development of a pelvic mass after pelvic surgery can indicate complications, such as postoperative

    _____, _____, or _____ formation.

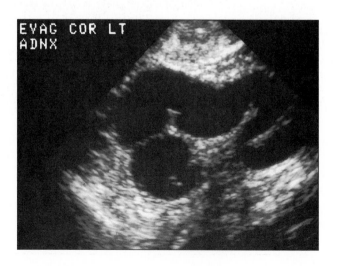

Exercise 3

Provide a short answer for each question after evaluating the images.

1. The patient presented with pelvic pain for 1 month. Describe your findings.

_____

_____

_____

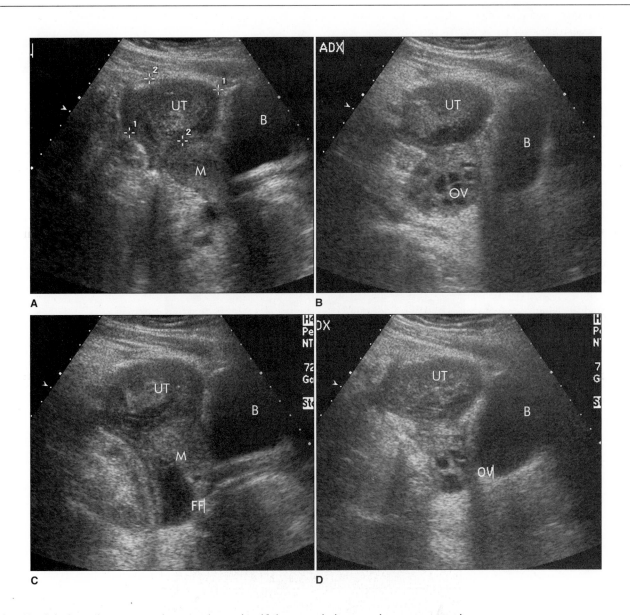

2. Explain how the sonographer can determine if the mass is intrauterine or extrauterine.

_____

_____

_____

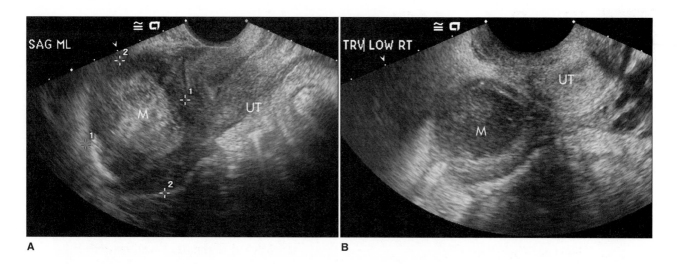

A   B

3. State whether this mass in the pelvis appears to be intrauterine or extrauterine.

_____

_____

_____

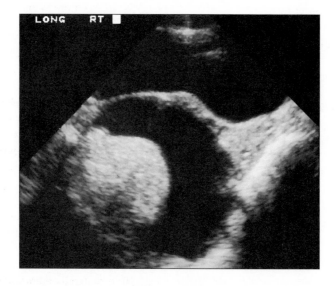

4. A 23-year-old female presented with fever, vaginal discharge, and acute pelvic pain for the past several days. Describe the ultrasound findings.

_____

_____

_____

40 The Role of Ultrasound in Evaluating Female Infertility

KEY TERMS

Exercise 1
Match the following female infertility terms with their definitions.

1. _____ assisted reproductive technology

2. _____ basal body temperature

3. _____ embryo transfer

4. _____ gamete intrafallopian transfer (GIFT)

5. _____ gonadotropins

6. _____ human chorionic gonadotropin

7. _____ intrauterine insemination

8. _____ in vitro fertilization (IVF)

9. _____ ovarian hyperstimulation syndrome (OHS)

10. _____ ovulation induction therapy

11. _____ postcoital test (PCT)

12. _____ zygote intrafallopian transfer (ZIFT)

A. A method of fertilizing the human ova outside the body by collecting the mature ova and placing them in a dish with a sample of spermatozoa

B. A technique that follows IVF in which the fertilized ova are injected into the uterus through the cervix

C. A syndrome that presents sonographically as enlarged ovaries with multiple cysts, abdominal ascites, and pleural effusions. Often seen in patients who have undergone ovulation induction postadministration of follicle-stimulating hormone or a GnRH analogue followed by hCG.

D. Technologies employed to assist the infertility patient to become pregnant. These methods include in vitro fertilization, gamete intrafallopian transfer, zygote intrafallopian transfer, and artificial insemination.

E. A clinical test done within 24 hours after intercourse to assess sperm motility in cervical mucus

F. A human fertilization technique in which the zygotes are injected through a laparoscope into the fimbriated ends of the fallopian tubes. Recently, this has been performed under ultrasound guidance.

G. The morning body temperature taken orally before the patient does any activity

H. A hormonal substance that stimulates the function of the testes and ovaries

I. The introduction of semen into the vagina or uterus by mechanical or instrumental means rather than by sexual intercourse

J. Controlled ovarian stimulation with clomiphene citrate or parenterally administered gonadotropins

K. A glycoprotein secreted from placental trophoblastic cells; this chemical component is found in maternal urine when pregnant.

L. A human fertilization technique in which male and female gametes are injected through a laparoscope into the fimbriated ends of the fallopian tubes. Recently, this has been performed under ultrasound guidance.

Exercise 2

Fill in the blank(s) with the word(s) that best completes the statements about female infertility.

1. Infertility is the inability to conceive within _____ months with regular coitus.

2. The cervix's role in fertility is to provide a _____ environment to harbor sperm.

3. The cervical mucus is evaluated by the _____ test.

4. The assessment of the endometrium should include: _____, and _____ characteristics, and

   _____ lesions.

5. The congenital anomalies most easily assessed with ultrasound are evaluation for the _____ uterus

   and uterus _____.

6. _____ uterus is associated with a low incidence of fertility complications.

7. The fallopian tubes can be examined by ultrasound to evaluate for a hydrosalpinx and assess _____ by
   injecting saline into the tube and looking for spillage of fluid into the cul-de-sac or by using contrast to evaluate
   for spillage.

8. A follicle is selected to develop into a _____ follicle in response to follicle-stimulating hormone
   (FSH) and an increase in estradiol.

9. The dominant follicle will grow at a rate of approximately 2 to 3 mm per day until it reaches an average diameter

   of _____ mm.

10. The best predictor of ovulation is the _____ .

11. If serum estradiol is _____ and a large ovarian cyst is present, then oral contraceptives may be indi-
    cated to suppress follicular activity before starting ovarian stimulation therapy.

12. A normal endometrial response associated with ovarian stimulation is an increasing thickness from 2 to 3 mm

    to _____ mm.

13. Complications associated with assisted reproductive technologies include ovarian _____ syndrome,

    multiple _____, and _____ pregnancy.

14. _____ is a syndrome that presents sonographically as enlarged ovaries with multiple cysts, abdominal
    ascites, and pleural effusions.

15. An ectopic pregnancy coexisting with a pregnancy is a(n) _____ pregnancy.

Exercise 3

Provide a short answer for each question after evaluating the images.

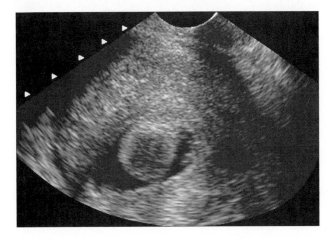

1. Identify what abnormality is demonstrated in this infusion sonography image.

_____

_____

_____

2. Identify what abnormality is demonstrated in this infusion sonography image, which may interfere with implantation.

_____

_____

_____

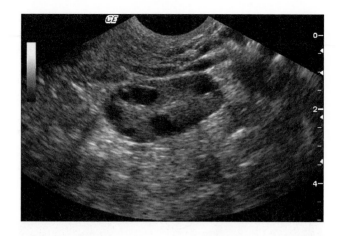

3. Identify the phase of the ovary shown in this image.

_____

_____

_____

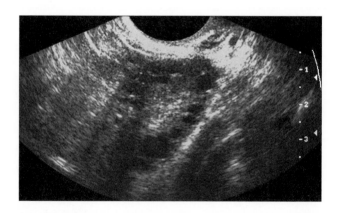

4. This condition is associated with infertility. Name the syndrome associated with this condition.

_____

_____

_____

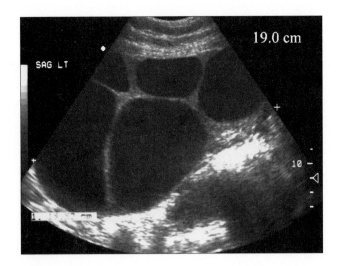

5.   This image represents a complication of this syndrome.

_____

_____

_____

41 The Role of Ultrasound in Obstetrics

KEY TERMS

Exercise 1

Match the following obstetric and gynecologic terms with their definitions.

1. __F__ abruptio placentae
2. __J__ amniocentesis
3. __D__ anencephaly
4. __H__ cerclage
5. __C__ cordocentesis
6. __A__ embryonic age (or conception age)
7. __B__ gestational age
8. __L__ hydatidiform mole
9. __G__ incompetent cervix
10. __I__ intrauterine growth restriction (IUGR)
11. __K__ macrosomia
12. __E__ maternal serum alpha fetoprotein (MSAFP)
13. __P__ oligohydramnios
14. __N__ placenta
15. __M__ placenta previa
16. __O__ polyhydramnios

A. Age of embryo stated as time from day of conception
B. Length of pregnancy defined in the United States as number of weeks from first day of last normal menstrual period (LNMP)
C. Insertion under sonographic guidance of a thin needle into the vessels of the umbilical cord usually at the site of placental insertion to obtain a fetal blood sample, deliver fetal drug therapy, or assess fetal well-being
D. A neural tube defect where absence of the brain, including the cerebrum, the cerebellum, and basal ganglia, may be present
E. One of several biochemical tests used to assess fetal risk for aneuploidy or fetal defect; a component of the "triple screen," the normal value of MSAFP varies with gestational age, and assessment of gestational age is essential for accurate interpretation of results
F. Bleeding from a normally situated placenta as a result of its complete or partial detachment after the twentieth week of gestation
G. A condition in which the cervix dilates silently during the second trimester; without intervention, the membranes bulge through the cervix, rupture, and the fetus drops out resulting in a premature preterm delivery
H. The ligatures around the cervix uteri to treat cervical incompetence during pregnancy
I. Reduced growth rate (symmetrical IUGR) or abnormal growth pattern (asymmetrical IUGR) of the fetus, resulting in a small for gestational age (SGA) fetus
J. Aspiration of a sample of amniotic fluid through the mother's abdomen for diagnostic analysis of fetal genetics, maturity, and/or disease
K. Exceptionally large infant with excessive fat deposition in the subcutaneous tissue; most frequently seen in fetuses of diabetic mothers
L. Abnormal conception in which there is partial or complete conversion of the chorionic villi into grape-like vesicles
M. Placental implantation encroaches upon the lower uterine segment; if the placenta presents first in late pregnancy, bleeding is inevitable
N. Organ of communication where nutrition and products of metabolism are interchanged between the fetal and maternal blood systems; forms from the chorion frondosum with a maternal decidual contribution
O. Excessive amount of amniotic fluid
P. Reduced amount of amniotic fluid

Exercise 2

Match the following ultrasound examination and safety terms with their definitions.

1. __H__ amnion
2. __E__ cervix
3. __A__ chorion
4. __D__ corpus luteum
5. __C__ ductus venosum
6. __G__ embryo
7. __L__ gestational sac
8. __I__ lower uterine segment
9. __K__ trimester
10. __F__ umbilical cord
11. __J__ yolk sac
12. __B__ zygote

A. Cellular, outermost extraembryonic membrane, composed of trophoblast lined with mesoderm; the outer chorion (villous chorion) develops villi, which are vascularized by allantoic vessels and give rise to the placenta; the inner chorion (the smooth chorion) is fused with the amnion except at the placental cord insertion

B. Products of conception from fertilization through implantation; the zygotic stage of pregnancy lasts for approximately 12 days after conception

C. Vascular structure within the fetal liver that connects the umbilical vein to the inferior vena cava and allows oxygenated blood to bypass the liver and return directly to the heart

D. A functional structure within the normal ovary, which is formed from cells lining the graafian follicle after ovulation; it produces estrogen and progesterone and may become enlarged and appear cystic during early pregnancy

E. Inferior segment of the uterus, which is normally more than 3.5 cm long during pregnancy, decreasing in length during labor

F. Connecting lifeline between the fetus and placenta; it contains two umbilical arteries, which carry deoxygenated fetal blood, and one umbilical vein, which carries oxygenated fetal blood encased in Wharton's jelly

G. Developing individual from implantation to the end of the ninth week of gestation

H. Smooth membrane enclosing the fetus and amniotic fluid; it is loosely fused with the outer chorionic membrane except at the placental insertion of the umbilical cord where it is contiguous with the membranes surrounding the umbilical cord

I. Thin expanded lower portion of the uterus that forms in the last trimester of pregnancy

J. A circular structure within the gestational sac seen sonographically between 4 and 10 weeks gestational age; the yolk sac supplies nutrition, facilitates waste removal, and is the origin of early hematopoietic stem cells in the embryo; it lies between the chorion and the amnion

K. A 40-week pregnancy is divided into three 13-week periods from the first day of the last normal menstrual period (weeks 1 through 12, first trimester; weeks 13 through 26, second trimester; week 27 to term, third trimester)

L. Structure lined by the chorion that normally implants within the uterine decidua and contains the developing embryo

Z E F

SONOGRAPHIC EVALUATION

Exercise 3

List the recommended indications for obstetric sonographic examinations.

1. gest. age
2. fetal growth
3. vag. bleeding
4. determination of fetal presentation
5. suspected mult. gest.
6. w/ amnio
7. discrepency b/t ut. size + clin. dates
8. pelvic mass
9. HYDATIDIFORM mole
10. w/ cerclage placemt.
11. susp. ectopic
12. w/ spec. proc like cordocentesis, IVF, etc.
13. susp. fetal death
14. susp. ut. abnormality
15. IUCD localization
16. ov. follicle developmt surveillance
17. Biophysical for fetal well being after 28 wks
18. observation of intra partum events
19.
20.
21.
22.
23.

24. _____

25. _____

26. _____

MATERNAL RISK FACTORS

Exercise 4

Fill in the blank(s) with the word(s) that best completes the statements or provide a short answer about the maternal risk factors and patient information.

1. List the maternal risk factors that increase the chances of producing a fetus with congenital anomalies.

   inc'd mat age

   abn'l triple screen

   mat disease

   ut. too small or lg for date

2. Other risk factors include a previous child born with a _chromosomal_ disorder or exposure to a known _teratogenic_ drug or infectious agent known to cause birth defects.

3. There are several important questions the sonographer should ask the patient before beginning the obstetric sonography evaluation. List these questions.

   a. _clinical dates_

   b. _latex all_

   c. _LMP_

   d. _any meds_

   e. _bleeding, pelvic pain, ↓ fetal mvnt,_

   f. _prev. preg. probs_

QUALITY STANDARDS

Exercise 5

Fill in the blank(s) with the word(s) that best completes the statements or provide a short answer about the quality standards for the obstetric examination.

1. Quality standards include not only the components of the examination protocol but also include the following:

   a. _qualit of sonog._

   b. _documentation_

   c. _eqpmt. specs_

   d. _fetal safety_

e. qual cont

f. Safety, inf cont,

g. Pt educ concerns

2. The purpose of a national Certification or registry is to assure the public that the person performing sonography has necessary knowledge, skills, and experience to provide this service.

3. Documentation standards require that there is a Permanent record maintained of the measurements and anatomic findings.

4. Images need to be labeled with the Pt's name, date, and image orientation if appropriate.

5. Describe the ultrasound protocol for the first-trimester pregnancy.

a. ut + adnx for gs, ys + embryo

b. +/- of card. act,

c. fet #

d. eval of ut + adnx'l structures + cds

6. Describe the ultrasound protocol for the second- and third-trimester pregnancies.

a. fetal life, #, presentation + activity

b. AFI quantity

c. placental loc, appearance + r/ship to cerv. os

d. things used to est gest age (IC, BPD, HC, AC, FL)

e. ut, adnx + cervical eval for masses

f. fetal anatomy after 18 wks

7. List the normal anatomic structures that should be recorded in a standard obstetric examination in each region during the second or third trimester.
a. Head and neck

cereb, choroid plexus, cist mag, lat cerebral vents, midline falx, cavum septum pellucid,

b. Chest

4ch heart + if poss both ~~fetal~~ outflow tracts

c. Abdomen

stomach (presence, size + situs), kidneys, bladders, CI, 3 vessel cord

d. Spine

cerv, thorac, lumbar, sacral

e. Extremities

+/−

f. Gender

only 4 assessment of mult preg

42 Clinical Ethics for Obstetric Sonography

KEY TERMS

Exercise 1
Match the following clinical ethics terms with their definitions.

1. _____ autonomy

2. _____ beneficence

3. _____ confidentiality

4. _____ ethics

5. _____ informed consent

6. _____ integrity

7. _____ justice

8. _____ morality

9. _____ nonmaleficence

10. _____ respect for persons

11. _____ veracity

A. The study of what is good and bad and of moral duty and obligation; systematic reflection on and analysis of morality

B. Bringing about good by maximizing benefits and minimizing possible harm

C. Truthfulness, honesty

D. Refraining from harming oneself or others

E. Incorporates both respect for the autonomy of individuals and the requirement to protect those with diminished autonomy

F. Self-governing or self-directing freedom and especially moral independence; the right of persons to choose and to have their choices respected

G. Adherence to moral and ethical principles

H. The protection of cherished values that relate to how persons interact and live in peace

I. Holding information in confidence; respect for privacy

J. The ethical principle that requires fair distribution of benefits and burdens; an injustice occurs when a benefit to which a person is entitled is withheld or when a burden is unfairly imposed

K. Providing complete information and ensuring comprehension and voluntary consent by a patient or subject to a required or experimental medical procedure

PRINCIPLES OF MEDICAL ETHICS

Exercise 2
Fill in the blank(s) with the word(s) that best completes the statements about medical ethics.

1. Ethics is defined as systematic reflection on and analysis of _____.

2. Morality concerns _____ conduct (what we ought or ought not do) and _____ character (the kinds of persons we should become and the virtues we should cultivate in doing so).

3. Morality reflects duties and _____.

4. To demonstrate values, a person has to have rights of expression, so _____ and _____ are also integral parts of morality.

5. Discussion, reflection, and discourse on morality are known as _____.

6. Hippocrates cautioned his students to *primum non nocere,* which means, "_____."

7. The principle of _____ directs the sonographer to not cause harm.

8. The application of the principle of nonmaleficence requires the sonographer to obtain appropriate

   _____ and clinical skills to ensure competence in performing each examination required.

9. The use of obstetric ultrasound must be justified by the goal of seeking the greater balance of clinical "goods" over "harms," not simply preventing harm to the patient at all cost. This ethical principle is called

   _____ and is a more comprehensive basis for ethics in sonography than is nonmaleficence.

10. Beneficence encourages sonographers to go beyond the _____ standard protocol and to seek additional images and information if achievable and in the best interests of patients.

11. Beneficence requires sonographers to focus on small comforts for the patient, respecting their _____ and the inclusion of family.

12. Beneficence, like nonmaleficence, requires _____, _____, and excellent

   _____ skills to ensure that the patient and the fetus receive the greatest benefit of the examination.

13. A person's capacity to formulate, express, and carry out value-based preferences is referred to as _____.

14. Informed _____ is an autonomy-based right. Each health professional has autonomy-based obligations regarding this process.

15. If a practitioner asks a sonographer to perform an examination that he or she is not competent to do, it is essential for

   the sonographer to be truthful about his or her limitations to protect the patient. This is an example of

   _____.

16. _____ means simply that sonographers must strive to treat all patients equally.

17. Justice and autonomy are the ethical principles that determine the _____ of routine obstetric sonography examinations.

18. The obligation of confidentiality derives from the principles of _____ (the patients will be more forthcoming) and respect for autonomy (the patient's privacy rights are protected).

43 The Normal First Trimester

KEY TERMS

Exercise 1

Match the following early development and gestational terms with their definitions.

1. __E__ diamniotic
2. __A__ dichorionic
3. __D__ embryologic age /conceptual age
4. __I__ menstrual age /gestation age
5. __G__ monoamniotic
6. __B__ monochorionic
7. __F__ primary yolk sac
8. __C__ secondary yolk sac
9. __H__ zygote
10. __J__ corpus luteum cyst

A. Multiple pregnancy with two chorionic sacs
B. Multiple pregnancy with one chorionic sac
C. Formed at 23 days when the primary yolk sac is pinched off by the extra embryonic coelom
D. Age calculated from when conception occurs
E. Multiple pregnancy with two amniotic sacs
F. First site of formation of red blood cells that will nourish the embryo
G. Multiple pregnancy with one amniotic sac
H. Fertilized ovum resulting from union of male and female gametes
I. Length of time calculated from the first day of the last normal menstrual period to the point at which the pregnancy is being assessed
J. The small yellow endocrine structure that develops within a ruptured ovarian follicle and secretes progesterone and estrogen

Exercise 2

Match the following laboratory values and sonographic technique terms with their definitions.

1. __K__ amniotic cavity
2. __C__ chorionic cavity
3. __G__ crown-rump length
4. __M__ decidua basalis
5. __B__ decidua capsularis
6. __J__ double decidual sac sign
7. __E__ embryonic period
8. __A__ endovaginal transducer
9. __H__ hematopoiesis
10. __D__ human chorionic gonadotropin

A. High-frequency transducer that is inserted into the vaginal canal to obtain better definition of first-trimester pregnancy
B. The villi surrounding the chorionic sac
C. Surrounds the amniotic cavity
D. Hormone secreted by the trophoblastic cells of the blastocyst; laboratory test indicates pregnancy when values are elevated
E. Time between 6 and 12 weeks of gestation
F. The umbilical duct connecting the yolk sac with the embryo
G. Most accurate measurement of the embryo in the first trimester
H. Production and development of blood cells
I. Mean sac diameter
J. Interface between the decidua capsularis and the echogenic, highly vascular endometrium

11. ___L___ IUP

12. ___I___ MSD

13. ___E___ yolk stalk

K. Cavity in which the fetus exists; forms early in gestation; fills with amniotic fluid to protect the fetus

L. Intrauterine pregnancy

M. The villi on the maternal side of the placenta or embryo; unites with the chorion to form the placenta

---

ANATOMY

Exercise 3

Label the following illustrations.

1. Diagram illustrates normal conception. (43-1)

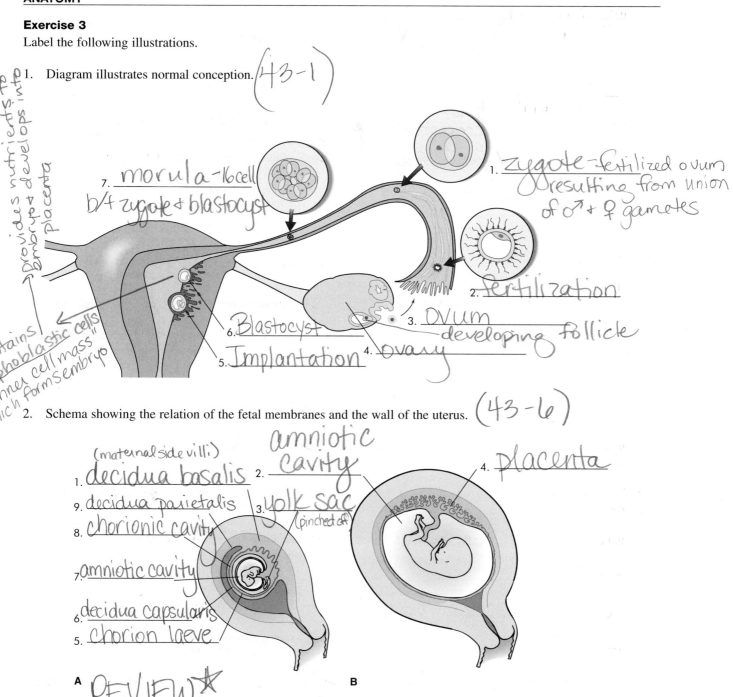

Provides nutrients to embryo & develops into placenta →

Contains "trophoblastic cells" + "inner cell mass" which forms embryo

7. morula - 16 cell b/4 zygote & blastocyst

1. zygote - fertilized ovum resulting from union of ♂ + ♀ gametes

2. fertilization

3. ovum developing follicle

4. ovary

5. Implantation

6. Blastocyst

2. Schema showing the relation of the fetal membranes and the wall of the uterus. (43-6)

(maternal side villi)
1. decidua basalis

2. amniotic cavity

3. yolk sac (pinched off)

4. placenta

9. decidua parietalis

8. chorionic cavity

7. amniotic cavity

6. decidua capsularis

5. chorion laeve

A   REVIEW ⭐

B

3. Schematics demonstrating the development of amnion, yolk sac, and embryo. (43-12)

1. amnion
2. connecting stalk
3. embryonic disc
4. yolk sac
5. chorion

6. chorionic cavity
7. amniotic sac
8. umbilical cord
9. yolk sac

10. amnion
11. connecting stalk
12. yolk sac
13. chorionic cavity

14. smooth chorion
15. amnion
16. amniotic sac
17. umbilical cord
18. yolk sac remnant

FIRST TRIMESTER

Exercise 4

Fill in the blank(s) with the word(s) that best completes the statements about the early development in the first trimester.

1. Clinicians and sonographers use gestational age aka menstrual age to date the pregnancy, with the first day of the last menstrual period as the beginning of the gestation.

2. In the first 9 menstrual weeks, the conceptus is called an embryo.

3. For the time after the first 9 weeks, the embryo is called a fetus.

4. The gestational age (age known as postmenstrual age) is calculated by adding 2 or 14 days weeks to conceptional age.

5. The fertilized ovum, which should now be referred to as a zygote, undergoes rapid cellular division to form the 16-cell morula.

6. The blastocyst typically enters the uterus 4 to 5 days after fertilization, with implantation occurring 7 to 9 days after ovulation.

7. Although the organ function remains as minimal, the cardiovascular system is the first organ to develop rapidly, with the first heart beats between 5.5 and 6 weeks.

8. Gestational sac size and hCG levels increase proportionately until 8 menstrual weeks.

9. After 8 weeks, hCG levels plateau and subsequently decline while the gestational sac continues to grow.

10. A normal gestational sac can be consistently demonstrated when the hCG level ranges between 1000 + 2000 mIU/mL.

11. The sonographer must be aware that when the hCG level is elevated and the gestational sac is not seen within the uterus, a(n) _ectopic_ pregnancy should be considered.

12. The interface between the decidua capsularis and the echogenic, highly vascularized endometrium forms the double decidual sac sign, which has been reported to be a reliable sign of a viable gestation.

13. The gestational sac size grows at a predictable rate of _1_ mm per day in early pregnancy.

14. The first intragestational sac anatomy seen is the sonographic _yolk (secondary yolk sac)_ sac, which is routinely visualized between 5 and 5.5 weeks' gestation.

15. The limb buds are embryologically recognizable during the _6th_ week of gestation.

16. The spine is also developing during the embryonic period, particularly in the _5th – 7th_ week(s) of gestation.

17. The embryonic face undergoes significant evolution starting in the 5th week of gestation, with palate fusion beginning around the _12th_ week of gestation.

18. At approximately 10 weeks of gestation, the midgut loop continues to grow and rotate before it descends into the fetal abdomen at about the _11th_ week.

19. The cystic rhomboid fossa can sonographically be imaged routinely from the _8th to 11th_ week of gestation.

20. It is important to note that the _lateral_ ventricles completely fill the cerebral vault at this time in gestation.

Exercise 5

Fill in the blank(s) with the word(s) that best completes the statements about the first trimester of pregnancy.

1. Sonographically the gestational sac size or mean sac diameter is determined by the average sum of the _length_, _width_, and _height_ of the gestational sac.

2. Failure to visualize the yolk sac, with a minimum of _8_ mm MSD, using endovaginal sonography, should provoke suspicion of abnormal pregnancy.

3. Transabdominal studies have shown that the yolk sac should be seen within mean sac diameters of _10–15_ mm and should always be visualized with a mean sac diameter of 20 mm.

4. The growth rate of the yolk sac has been reported to be approximately _1_ mm per millimeter of growth of the MSD when the MSD is less than 15 mm.

Exercise 6

Fill in the blank(s) with the word(s) that best completes the statements about multiple gestations.

1. Using endovaginal sonography, multiple gestations can readily be diagnosed at very early stages, between _5.5 – 6.5_ weeks.

2. Sonographically, dichorionic and diamniotic twins appear as _____2_____ separate gestational sacs with individual trophoblastic tissue, which allows the appearance of a thick dividing membrane.

3. Monochorionic-diamniotic twins appear to be contained within _____one_____ chorionic sac;

_____2_____ amnion(s), _____2_____ yolk sac(s), and _____2_____ embryos are identified.

4. The monozygotic, monoamniotic-monochorionic twin gestation shows _____one_____ gestational sac with

_____one_____ amniotic membrane, which may contain one or two yolk sacs and two embryos within the single amniotic membrane.

Exercise 7

Provide a short answer for each question after evaluating the images.

A   B   C

1. Identify the age and appearance of the gestational sac in images **A** through **C**.

4 week   5 week   6 week

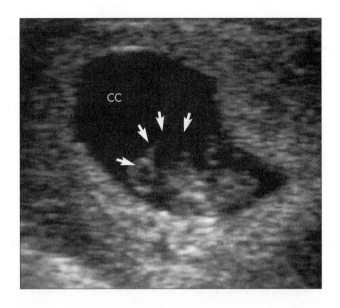

2. Identify the structure the arrows are pointing to in this 7.5-week gestation.

amniotic membrane

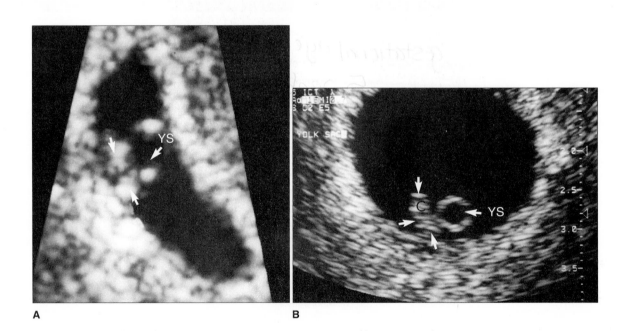

A   **B**

3. Identify the disklike structure adjacent to the yolk sac in image **A.** Identify what the letter C represents in image **B.**

embryo   *embryonic cranium*

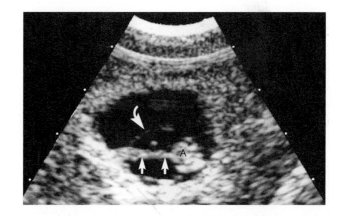

4. In this 8-week gestation, name the structure that the curved arrow is pointing to. Name the structure that the straight arrows are pointing to.

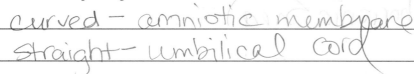

curved — amniotic membrane
straight — umbilical cord

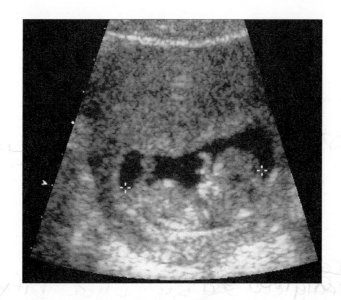

5. This image represents this important fetal measurement.

crown-rump length

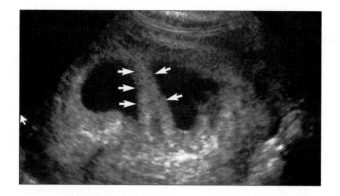

6. Name the type of multiple gestations you would predict from this image.

fraternal twins
(diamniotic, dichorionic preg)

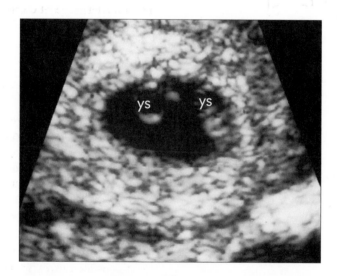

7. Name the type of multiple gestations you would expect from this sonogram.

conjoined twins
(monoamniotic, monochorionic preg)

44 First-Trimester Complications

KEY TERMS

Exercise 1

Match the following embryonic abnormality terms with their definitions.

1. ___I___ acrania

2. ___C___ anencephaly

3. ___F___ bowel herniation

4. ___B___ cephalocele [handwritten: midline cranial defect -herniation of brain + meninges]

5. ___J___ cystic hygroma

6. ___E___ gastroschisis

7. ___K___ holoprosencephaly

8. ___G___ iniencephalus [handwritten: extreme retroflexion of spine -open spinal defect]

9. ___A___ omphalocele

10. ___D___ Turner's syndrome

11. ___H___ ventriculomegaly

A. Congenital hernia of the umbilicus that is covered with a membrane; the cord may be seen in the middle of the mass

B. Protrusion of the brain from the cranial cavity

C. Congenital absence of the brain and cranial vault with the cerebral hemispheres missing or reduced to small masses

D. A nonlethal genetic abnormality in which chromosomal makeup is 45 XO instead of the normal 46 XX or XY

E. Congenital fissure that remains open in the wall of the abdomen just to the right of the umbilical cord; bowel and other organs may protrude outside the abdomen from this opening

F. During the first trimester, the bowel normally herniates outside the abdominal cavity between 8 and 12 weeks

G. A congenitally deformed fetus in which the brain substance protrudes through a fissure in the occiput so that the brain and spinal cord occupy a single cavity

H. Dilation of the ventricular system without enlargement of the cranium

I. Partial or complete absence of the cranium

J. Fluid-filled structure, initially surrounding the neck; may extend upward to the head or laterally to the body

K. Failure of forebrain to divide into cerebral hemispheres, which results in a single large ventricle with varying amounts of cerebral cortex that has been known to occur with trisomies 13 to 15 and trisomy 18

[handwritten: holoprosencephaly → (however, before 9 weeks, the normal fetal brain appears to have a "single" ventricle)]

Exercise 2

Match the following first-trimester terms with their definitions.

1. __D__ anembryonic pregnancy/blighted ovum
2. __H__ complete abortion
3. __B__ corpus luteum cyst
4. __E__ ectopic pregnancy
5. __I__ gestational trophoblastic disease
6. __C__ heterotopic pregnancy
7. __F__ incomplete abortion
8. __A__ interstitial pregnancy
9. __G__ pseudogestational sac

A. Pregnancy occurring in the fallopian tube near the cornu of the uterus

B. A physiologic cyst that develops within the ovary after ovulation and that secretes progesterone and prevents menses if fertilization occurs; may persist until the 16th to 18th week of pregnancy

C. Simultaneous intrauterine and extrauterine pregnancy

D. Ovum without an embryo

E. Pregnancy outside the uterus

F. Retained products of conception

G. Decidual reaction that occurs within the uterus in a patient with an ectopic pregnancy

H. Complete removal of all products of conception, including the placenta

I. Condition in which trophoblastic tissue overtakes the pregnancy and propagates throughout the uterine cavity

FIRST-TRIMESTER COMPLICATIONS

Exercise 3

Fill in the blank(s) with the word(s) that best completes the statements or provide a short answer about the abnormal first trimester.

1. The dominant structure seen within the embryonic cranium within the first trimester is that of the choroid plexus, which fills the lateral ventricles that in turn fill the cranial vault.

2. Ossification of the cranial vault is not complete in the first trimester; the resulting false cranial border definition may give rise to a false-negative diagnosis.

3. An abnormality that may be seen near the end of the first trimester when there is absence of the cranium superior to the orbits with preservation of the base of the skull and facial features with the brain projected from the open cranial vault is anencephaly.

4. In ventriculo-megaly the choroid plexus is shown to be "dangling" in the dilated dependent lateral ventricle.

5. On sonography a large posterior fossa cyst that is continuous with the fourth ventricle, an elevated tentorium, and dilatation of the third and lateral ventricles may be seen in a fetus with Dandy-Walker malformation.

6. The fetal urinary bladder becomes sonographically apparent at 10 to 12 weeks of gestation.

7. One of the most common abnormalities seen sonographically in the first trimester is cystic hygroma.

8. A potential diagnostic pitfall for the sonographer is misinterpreting the hypoechoic or sonolucent embryonic skin surface in the region of the posterior neck. This has been described as the _pseudomembrane_ sign and should not be confused with cystic hygroma, encephalocele, cervical meningomyelocele, teratoma, or hemangioma.

9. Sonographically, placental hematomas may be difficult to distinguish from _subchorionic_ hemorrhages.

10. By far the most common ovarian mass seen in the first trimester of pregnancy is a(n) _corpus luteum_ cyst.

11. List the associated risk factors for ectopic pregnancy. _history of ectopic pregnancy_
previous pelvic infections
IUCD use
fallopian tube surgeries
infertility treatments

12. The most important finding when scanning for ectopic pregnancy is to determine if there is a normal intrauterine gestation (~~thus ruling out the possibility~~ _reducing the probability_ of an ectopic pregnancy) or if the uterine cavity is _empty_ and an adnexal _mass_ is present.

13. As many as 20% of patients with ectopic pregnancy demonstrate an intrauterine saclike structure known as the _pseudogestational sac_.

14. Cornual pregnancy, or _interstitial pregnancy_, is potentially the most life-threatening of all ectopic gestations.

15. Embryonic cardiac rates of less than _90_ beats per minute at any gestational age within the first trimester have been shown to be a poor prognostic finding.

16. The most common occurrence of bleeding in the first trimester is from _subchorionic_ hemorrhage.

17. Characteristics for the sonographic diagnosis of _complete_ abortion consist of an empty uterus with no adnexal masses or free fluid and positive hCG levels.

18. Several sonographic findings may be shown with _incomplete_ abortion, ranging from an intact gestational sac with a nonliving embryo to a collapsed gestational sac that is grossly misshapen.

19. A proliferative disease of the trophoblast after a pregnancy is _gestational trophoblastic_ disease.

20. In the above condition, the serum levels of beta-hCG are dramatically _elevated_, often greater than 100,000 IU/mL.

21. The characteristic "_snowstorm_" appearance of hydatidiform mole, which includes a moderately echogenic soft tissue mass filling the uterine cavity and studded with small cystic spaces representing hydropic chorionic villi, may be seen on ultrasound.

22. Bilateral _theca lutein_ cysts have been reported in as many as half of the molar pregnancies.

Exercise 4

Provide a short answer for each question after evaluating the images.

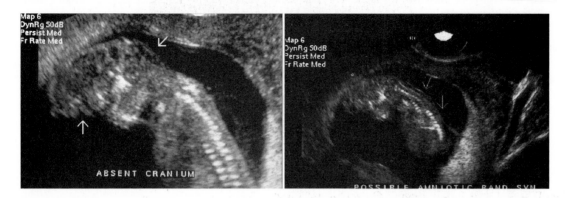

1. The mother presented with an elevated maternal serum alpha fetoprotein level. Describe the sonographic findings in this fetus.

Acrania in pt. w/ elevated maternal serum alpha-fetoprotein level. Amnion along back of fetus → amniotic band syndrome probable cause of acrania

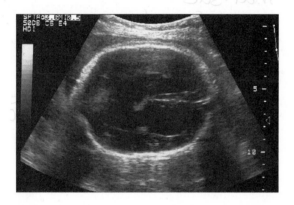

2. The fetus was known to have spina bifida. Describe the findings in the fetal head.

Ventriculomegaly caused by spina bifida. The near field lateral ventricles choroid plexus "dangles" into the far field dilated ventricle.

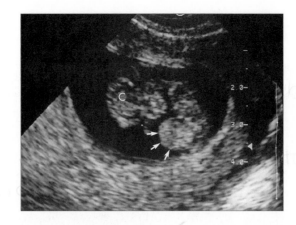

3. Sonogram of a 9-week fetus demonstrates this condition.

herniated liver contents into the base of the
umbilical cord, consistent w/ 1st trimester
omphalocele (could just be normal bowel
migration, but a membrane is seen)

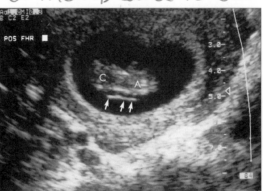

C=cranium
A=abdomen

4. Name the structure that the arrows are pointing to in this 9-week embryo.

embryo lying on amniotic membrane —
   gives false impression of cystic hygroma/nuchal
      thickening

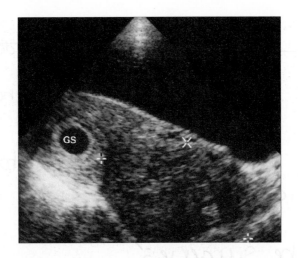

5. The size of the uterus on palpation was larger than dates in this 8-week pregnancy. Describe the sonographic findings.

IUP of 8 weeks w/ fibroid/leiomyoma in LUS

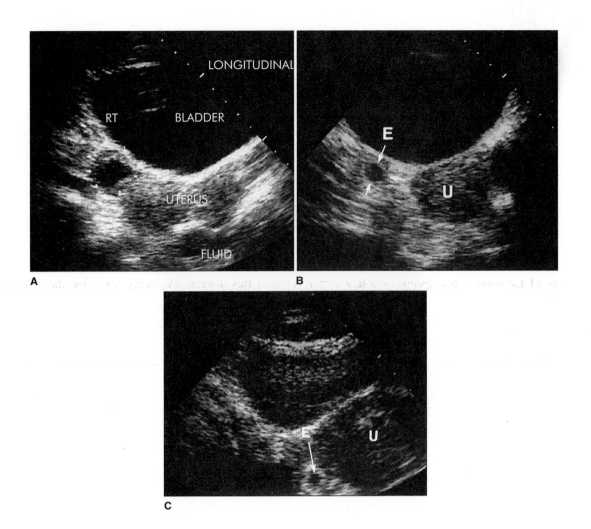

6. Patient presented with positive pregnancy test, bleeding, and cramping for 2 days. Describe the sonographic findings.

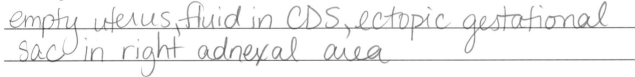

empty uterus, fluid in CDS, ectopic gestational sac in right adnexal area

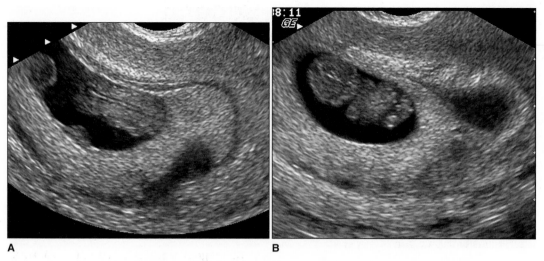

From Henningsen C: *Clinical guide to ultrasonography,* St Louis, 2004, Mosby.

7. The mother experienced mild pain in her first trimester. Describe the sonographic findings.

subchorionic hemorrhage of the placenta

45 Sonography of the Second and Third Trimesters

KEY TERMS

Exercise 1
Match the following obstetric parameter terms with their definitions.

1. _____ gravidity

2. _____ human chorionic gonadotropin

3. _____ menstrual age

4. _____ parity

5. _____ trimester

A. Duration of pregnancy determined from the last menstrual period
B. Pregnancy is divided into three 13-week segments
C. Hormone within the maternal urine and serum
D. Number of live births
E. Total number of pregnancies

Exercise 2
Match the following fetoplacental anatomic terms with their definitions.

1. _____ apex

2. _____ breech

3. _____ ductus arteriosus

4. _____ ductus venosus

5. _____ frontal bossing

6. _____ micrognathia

7. _____ midline echo

8. _____ nomogram

9. _____ normal situs

10. _____ transverse fetal lie

11. _____ vertex

A. Linear echoes located centrally in the fetal head that are produced by the borders of the opposing cerebral hemispheres
B. Structure that carries oxygenated blood from the umbilical vein to the inferior vena cava
C. Indicates fetus is lying transversely in the uterus, horizontal or perpendicular to the maternal sagittal axis
D. Structure that carries oxygenated blood from the pulmonary artery to the descending aorta
E. Typical position of the abdominal organs with the liver and IVC on the right, stomach on the left, and the apex of the heart directed toward the left
F. Where the ventricles of the heart come to a point; directed toward the left hip
G. Abnormally small chin
H. Protrusion to bulging of the forehead that results from hydrocephalus
I. Indicates that the fetus is positioned head down in the uterus
J. Indicates that the fetal head is toward the fundus of the uterus
K. Written representation by graphs, diagrams, or charts of the relationship between numerical variables

Exercise 3

Provide a short answer that best completes the statements about the protocol and guidelines for the second and third trimester.

1. The second and third trimester sonography examination should include the following:

a. _____

b. _____

c. _____

d. _____

e. _____

f. _____

g. _____

h. _____

i. _____

j. _____

k. _____

OBSTETRIC PARAMETERS

Exercise 4

Fill in the blank(s) with the word(s) that best completes the statements about the obstetric parameters, gravidity, and parity of the first, second, and third trimesters.

1. Pregnancy can be clinically verified approximately 6 to 8 days after ovulation by the presence of _____ within the maternal urine or serum.

2. The number of pregnancies, including the present one is _____.

3. A numeric system that describes all possible pregnancies is used to report _____.

4. A G4P2103 describes a patient undergoing her fourth pregnancy. She has had _____ full-term deliveries, _____ premature births, _____ early pregnancy losses, and _____ living children.

Exercise 5

Fill in the blank(s) with the word(s) that best completes the statements about the normal fetoplacental anatomy of the second and third trimesters.

1. The sonographer should initially determine the position of the fetus in relationship to the position of the

   _____.

2. It is important to remember to view _____ activity at the beginning of each study to ensure that the fetus is alive.

3. After fetal position is conceptualized, the sonographer determines the _____ of the fetus.

4. The fetal position changes less frequently after _____ weeks.

5. If the fetus is lying perpendicular to the long axis of the mother, it is described as a _____ fetal lie.

6. If the fetus is lying longitudinal or parallel to the maternal long axis, it is described as a _____ (head down) presentation or _____ (head up) presentation.

7. A _____ breech is found when the hips are extended and one (single footling) or both feet (double footling) are the presenting parts closest to the cervix.

8. If the fetus is in a vertex presentation with the fetal spine toward the maternal right side, the right side of the fetus

   is _____, and the left side is _____.

Exercise 6

Fill in the blank(s) with the word(s) that best completes the statements about the normal fetoplacental anatomy of the cranium of the fetus.

1. Fetal brain tissue, a solid structure, may appear _____ or cystic because of the low density of the tissue.

2. As the brain develops, structures change their sonographic appearances (e.g., the choroid plexuses

   seem_____early in pregnancy), but as the brain grows, these structures appear small in relationship to the entire brain.

3. By the 12th week of gestation, the cranial bones _____.

4. Two types of brain tissues are highly echogenic, the _____ and the _____, which cover the inner and outer brain surfaces.

5. In a transverse plane, at the most cephalad level within the skull, the contour of the skull should be

   _____ (depending on exact level) and should have a _____ surface.

6. At this level, the interhemispheric fissure, or _____, is observed as a membrane separating the brain into two equal hemispheres.

7. The fetal ventricles are important to assess because ventriculomegaly or hydrocephalus (dilated ventricular system) is a sign of _____ system abnormalities.

8. If the _____ appears to float or dangle within the cavity, measurements of ventricular size are recommended to exclude abnormally enlarged or dilated ventricles (ventriculomegaly).

9. Any ventricle measuring greater than _____ mm is considered outside of normal error ranges and is therefore abnormal, warranting further consultation and prenatal testing.

10. The widest transverse diameter of the skull is the _____ and is therefore the proper level at which to measure the biparietal diameter and to assess the development of the midline brain structures.

11. Between the thalamic structures lies the cavity of the _____ ventricle.

12. The circle of _____ may be seen anterior to the midbrain and appears as a triangular region that is highly pulsatile as a result of the midline-positioned anterior cerebral artery and lateral convergence of the middle cerebral arteries.

13. The _____ is located in back of the cerebral peduncles within the posterior fossa.

14. The _____ (a posterior fossa cistern filled with CSF) lies directly behind the cerebellum.

15. The normal cisterna magna measures _____ mm, with an average size of 5 to 6 mm.

16. In second trimester sonographic examinations, the thickness of the nuchal skin fold is measured in a plane containing the cavum septi pellucidi, the _____, and the cisterna magna.

Exercise 7
Fill in the blank(s) with the word(s) that best completes the statements or provide a short answer about the face, spine, and thorax of the fetus.

1. Facial morphology becomes more apparent in the second trimester, but visualization is heavily dependent on

   fetal _____, adequate amounts of _____, and excellent _____ window.

2. In a normally proportioned face, the segments containing the forehead, the eyes and nose, and the mouth and chin

   each form approximately _____ of the profile.

3. The oral cavity and tongue are frequently outlined during fetal _____.

4. Fetal hair is often observed along the _____ of the skull and must not be included in the biparietal diameter measurement.

5. The standard antepartum obstetric examination guidelines require the sonographer to image and record

   the _____, _____, _____, and _____ spine.

6. There are _____ ossification points in each vertebra.

7. The double line appearance of the spine is referred to as the "_____ sign" and is generated by echoes from the posterior and anterior laminae and spinal cord.

8. In a transverse plane, all three ossification points are visible; the points are spaced _____, and the spinal column appears as a closed circle, indicating closure of the neural tube.

9. Three echoes form a circle that represents the _____ of the vertebral body and the posterior elements (laminae or pedicles).

10. Optimal viewing of the spine occurs when the fetus is lying on its side in a _____ direction with its back a slight distance from the uterine wall.

11. The fluid-filled fetal lungs are observed as solid, _____ masses of tissue bordered medially by the heart, inferiorly by the diaphragm, and laterally by the rib cage.

12. List the criteria that are used to assess the fetal heart.

_____

_____

_____

_____

Exercise 8

Fill in the blank(s) with the word(s) that best completes the statements about the diaphragm, fetal circulation, and abdomen.

1. The diaphragm is the muscle that separates the thorax and abdomen and is commonly viewed in the

   _____ plane.

2. The esophagus and oropharynx help determine the location of the carotid arteries and are outlined when amniotic

   fluid is _____ by the fetus.

3. The sonographer should recognize the characteristic arterial _____ from the aorta and its branches.

4. The inferior vena cava is identified coursing to the _____ and parallel with the aorta.

5. Fetal _____ occurs in the placenta where small fetal vessels on the surface of the villi are bathed by maternal blood within the intervillous spaces.

6. Concentrations of waste products, such as urea and creatinine, are _____ in fetal blood, and these products diffuse into the maternal circulation.

7. Fetal circulation _____ the lungs since the fetal lungs do not oxygenate blood.

8. The ductus arteriosus shunts blood _____ from the lungs.

9. Fetal circulation shunts oxygenated blood arriving from the placenta away from the abdomen _____ to the heart and then to the brain.

10. The hepatobiliary system serves the important function of shunting oxygen-rich blood arriving from the placenta

    directly to the heart through the _____.

11. Oxygenated blood from the placenta flows through the _____ vein, within the umbilical cord, to the fetal cord insertion, where it enters the abdomen.

12. From the umbilicus, the umbilical vein courses cephalad along the _____ ligament to the liver, where it connects with the left portal vein.

13. This blood then filters into the liver sinusoids, returning to the inferior vena cava by drainage into the

    _____ veins.

14. Inferior vena cava blood flows from the right atrium through the left atrium by way of the _____ ovale.

15. After birth the _____, the _____, and the _____ close, and fetal circulation converts to the pattern seen throughout the rest of life.

16. The _____ lobe of the liver is larger than the right lobe because of the large quantity of oxygenated blood flowing through the left lobe.

17. The fetal _____ appears as a cone-shaped or teardrop-shaped cystic structure located in the right upper abdomen just below the left portal vein.

18. The spleen may be observed by scanning transversely and posteriorly to the left of the _____.

19. The stomach becomes apparent as early as the _____ week of gestation as swallowed amniotic fluid

    fills the stomach cavity. The full stomach should be seen in all fetuses beyond the _____ week of gestation.

20. The large bowel typically contains _____ particles and may measure up to 20 mm in the preterm fetus and even larger near the time of birth or in the postdate fetus.

21. The kidneys are located on either side of the spine in the posterior abdomen and are apparent as early as

    the _____ week of pregnancy.

22. The _____ center may be difficult to define in early pregnancy, whereas with continued maturation of the kidneys, the borders become more defined and the renal pelvis becomes more distinct.

23. A renal pelvis that measures greater than _____ mm beyond 20 weeks of gestation is considered abnormal.

24. The center of the adrenal gland appears as a central _____ line surrounded by tissue that is less echogenic.

25. A fetus generally voids at least _____ an hour, so failure to see the bladder should prompt the investigator to recheck for bladder filling.

26. The bladder should be visualized in all _____ fetuses and is an important indicator of renal function.

27. Identification of the male and female genitalia is possible provided the fetal legs are _____ and a sufficient quantity of amniotic fluid is present.

28. The gender of the fetus may be appreciated as early as _____ weeks of gestation, although clear

    delineation may not be possible until the _____ weeks.

29. The male genitalia may be differentiated as early as the _____ week of pregnancy.

30. The scrotal sac is seen as a mass of _____ between the hips with the scrotal septum.

Exercise 9

Fill in the blank(s) with the word(s) that best completes the statements about the musculoskeletal system of the fetus.

1. The sonographer must attempt to not only measure fetal limb bones but also survey the anatomic configurations of

   the individual bones whenever possible for evidence of _____, _____, or demineralization, as seen in several common forms of skeletal dysplasias.

2. The _____ is found in a sagittal plane by moving the probe laterally away from the ribs and scapula.

3. Epiphyseal ossification centers may be apparent around the _____ week of pregnancy.

4. The laterally positioned _____ projects deeper into the elbow, which is helpful in differentiating this bone from the medially located radius.

5. Coronally the hands and fingers may be viewed when _____.

6. The distal femoral epiphysis is seen within the cartilage at the knee, and this signifies a gestational age

   beyond _____ weeks of gestation.

Exercise 10

Provide a short answer for each question after evaluating the images.

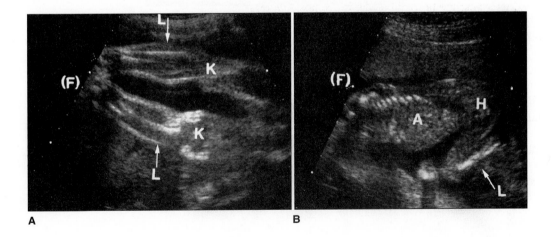

A   B

1. The fetus is lying in this position.

_____

_____

_____

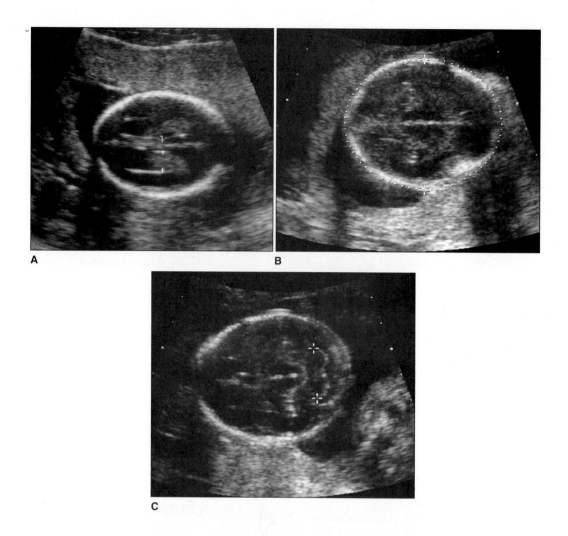

A

B

C

2. In image **A,** name the echogenic structure within the ventricle. In image **B,** name the hypoechoic structure in the center of the fetal head. In image **C,** name the structure that is being measured. Identify the level at which the biparietal diameter should be measured.

_____

_____

_____

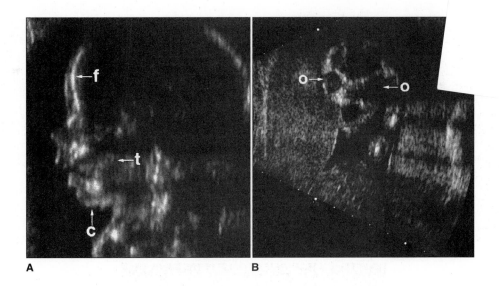

A   B

3. Identify the anatomic parts denoted by *f, t,* and *c*.

_____

_____

_____

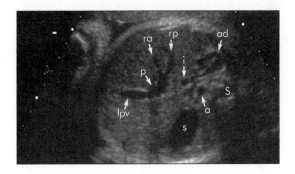

4. Name the fetal side lying closest to the transducer.

_____

_____

_____

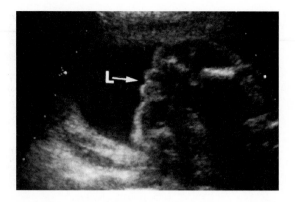

5. Identify what the letter L is pointing to in this fetus.

_____

_____

_____

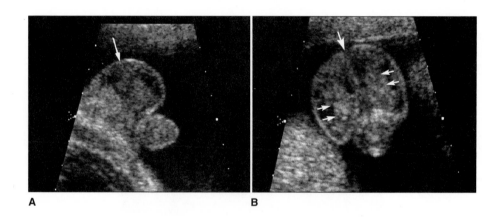

A   B

6. Identify the structure demonstrated in this fetus.

_____

_____

_____

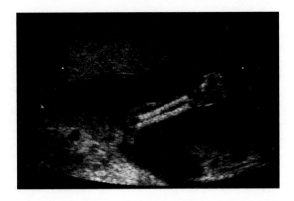

7. Name the two echogenic structures demonstrated in this fetus.

_____

_____

_____

46 Obstetric Measurements and Gestational Age

KEY TERMS

Exercise 1

Match the following obstetric and gestational terms with their definitions.

1. __K__ average age
2. __D__ biparietal diameter
3. __H__ Chiari's malformations
4. __F__ "lemon" sign
5. __C__ crown-rump length
6. __J__ embryonic heart rate
7. __A__ gestational sac
8. __L__ growth-adjusted sonar age
?. ☆ 9. __I__ hypertelorism
10. __M__ intrauterine growth restriction
11. __E__ microphthalmos
12. __B__ platycephaly
13. __G__ spina bifida

A. Structure that is normally found within the uterus and contains the developing embryo
B. Flattening of the skull
C. Most accurate measurement for determining gestational age; made in the first trimester
D. Fetal transverse cranial diameter at the level of the thalamus and cavum septi pellucidi
E. Small eyes
F. Occurs with spina bifida; frontal bones collapse inward
G. Failure of the vertebrae to close
H. Associated with spinal defects
I. Condition in which the orbits are ~~close together~~ *spaced far apart*
J. The heart rate before the early 9th week of gestation
K. Average of multiple fetal parameters' ages
L. The method whereby the fetus is categorized into small, average, or large growth percentile
M. Condition in which the fetus is not growing as fast as normal, usually considered being malnourished or abnormal

Exercise 2

Match the following obstetric and gestational terms with their definitions.

1. __J__ binocular distance
2. __G__ brachycephaly
3. __A__ "banana" sign
4. __D__ dolichocephaly
5. __H__ femur length
6. __B__ gestational sac diameter

A. Refers to the shape of the cerebellum when a spinal defect is present
B. Used in the first trimester to estimate appropriate gestational age with menstrual dates
C. The condition of having a malformed cranial vault with a high or peaked appearance and a vertical index above 77. It is caused by premature closure of the coronal, sagittal, and lambdoidal sutures.
D. Fetal head is relatively narrow in the transverse plane and elongated in the anteroposterior plane
E. A normal but small fetus

397

7. ___K___ humeral length

8. ___F___ hypotelorism

9. ___I___ last menstrual period

10. ___C___ oxycephaly, acrocephaly

11. ___E___ small for gestational age

F. Condition in which the orbits are close together

G. Fetal head is relatively wide in the transverse diameter and shortened in the anteroposterior diameter

H. Measurement of the femoral diaphysis

I. The first day of the LMP is used as the start date for human pregnancies

J. Measurement that includes both fetal orbits at the same time to predict gestational age

K. Measurement from the humeral head to the distal end of the humerus

GESTATIONAL AGE ASSESSMENT: FIRST TRIMESTER

Exercise 3

Fill in the blank(s) with the word(s) that best completes the statements about the gestational age assessment in the first trimester.

1. Sonographically the earliest sign of intrauterine pregnancy is the _thickening of the decidua_ that appears as an echogenic, thickening filling of the fundal region of the endometrial cavity occurring at approximately 3 to 4 weeks of gestation.

2. At 5 weeks the average of the three perpendicular internal diameters of the gestational sac, calculated as the mean of the _anteroposterior_ diameter, the _transverse_ diameter, and the _longitudinal_ diameter, can provide an adequate estimation of menstrual age.

3. The sac grows rapidly in the first _10_ weeks, with an average increase of 1 mm per day.

4. When the gestational sac exceeds _8_ mm in mean internal diameter, a yolk sac should be seen.

5. Normal yolk sac size should be less than _6_ mm; greater than _8_ mm has been associated with poor pregnancy outcome.

6. When the mean gestational sac diameter exceeds _16_ mm, an embryo with definite cardiac activity should be well visualized with endovaginal scanning.

7. The embryonic echoes can be identified as early as 38 to 39 days of menstrual age, and the crown-rump length is usually _1 to 2_ mm at this stage.

8. The most accurate sonographic technique for establishing gestational age in the first trimester is _crown-rump length_

9. In general the CRL should increase at a rate of _8_ mm per day.

10. Absence of an embryo by 7 to 8 weeks of gestation is consistent with an embryonic demise or an _anembryonic_ pregnancy. (blighted ovum)

11. If a nomogram is not readily available to identify gestational age, a convenient formula is gestational age in weeks equals _CRL in cm + 6_.

Exercise 4

Fill in the blank(s) with the word(s) that best completes the statements about the gestational age assessment in the second and third trimester.

1. In the second trimester, the gestational age parameters extend to the _____ diameter, _____ circumference, _____ circumference, and _____ length.

2. The reproducibility of the BPD is ± _____ mm (±2 standard deviations).

3. The growth of the fetal skull slows from _____ mm per week in the second trimester to _____ mm per week in the third trimester.

4. The fetal head should be imaged in a transverse _____ section, ideally with the fetus in a direct occiput transverse position.

5. The BPD should be measured perpendicular to the fetal skull at the level of the _____ and the _____ .

6. Intracranial landmarks should include the _____ anteriorly and posteriorly, the _____ anteriorly in the midline, and the _____ in the atrium of each lateral ventricle.

7. The head shape should be _____ not round (brachycephaly) because this can lead to overestimation of gestational age, just as a flattened or compressed head (dolichocephaly) can lead to underestimation of gestational age.

8. The calipers should be placed from the _____ edge of the parietal bone to the _____ edge of the opposite parietal bone, or "outer edge to inner edge."

9. The _____ head circumference is less affected than BPD by head compression; therefore the head circumference (HC) is a valuable tool in assessing gestational age.

10. The proper coronal view should be _____ to the standard transverse HC view passing through the thalamus.

11. One can _____ gestational age from a dolichocephalic head or _____ with brachycephaly.

12. The AC is very useful in monitoring normal fetal growth and detecting fetal growth disturbances, such as intrauterine growth restriction (IUGR) and macrosomia; however, it is more useful as a _____ than in predicting gestational age.

13. The fetal abdomen should be measured in a transverse plane at the level of the _____ where the _____ vein branches into the left portal sinus.

14. The abdomen should be more _____ than oval because an oval shape indicates an oblique cut resulting in a false estimation of size.

15. An especially useful parameter that can be used to date a pregnancy when a fetal head cannot be measured because of position or when there is a fetal head anomaly is the _____ length.

16. Often an echo from the near side of the cartilaginous distal femoral condyles will be seen, called the "_____," and should not be included in the measure of the diaphysis.

17. The tibia and fibula can be measured by first identifying the _____, then following it down until the two parallel bones can be identified.

18. Humerus length is sometimes more difficult to measure than femur length because the humerus is usually found very close to the fetal _____, but can exhibit a wide range of motion.

19. The ulna can be distinguished from the radius because it penetrates much deeper into the _____.

OBSTETRIC MEASUREMENTS AND GESTATIONAL AGE

Exercise 5
Provide a short answer for each question after evaluating the images.

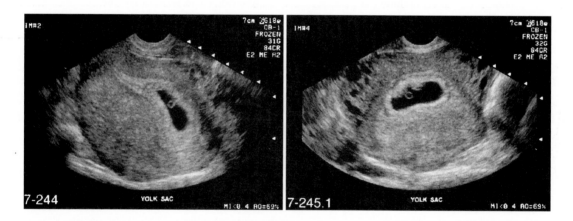

1. Identify the small sonolucent structure within the gestational sac and estimate the gestational age.

_____

_____

_____

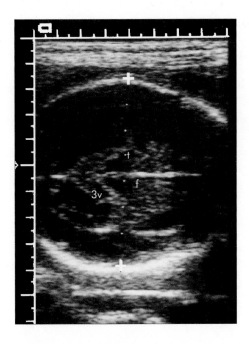

2. Identify *f, t,* and *3v* in this image of the fetal biparietal diameter.

_____

_____

_____

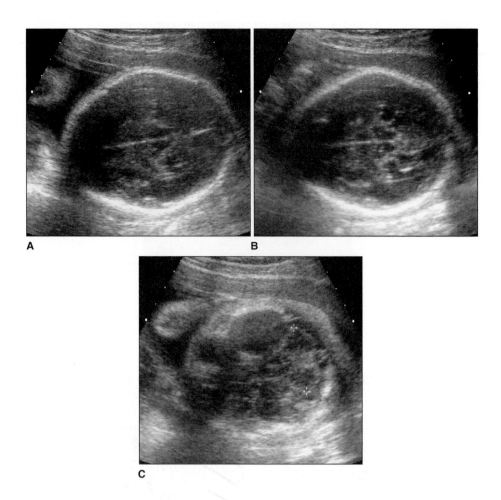

A

B

C

3. Name the image that shows the cerebellum.

_____

_____

_____

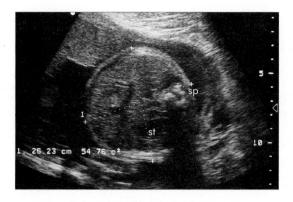

4. Identify *sp* and *st*. This measurement should be made at this level.

_____

_____

_____

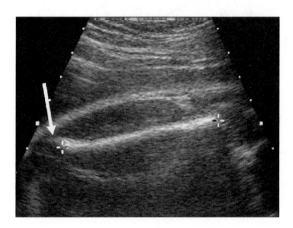

5. Name the structure the arrow is pointing to. Name the structure being measured.

_____

_____

_____

47 Fetal Growth Assessment by Ultrasound

KEY TERMS

Exercise 1

Match the following fetal growth terms with their definitions.

1. _____ amniotic fluid index

2. _____ biophysical profile

3. _____ Doppler

4. _____ estimated fetal weight

5. _____ intrauterine growth restriction

6. _____ large for gestational age

7. _____ macrosomia

8. _____ nonstress test

9. _____ placental grade

10. _____ postterm

11. _____ preterm

12. _____ systolic to diastolic ratio

13. _____ small for gestational age

A. A change in the frequency of a sound wave when either the source or the listener is moving relative to one another

B. Doppler determination of the peak-systolic velocity divided by the peak-diastolic velocity

C. Technique of grading the placenta for maturity

D. Decreased rate of fetal growth; may be symmetric or asymmetric

E. Fetus born earlier than the normal 38- to 42-week gestational period

F. Assessment of fetus to determine fetal well-being; includes evaluation of cardiac nonstress test, fetal breathing movement, gross fetal body movements, fetal tone, and amniotic fluid volume

G. Birth weight greater than 4000 g or above the 90th percentile for the estimated gestational age

H. Fetus born later than the 42-week gestational period

I. Incorporation of all fetal growth parameters

J. Fetus measures smaller than dates

K. Uses Doptone to record the fetal heart rate and its reactivity to the stress of uterine contraction

L. Sum of the four quadrants of amniotic fluid

M. Fetus measures larger than dates

FETAL GROWTH ASSESSMENT

Exercise 2

Fill in the blank(s) with the word(s) that best completes the statements or provide a short answer about intrauterine growth restriction.

1. Intrauterine growth restriction is most commonly defined as a fetal weight at or below _____ % for a given gestational age.

2. Identify the most significant maternal factors for IUGR.

_____

_____

_____

_____

3. Identify the structures that should be measured to determine gestational age during the second or third trimester.

_____

_____

_____

_____

4. _____ IUGR is usually the result of a first-trimester insult, such as a chromosomal abnormality or infection.

5. _____ IUGR begins late in the second or third trimester and usually results from placental insufficiency.

6. Symmetric growth restriction is characterized by a fetus that is _____ in all physical parameters (e.g., BPD, HC, AC, and FL).

7. Asymmetric IUGR is characterized by an appropriate BPD and HC and a disproportionately small _____.

Exercise 3
Fill in the blank(s) with the word(s) that best completes the statements or provide a short answer about ultrasound diagnostic criteria for fetal growth parameters.

1. The fetal blood is shunted away from other vital organs to nourish the fetal brain, giving the fetus an appropriate

   BPD (± 1 standard deviation) for the true gestational age in the _____ theory.

2. A problem with using the biparietal diameter as a predictor of IUGR is the potential alteration in fetal

   _____ shape secondary to oligohydramnios.

3. In IUGR the fetal _____ is one of the most severely affected body organs, which alters the circumference of the fetal abdomen.

4. The association between IUGR and _____ is well recognized and also has been associated with fetal renal anomalies, rupture of the intrauterine membranes, and postdate pregnancy.

Exercise 4

Fill in the blank(s) with the word(s) that best completes the statements or provide a short answer about the biophysical profile and intrauterine growth restriction.

1. List the five requirements in the biophysical profile.

   _____

   _____

   _____

   _____

2. Doppler ultrasound has shown that in fetuses with asymmetric IUGR, the vascular resistance _____ in the aorta and umbilical artery and _____ in the fetal middle cerebral artery.

3. In the umbilical circulation, extreme cases of elevated _____ causing absent or reverse end-diastolic flow velocity waveforms are associated with high rates of morbidity and mortality.

4. Macrosomia has classically been defined as a birth weight of _____ g or greater or above the 90th percentile for estimated gestational age.

5. Macrosomia is also a common result of poorly controlled maternal _____.

Exercise 5

Provide a short answer for each question after evaluating the images.

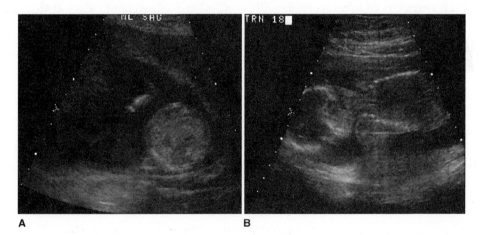

A   B

1. An 18-week fetus with trisomy 18 showed symmetric intrauterine growth restriction. Assess whether this can be determined from one ultrasound examination.

   _____

   _____

   _____

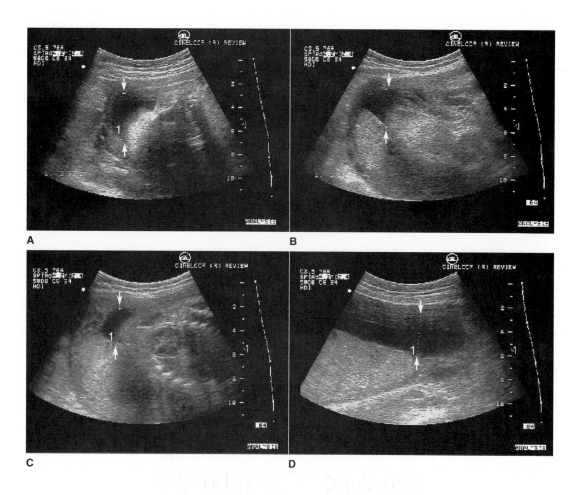

A   B

C   D

2. Name the assessment that these images are demonstrating.

_____

_____

_____

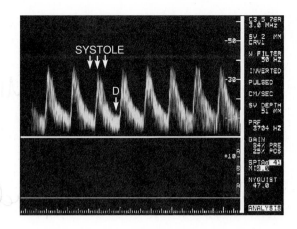

3. State whether this flow velocity pattern of the fetal umbilical artery represents normal or abnormal flow.

_____

_____

_____

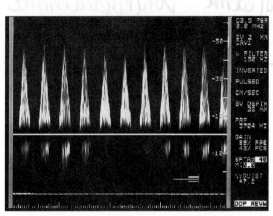

4. Determine whether this flow velocity pattern represents a high-resistance or low-resistance profile. Describe the complications for this fetus.

_____

_____

_____

48 Ultrasound and High-Risk Pregnancy

KEY TERMS

Exercise 1

Match the following ultrasound terms with their definitions.

1. __T__ acardiac anomaly

2. __L__ anasarca

3. __D__ caudal regression syndrome

4. __J__ conjoined twins

5. __B__ dizygotic

6. __P__ eclampsia

7. __H__ fetus papyraceus

8. __O__ hydrops fetalis

9. __R__ hyperemesis gravidarum

10. __E__ maternal serum alpha fetoprotein

11. __N__ maternal serum quad screen

12. __I__ monozygotic

13. __A__ nonimmune hydrops

14. __K__ oligohydramnios

15. __Q__ polyhydramnios

16. __F__ preeclampsia

17. __S__ Rh blood group

18. __C__ Spalding's sign

19. __M__ systemic lupus erythematosus

20. __G__ twin-twin transfusion syndrome

A. Term that describes a group of conditions in which hydrops is present in the fetus, but is not a result of fetomaternal blood group incompatibility

B. Twins that arise from two separately fertilized ova

C. Overlapping of the skull bones; indicates fetal death

D. Lack of development of the caudal spine and cord that may occur in the fetus of a diabetic mother

E. An antigen present in the fetus

F. A complication of pregnancy characterized by increasing hypertension, proteinuria, and edema

G. Monozygotic twin pregnancy with single placenta and arteriovenous shunt within the placenta

H. Fetal death that occurs after the fetus has reached a certain growth that is too large to resorb into the uterus

I. Twins that arise from a single fertilized egg, which divides to produce two identical fetuses

J. Occurs when the division of the egg occurs after 13 days

K. Too little amniotic fluid; fluid measures less than 5 on the amniotic fluid index

L. Severe generalized massive edema often seen with fetal hydrops

M. Inflammatory disease involving multiple organ systems

N. A blood test conducted during the second trimester to identify pregnancies at a higher risk for chromosomal anomalies and neural tube defects

O. Fluid occurring in at least two areas; pleural effusion, pericardial effusion, ascites, or skin edema

P. Coma and seizures in the second- and third-trimester patient secondary to pregnancy-induced hypertension

Q. Too much amniotic fluid; fluid measures greater than 22 on the amniotic fluid index

R. Excessive vomiting that leads to dehydration and electrolyte imbalance

S. System of antigens that may be found on the surface of red blood cells

T. A rare anomaly in monochorionic twins in which one twin develops without a heart and often without an upper half of the body

Exercise 2

Fill in the blank(s) with the word(s) that best completes the statements or provide a short answer about infertility.

1. A patient who will be 35 or older at the time of delivery is referred to as _AMA – advanced maternal age_

2. In the first trimester, testing is performed by looking for the pattern of biochemical markers associated with plasma protein A (PAPP-A) and free βhCG3. These lab values are used in conjunction with an ultrasound (performed between 11 to 14 weeks) to measure the _nuchal_ translucency.

3. Second trimester screening can be performed with the maternal serum _quad_ screen lab value and a targeted ultrasound exam.

4. A detailed evaluation of all fetal anatomy that can be seen at the time between 18 to 20 weeks of gestation is the _targeted_ ultrasound.

5. A condition in which excessive fluid accumulates within the fetal body cavities is _hydrops fetalis_

6. The excessive fluid accumulation may result in _anasarca_ _severe generalized edema_, _ascites_, _pericardial effusion_, _pleural effusion_, _placental edema_, and _polyhydramnios_

7. Any substance that elicits an immunologic response, such as production of an antibody to that substance, is a(n) _antigen_.

8. Ultrasound findings of hydrops are _scalp_ edema, _pericardial_ effusion, _pleural_ effusion, _ascites/polyhydramnios_, and _thickened_ placenta.

9. A procedure in which a needle is placed into the fetal umbilical vein and a blood sample obtained is _cordocentesis_

10. Infants born with _thrombocytopenia_ are at increased risk for intracerebral hemorrhage in utero and spontaneous bleeding.

11. A group of conditions in which hydrops is present in the fetus but is not a result of fetomaternal blood group incompatibility is _nonimmune hydrops_

12. Cardiovascular lesions are often the most frequent causes of NIH. Congestive heart failure may result from _functional_ cardiac problems, such as dysrhythmias, tachycardias, and myocarditis, and from _structural_ anomalies, such as hypoplastic left heart and other types of congenital heart disease.

13. If glucose levels are very high and uncontrolled, the fetus may also become _macrosomic_ _maternal diabetes_

14. If delivery is accomplished vaginally, however, the physician may have difficulty delivering the shoulders of the baby after the head has delivered. This is termed _shoulder_ dystocia

15. Anomalies associated with diabetes include congenital heart and neural tube defects. The most common cardiac problems in the diabetic fetus include _transposition of the great arteries_ and _tetralogy of Fallot_

16. Caudal regression syndrome (lack of development of the caudal spine and cord) is seen almost exclusively in _diabetic_ individuals.

17. Hypertensive pregnancies may be associated with _small_ placentas because of the effect of the hypertension on the blood vessels.

18. The occurrence of seizures or coma in a preeclamptic patient is representative of _eclampsia_

19. A chronic autoimmune disorder that can affect almost all organ systems in the body is _SLE (systemic lupus erythematosus)_

20. _Hyperemesis Gravidarum_ exists when a pregnant woman vomits so much that she develops dehydration and electrolyte imbalance.

21. Identify the combination of effects that may cause hydronephrosis. _in mother_
Progesterone has a dilatory effect on the smooth muscle of the ureter, and enlarging uterus compresses the ureters at the pelvic brim = hydro

PREGNANCY COMPLICATIONS

Exercise 3
Fill in the blank(s) with the word(s) that best completes the statements or provide a short answer about complications of pregnancy.

1. Intrauterine fetal death accounts for roughly _half_ of all perinatal mortality.

2. Fetal heart tones should be heard with Doppler at approximately _10-12_ weeks of gestation.

3. At 20 weeks of gestation, the uterine fundal height should have risen to the umbilicus, and the uterus should measure approximately _20_ cm above the symphysis pubis.

4. The mother should also perceive fetal movements on a daily basis beginning between _16-20_ weeks of gestation.

5. Identify the ultrasound findings that are associated with fetal death.
1) absent heart beat   2) absent fetal movement
3) overlap of skull bones (Spalding's sign)
4) exaggerated curvature of fetal spine
5) gas in the fetal abdomen

Exercise 4

Fill in the blank(s) with the word(s) that best completes the statements about multiple gestation pregnancy.

1. The mother with a multiple gestation is at increased risk for obstetric complications, such as _preeclampsia_, _third-trimester_ bleeding, and _prolapsed_ cord.

2. A twin has a _5_ times greater chance of perinatal death than a singleton fetus.

3. During the first trimester, multiple pregnancy can be identified by visualizing more than one _gestational_ sac within the uterus.

4. _Dizygotic_ twins arise from two separately fertilized ova. Each ovum implants separately in the uterus and develops its own placenta, chorion, and amniotic sac (_diamniotic_, _dichorionic_).

5. Identical or _monozygotic_ twins arise from a single fertilized egg, which divides, resulting in two genetically identical fetuses.

6. Depending on whether the fertilized egg divides _early_ or _late_, there may be one or two placentas, chorions, and amniotic sacs.

7. If the division occurs _early_, 0 to 4 days postconception, there will be two amnions and two chorions (dichorionic, diamniotic).

8. If the division occurs at _4-8_ days, there will be one chorion and two amniotic sacs (monochorionic, diamniotic).

9. If the division occurs after 8 days, two fetuses will be present but only one chorion and one amnion (_mono_ chorionic, _mono_ amniotic).

10. If the division occurs after 13 days, the division may be incomplete and _conjoined_ twins may result.

11. Stuck twin syndrome, or _poly-oli_ sequence, is characterized by a diamniotic pregnancy with polyhydramnios in one sac and severe oligohydramnios and a smaller twin in the other sac.

12. Twin-to-twin transfusion syndrome exists when there is an _arteriovenous_ shunt within the placenta.

13. By definition a rare anomaly occurring in monochorionic twins in which one twin develops without a heart and often absence of the upper half of the body is _acardiac_ anomaly.

14. When scanning multiple gestations, the sonographer should always attempt to determine whether there are one or two _amniotic_ sacs by locating the membrane that separates the sacs.

15. It is important to keep in mind that a fetus from a multiple gestation is usually _smaller_ than a singleton fetus.

16. No flow or _reverse_ flow during diastole are signs of fetal jeopardy and may prompt the obstetrician to do further fetal well-being testing or even deliver the fetuses.

Exercise 5

Provide a short answer for each question after evaluating the images.

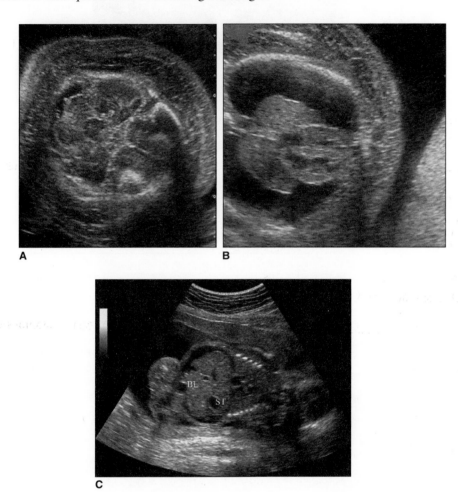

A

B

C

1. Erythroblastosis fetalis is a condition marked by several sonographic findings. In images **A** through **C,** identify which abnormality is shown.

   A=scalp edema

   B=pleural effusion

   C=abd'l ascites

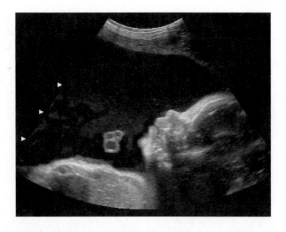

2. Name the abnormality demonstrated in this image.

   Polyhydramnios

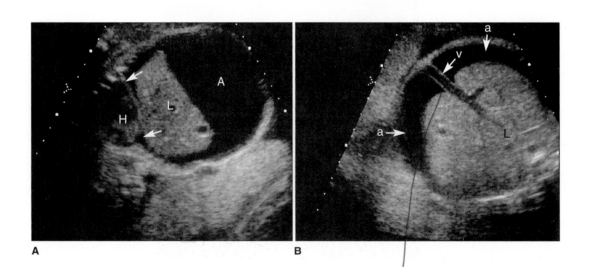

A   B

3. Identify the abnormality demonstrated in this fetus with nonimmune hydrops. Name *v* in image **B.**

   A = abd'l ascites

   V = umbilical vein

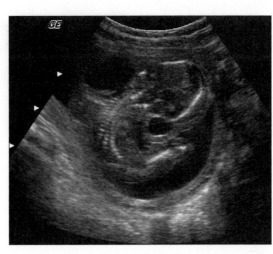

fetal demise w/ fetus curled up; no cardiac activity or fetal motion is noted; scalp edema is present

4. The mother did not feel fetal movement for 36 hours. Describe the ultrasound findings. Describe the other findings that you should look for.

FOUND - overlap of skull bones (Spalding's sign), exaggerated curvature of fetal spine,

SHOULD LOOK FOR - absent FHT + movement

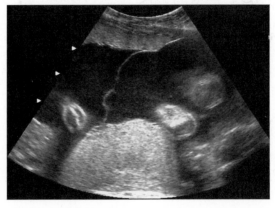

5. This sonogram represents this type of twin gestation.

Dichorionic, diamniotic

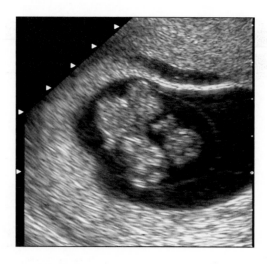

6. This sonogram depicts this type of twinning.

Monochorionic, monoamniotic

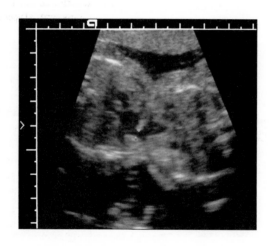

7. This patient presented with a gestation larger than dates. Describe the sonographic findings.

Conjoined twins at the thorax
?

49 Prenatal Diagnosis of Congenital Anomalies

KEY TERMS

Exercise 1

Match the following prenatal diagnosis terms with their definitions.

1. _____ alpha fetoprotein

2. __B__ amniocentesis

3. _____ cystic hygroma

4. _____ hypertelorism

5. _____ hypoplasia

6. _____ hypotelorism

7. _____ intrauterine growth restriction

8. _____ micrognathia

9. _____ omphalocele

10. _____ polydactyly

11. __D__ TORCH

A. Abnormally small chin; commonly associated with other fetal anomalies

B. Transabdominal removal of amniotic fluid from the amniotic cavity using ultrasound

C. Underdevelopment of a tissue, organ, or body

D. An acronym originally coined from the first letters of toxoplasmosis, rubella, cytomegalovirus, and herpesvirus type 2

E. Dilation of jugular lymph sacs because of improper drainage of the lymphatic system into the venous system

F. Anterior abdominal wall defect in which abdominal organs are atypically located within the umbilical cord; highly associated with cardiac, central nervous system, renal, and chromosomal anomalies

G. Abnormally wide-spaced orbits usually found in conjunction with congenital anomalies and mental retardation

H. Abnormally closely spaced orbits; association with holoprosencephaly, chromosomal and central nervous system disorders, and cleft palate

I. Anomalies of the hands or feet in which there is an addition of a digit; may be found in association with certain skeletal dysplasias

J. A decreased rate of fetal growth, usually a fetal weight below the 10th percentile for a given gestational age

K. Protein manufactured by the fetus, which can be studied in amniotic fluid and maternal serum

GENETIC TESTING

Exercise 2

Fill in the blank(s) with the word(s) that best completes the statements about genetic testing.

1. A major congenital anomaly is found in _____ of every 100 births, and an additional 10% to 15% of births are complicated by minor birth defects.

2. An ultrasound-directed biopsy of the placenta or chorionic villi (chorion frondosum) is _____.

3. A specialized prenatal test that permits the direct viewing of the developing embryo using a transcervical endoscope inserted into the extracoelomic cavity during the first trimester of pregnancy is _____.

4. First used as a technique to relieve polyhydramnios, to predict Rh isoimmunization, and to document fetal

   lung maturity is _____.

5. The amniocentesis technique for multiple gestations is similar to the singleton method, except that

   _____ fetal sac is entered.

6. Another method in which chromosomes are analyzed is _____.

7. The major protein in fetal serum and also produced by the yolk sac in early gestation and later by the fetal liver

   is _____.

8. AFP is transported into the _____ by fetal urination and reaches maternal circulation or blood through
   the fetal membranes.

9. Common reasons for high AFP levels are _____, such as anencephaly and open spina bifida.

10. Two common abdominal wall defects, _____ and _____, produce elevations of AFP.

11. It is expected that the AFP level in a _____ pregnancy will be twice that of a singleton pregnancy
    because two fetuses make twice the AFP.

12. The quadruple screen was formerly known as the triple test or triple screen; this biochemical screening test

    combined three serum markers: _____, _____, and _____ plus another
    maternal serum marker, dimeric inhibin.

MEDICAL GENETICS

Exercise 3
Fill in the blank(s) with the word(s) that best completes the statements about medical genetics.

1. A normal karyotype consists of _____ chromosomes, _____ pairs of autosomes, and a pair
   of sex chromosomes.

2. An abnormality of the number of chromosomes is _____.

3. One of the most common aneuploid conditions is _____ syndrome in which an individual has an extra
   chromosome number 21.

4. An inherited dominant disorder carries a _____ % chance that each time pregnancy occurs, the fetus
   will have the condition.

5. A recessive disorder is caused by a pair of defective genes, one inherited from each parent. With each pregnancy,

   the parents have a _____ % chance of having a fetus with the disorder.

6. X-linked disorders are inherited by _____ from their mothers.

7. The _____ of female carriers of X-linked disorders each has a 50% chance of being affected, and

   the _____ each has a 50% chance of being a carrier.

8. An abnormal event that arises because of the interaction of one or more genes and environmental factors is

   a(n) _____ condition.

9. The occurrence of a gene mutation or chromosomal abnormality in a portion of an individual's cells is

   _____. It is difficult to predict the types of problems that will occur when mosaicism is found.

CHROMOSOMAL ABNORMALITIES

Exercise 4
Fill in the blank(s) with the word(s) that best completes the statements or provide a short answer about chromosomal abnormalities.

1. An abnormal fluid collection behind the fetal neck has been strongly associated with _____.

2. A nuchal translucency of _____ mm or greater has been used in earlier literature to define an abnormal thickness.

3. The translucency should be oriented perpendicular to the ultrasound beam, and the measurement should be taken

   from inside the fetal _____ to inside the _____ membrane.

4. A measurement of _____ mm increases the risk of aneuploidy four times, and nuchal translucencies

   of _____ mm and greater carry an even greater risk.

5. List the ultrasound anomalies that may be identified with Down syndrome.

   _____

   _____

   _____

   _____

6. Identify the sonographic anomalies associated with Trisomy 18.

   _____

   _____

   _____

   _____

7. Identify the sonographic anomalies associated with trisomy 13.

_____

_____

_____

_____

8. List the sonographic anomalies associated with triploidy.

_____

_____

_____

_____

9. A genetic abnormality marked by the absence of the X or Y chromosome is _____ syndrome (45, X).

10. The most pathognomonic finding for the above disorder is _____. Other physical features include cardiac anomalies, which are commonly present, with _____ being the most common.

Exercise 5

Provide a short answer for each question after evaluating the images.

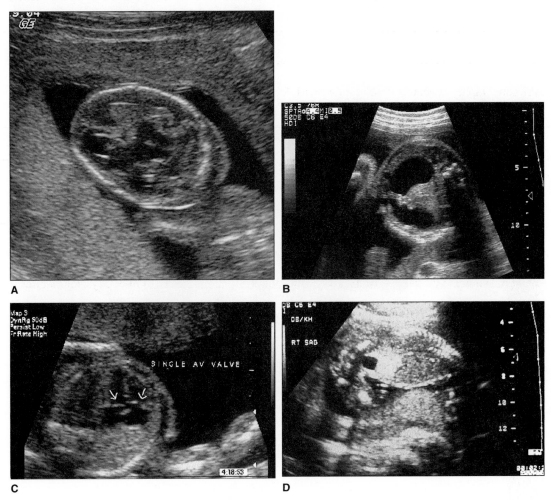

A B C D

From Henningsen C: *Clinical guide to ultrasonography,* St Louis, 2004, Mosby.
From Goreczky G, RDMS, Maternal Fetal Center at Florida Hospital, Orlando, Fla.

1. Describe the sonographic findings in these images in different fetuses with trisomy 21.

_____

_____

_____

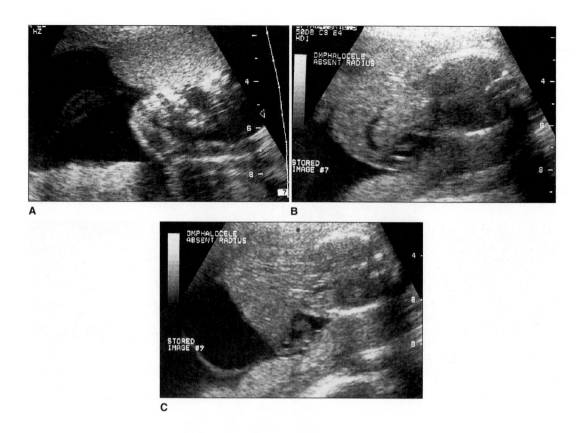

A

B

C

2. A fetus with trisomy 18 presented with radial aplasia and omphalocele. Describe the other sonographic findings.

_____

_____

_____

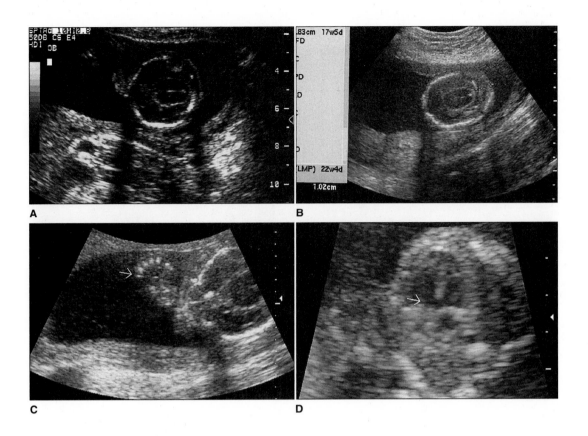

A

B

C

D

3. An 18-week fetus with trisomy 13 is presented. Describe the sonographic findings.

_____

_____

_____

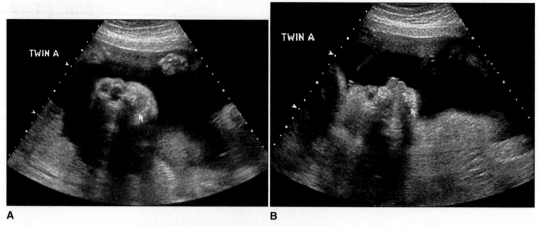

From Henningsen C: *Clinical guide to ultrasonography,* St Louis, 2004, Mosby.

4. A fetus with trisomy 13 is presented. Describe the sonographic findings.

_____

_____

_____

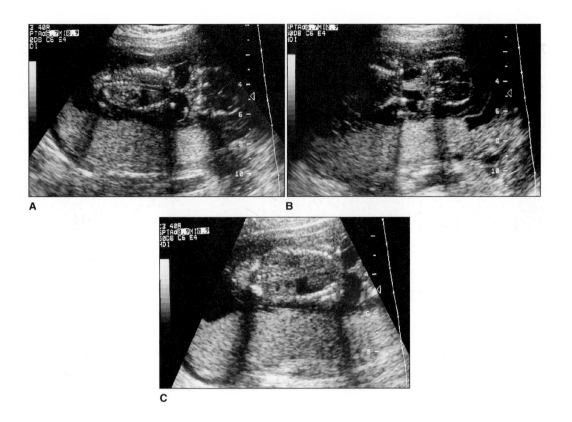

A

B

C

5. A fetus with Turner's syndrome is presented. Describe the sonographic findings.

_____

_____

_____

50 Sonographic 3-D and 4-D Evaluation of Fetal Anomalies

KEY TERMS

Exercise 1

Match the following fetal anomaly terms with their definitions.

1. _____ four-dimensional ultrasound

2. _____ free hand

3. _____ multiplanar imaging

4. _____ planar reconstruction

5. _____ ROI

6. _____ surface mode

7. _____ three-dimensional ultrasound

8. _____ transparent mode

9. _____ volume rendering

A. Permits collection and review of data obtained from a volume of tissue in multiple imaging planes and rendering of surface features

B. Ability to collect data from axial, coronal, and sagittal planes for reconstruction into 3-D format

C. Region of interest

D. Ability to reconstruct the 3-D image and see it in real time

E. In the surface-light mode, there are brighter image intensity values to structures that are closer to the viewer and darker image intensity values to structures that are farther from the viewer

F. Sometimes called x-ray mode, it is best for viewing a relatively low-contrast block of soft tissue

G. Movement of the intersection point of the three orthogonal image planes throughout the 3-D volume and rotation of the image planes

H. The volume is evaluated by rotating the volume data to standard orientation and then scrolling through parallel planes

I. System that uses a smooth sweeping motion in a single plane of acquisition

3-D IMAGING METHODS

Exercise 2

Fill in the blank(s) with the word(s) that best completes the statements about 3-D applications in sonography.

1. List the steps necessary to obtain the 3-D image.

_____

_____

_____

_____

2. The _____ transducer movement is more accurate than hand-controlled transducers because the mechanics and/or electronics of the transducer control the beam.

3. The system that uses both automatic and manual techniques has a hand-held B-mode transducer with the ability to "*sweep*" in a single plane of acquisition. This method is called "_____."

4. The controlled system that involves a single transducer that is moved by hand for position detection to produce a single line of ultrasound information is the _____ controlled system.

5. There are two different types of 3-D imaging, the _____ mode and the _____ mode.

6. Brighter image intensity values to structures that are closer to the viewer and darker image intensity values to structures that are farther from the viewer are characteristic of the _____ mode.

7. The x-ray mode, or the _____ mode, is best for viewing a relatively low-contrast block of soft tissues.

51 The Placenta

KEY TERMS

Exercise 1
Match the following terms relating to embryogenesis with their definitions.

1. __D__ basal plate
2. __G__ battledore placenta
3. __A__ chorion frondosum
4. __H__ chorionic plate
5. __C__ chorionic villi
6. __F__ decidua basalis
7. __E__ decidua capsularis
8. __B__ placenta previa

A. The portion of the chorion that develops into the fetal portion of the placenta
B. Placenta completely covers the lower uterine segment (internal os)
C. Vascular projections from the chorion
D. The maternal surface of the placenta that lies contiguous with the decidua basalis
E. The part of the decidua that surrounds the chorionic sac
F. The part of the decidua that unites with the chorion to form the placenta
G. Cord insertion into the margin of the placenta
H. Part of the chorionic membrane that covers the placenta

Exercise 2
Match the following terms with their definitions.

1. __M__ abruptio placentae
2. __D__ Braxton Hicks contractions
3. __O__ circummarginate placenta
4. __J__ circumvallate placenta
5. __L__ ductus venosus
6. __B__ ligamentum venosum
7. __G__ lower uterine segment (LUS)
8. __A__ molar pregnancy
9. __C__ placenta accreta
10. __I__ placenta increta
11. __N__ placenta percreta

A. Also known as gestational trophoblastic disease; abnormal proliferation of trophoblastic cells in the first trimester
B. Transformation of the ductus venosus in fetal life to closure in neonatal life
C. Growth of the chorionic villi superficially into the myometrium
D. Spontaneous painless uterine contractions described originally as a sign of pregnancy. They occur from the first trimester to the end of pregnancy.
E. Occurs when the intramembranous vessels course across the cervical os
F. The placenta is attached to the uterine wall. As the uterus enlarges, the placenta "moves" with it. Therefore a low-lying placenta may move out of the uterine segment in the second trimester.
G. Lowest segment of the uterus at the junction of the internal os and cervix
H. Mucoid connective tissue that surrounds the vessels within the umbilical cord

12. ___F___ placental migration

13. ___K___ succenturiate placenta

14. ___E___ vasa previa

15. ___H___ Wharton's jelly

I. Growth of the chorionic villi deep into the myometrium

J. A placental condition in which the chorionic plate of the placenta is smaller than the basal plate; the margin is raised with a rolled edge

K. One or more accessory lobes connected to the body of the placenta by blood vessels

L. Connection that is patent during fetal life from the left portal vein to the systemic veins (inferior vena cava)

M. Premature detachment of the placenta from the maternal wall

N. Growth of the chorionic villi through the myometrium

O. A placental condition in which the chorionic plate of the placenta is smaller than the basal plate, with a flat interface between the fetal membranes and the placenta

ANATOMY AND PHYSIOLOGY

Exercise 3

Label the following illustrations.

1. The placenta.

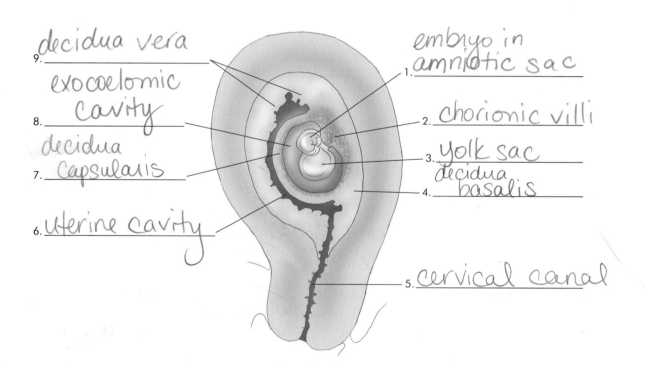

9. decidua vera

8. exocoelomic cavity

7. decidua capsularis

6. uterine cavity

1. embryo in amniotic sac

2. chorionic villi

3. yolk sac

4. decidua basalis

5. cervical canal

2. The chorionic villi.

LATER

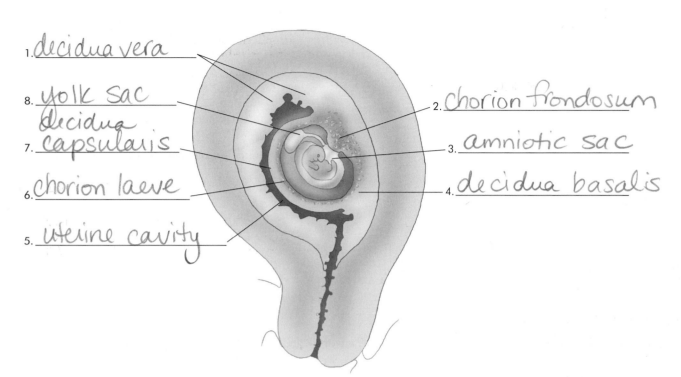

1. decidua vera
8. yolk sac
7. decidua capsularis
6. chorion laeve
5. uterine cavity
2. chorion frondosum
3. amniotic sac
4. decidua basalis

3. The major functioning unit of the placenta.

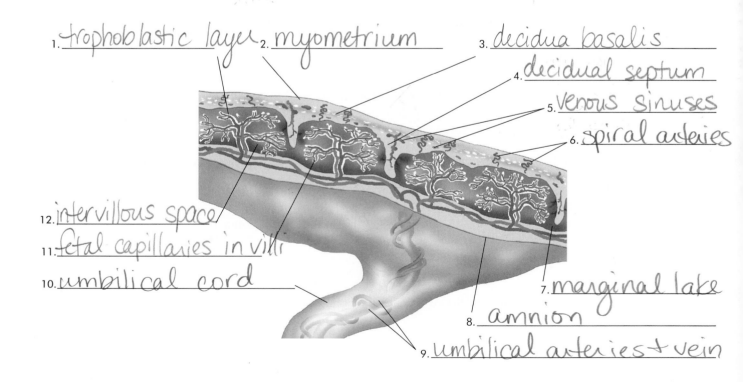

1. trophoblastic layer
2. myometrium
3. decidua basalis
4. decidual septum
5. venous sinuses
6. spiral arteries
12. intervillous space
11. fetal capillaries in villi
10. umbilical cord
7. marginal lake
8. amnion
9. umbilical arteries + vein

Exercise 4

Fill in the blank(s) with the word(s) that best completes the statements or provide a short answer about the anatomy and physiology of the placenta.

1. The major role of the placenta is to permit the exchange of _oxygenated_ maternal blood (rich in oxygen and nutrients) with _deoxygenated_ fetal blood.

2. Maternal vessels coursing _posterior_ to the placenta circulate blood into the placenta, whereas blood from the fetus reaches this point through the _umbilical cord_.

3. The fetal surface of the placenta, which is contiguous with the surrounding chorion, is termed the _chorionic plate_.

4. The maternal portion of the placenta that lies contiguous with the decidua basalis is termed the _basal plate_.

5. The major functioning unit of the placenta is the _chorionic villus_.

6. Before birth, the fetal membranes and placenta perform the following functions and activities: _(storage, hormone production)_ _protection_, _nutrition_, _respiration_, and _excretion_.

7. Oxygenated maternal blood is brought to the placenta through 80 to 100 end branches of the uterine arteries, the _spiral_ arteries.

8. The maternal placental circulation may be reduced by a variety of conditions that decrease uterine blood flow, such as severe _htn_, _renal_ disease, or _placental_ infarction.

9. List the three main functions of the placenta.

   metabolism

   endocrine

   transfer

   _____

10. The attachment of the cord is usually near the _center_ of the placenta.

11. Most of the amniotic fluid comes from the maternal _blood_ by diffusion across the amnion from the decidua parietalis and intervillous spaces of the placenta.

12. In the first trimester, the fetus begins to _excrete_ urine into the sac to fill the amniotic cavity; the fetus _swallows_ this fluid, and the cycle continues throughout pregnancy.

Exercise 5

Fill in the blank(s) with the word(s) that best completes the statements or provide a short answer about the pathology of the placenta.

1. The placenta is separated from the myometrium by a _Subplacental_ venous complex.

2. The placenta increases in size and volume with gestational age; however, the maximum thickness does not exceed _45-50_ mm.

3. The sonographer should always describe the _position_ of the placenta.

4. For the sonographer to visualize the internal os of the cervix, the patient should have a _full bladder_.

5. When the sonographer sees two separate parts of the placenta that do not appear to communicate, a _Succenturiate_ placenta should be considered.

6. Prior to 20 weeks, uterine artery Doppler typically shows a _high_ flow, _low_ resistance pattern, particularly for the uterine artery on the same side as the placenta.

7. Maternal diabetes and Rh incompatibility are primary causes for _Placentomegaly_.

8. Placenta _previa_ is the implantation of the placenta in the lower uterine segment in advance of the fetus.

9. With _Complete_ previa, the cervical internal os is completely covered by placental tissue.

10. The other approaches useful in evaluating the lower uterine segment with ultrasound when the definition of the placenta needs to be clarified include _transperineal_ and _translabial_.

11. A potentially life-threatening fetal complication of the placenta that occurs when large fetal vessels run in the fetal membranes across the cervical os is _vasa_ previa, which places them at risk of rupture and hemorrhage.

12. The abnormal adherence of part or all of the placenta with partial or complete absence of the decidua basalis is _placenta_ accreta.

13. The risk of placenta accreta increases in patients with placenta previa and uterine scar from previous _cesarean section_.

14. Placenta _increta_ results from underdeveloped decidualization of the endometrium.

15. The attachment of the placental membranes to the fetal surface of the placenta rather than to the placental margin is a(n) _circumvallate_ placenta.

16. The separation of a normally implanted placenta before term delivery is referred to as placental _abruption_.

17. ___Retroplacental___ abruption results from the rupture of spiral arteries and is a "high-pressure" bleed.

18. ___Marginal___ abruption results from tears of the marginal veins and represents a "low-pressure" bleed.

19. A focal discrete lesion caused by ischemic necrosis is placenta ___infarction___.

20. The sonogram shows a uterine size larger than dates, no identifiable parts, and an inhomogeneous texture with various sized cystic structures of the placenta that represent the multiple vesicular changes throughout the placenta in ___gestational trophoblastic___ disease.

21. The second most common tumor of the placenta is known as ___chorioangioma___

Exercise 6

Provide a short answer for each question after evaluating the images.

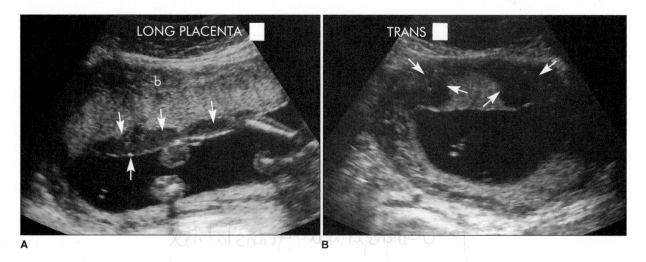

1. Describe and name the area that is outlined by the arrows in images **A** and **B**.

___intervillous lakes___

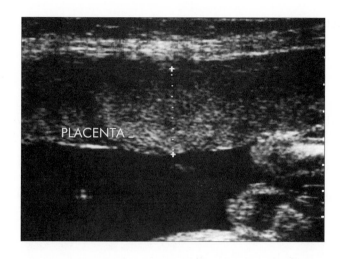

PLACENTA

2. The thickness of this placenta measured greater than 7 cm. Name the condition this may represent.

Placentomegaly edematous placenta

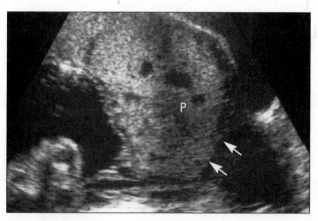

P

3. This is an image of the lower uterine segment in a patient who has been bleeding for 3 days with bright red blood. Describe the sonographic finding.

Placenta previa

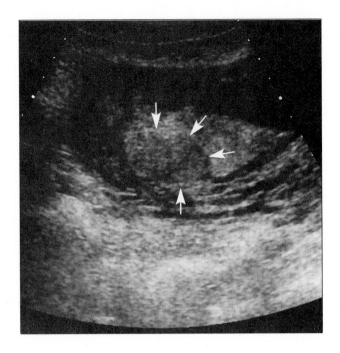

4. This patient experienced severe acute pain 36 hours previous to the sonogram. Describe the findings.

Retroplacental abruption

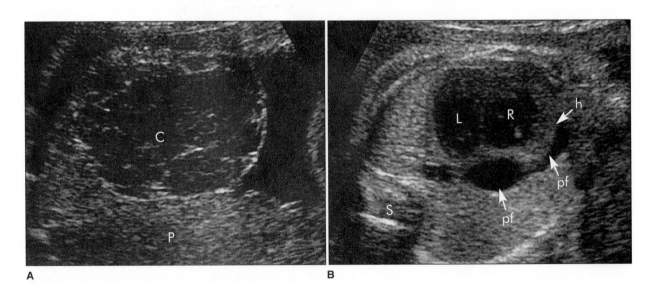

A   **B**

5. This patient presented with size larger than dates. A palpable "masslike" structure was noted on the left upper uterine area. Describe the findings.

Chorioangioma. Rt ♡ enlargement + pleural effusion

52 The Umbilical Cord

KEY TERMS

Exercise 1

Match the following with their definitions.

1. _H_ allantoic duct

2. _D_ battledore placenta

3. _C_ ductus venosus

4. _J_ false knots of the umbilical cord

5. _P_ gastroschisis

6. _M_ hemangioma of the cord

7. _A_ membranous or velamentous insertion of the cord

8. _L_ nuchal cord

9. _B_ omphalocele

10. _K_ omphalomesenteric cyst

11. _I_ single umbilical artery

12. _Q_ superior vesical arteries

13. _N_ true knots of the umbilical cord

14. _F_ umbilical herniation

15. _O_ vasa previa

16. _G_ Wharton's jelly

17. _E_ yolk stalk

A. Cord inserts into the membranes before it enters the placenta

B. Failure of the bowel, stomach, and liver to return to the abdominal cavity; completely covered by a peritoneal-amniotic membrane

C. The smaller, shorter, and posterior of the two branches into which the umbilical vein divides after entering the abdomen. It empties into the inferior vena cava.

D. Marginal or eccentric insertion of the umbilical cord into the placenta

E. Umbilical duct connecting the yolk sac with the embryo

F. Failure of the anterior abdominal wall to close completely at the level of the umbilicus

G. Myxomatous connective tissue that surrounds the umbilical vessels and varies in size

H. Elongated duct that contributes to the development of the umbilical cord and placenta during the first trimester

I. High association of congenital anomalies with this

J. Occurs when blood vessels are longer than the cord; they fold on themselves and produce nodulations on the surface of the cord

K. Cystic lesion of the umbilical cord

L. Occurs when the cord is wrapped around the fetal neck

M. Vascular tumor within the umbilical cord

N. Formed when a loop of cord is slipped over the fetal head or shoulders during delivery

O. Occurs when the umbilical cord vessels cross the internal os of the cervix

P. Anomaly in which part of the bowel remains outside the abdominal wall without a membrane

Q. After birth the umbilical arteries are known as these

Exercise 2

Fill in the blank(s) with the word(s) that best completes the statements about the development and normal anatomy of the umbilical cord.

1. The umbilical cord is the essential link for __Oxygen__ and important nutrients between the fetus, the placenta, and the mother.

2. The intestines grow at a faster rate than the abdomen and __herniate__ into the proximal umbilical cord at approximately 7 weeks and remain there until approximately 10 weeks.

3. The umbilical cord includes __2__ umbilical arteries and __one__ umbilical vein and is surrounded by a homogeneous substance called __Wharton's__ jelly.

4. The intraabdominal portions of the umbilical vessels degenerate after birth; the umbilical arteries become the lateral ligaments of the __bladder__, and the umbilical vein becomes the round ligament of the __liver__.

5. From the left portal vein, the umbilical blood flows either through the __ductus venosus__ to the systemic veins (inferior vena cava or hepatics) bypassing the liver or through the right portal sinus to the right portal vein.

6. The ductus venosus forms the conduit between the __portal__ system and the __systemic__ veins.

7. The ductus venosus is patent during fetal life until shortly after birth, when transformation of the ductus into the ligamentum __venosum__ occurs (beginning in the second week after birth).

8. The umbilical arteries run along the __lateral__ margin of the fetal bladder and are well imaged with color flow Doppler. In the postpartum stage, the umbilical arteries become the superior vesical arteries.

9. The diameter of the umbilical cord has been measured from __2.6-6.0__; variations in cord diameter are usually attributed to diffuse accumulation of Wharton's jelly.

PATHOLOGY

Exercise 3

Fill in the blank(s) with the word(s) that best completes the statements about the pathology of the umbilical cord.

1. __True__ knots of the umbilical cord have been associated with long cords, polyhydramnios, intrauterine growth restriction, and monoamniotic twins.

2. __False__ knots of the umbilical cord are seen when the blood vessels are longer than the cord.

3. The most common cord entanglement in the fetus is __nuchal__ cord.

4. The cord implants into the edge of the placenta (__battledore__ placenta) instead of into the middle of the placenta.

5. Membranous or __velamentous__ insertion of the cord occurs when the cord inserts into the membranes before it enters the placenta rather than inserting directly into the placenta.

6. When the cord lies below the presenting part, __prolapse__ of the umbilical cord occurs.

7. _Compression_ of the cord reduces or cuts off the blood supply to the fetus and may result in fetal demise.

8. The sonographic detection of a _single_ umbilical artery should prompt the investigation of further fetal anomalies.

Exercise 4

Provide a short answer for each question after evaluating the images.

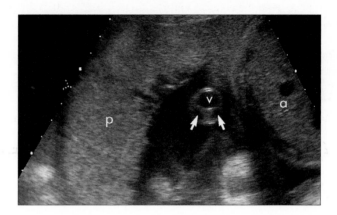

1. Name the structures that the two arrows are pointing to in this image.

Umb. arts

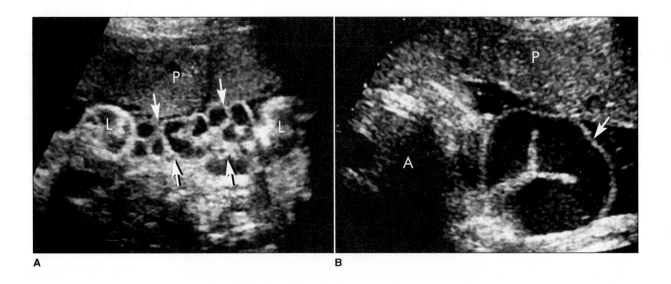

2. This mass was seen to project outside the fetal abdomen. The abnormality you suspect is:

Gastroschis

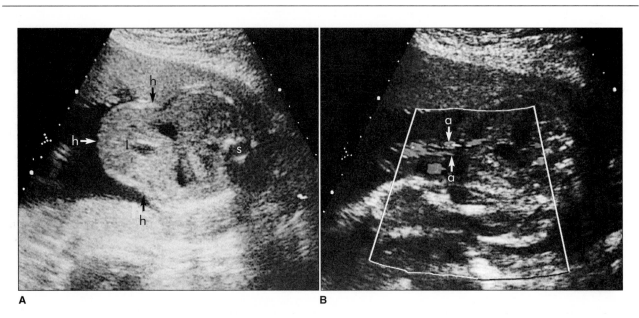

3. This abnormality is present on this fetal abdomen.

Umbilical hernia

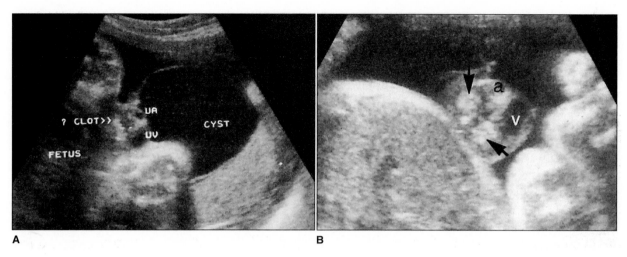

A   B

4. This omphalomesenteric cyst was found in a 34-week fetus with clot formation in one artery. Identify what the arrows are pointing to in image **B.**

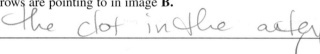

the clot in the artery

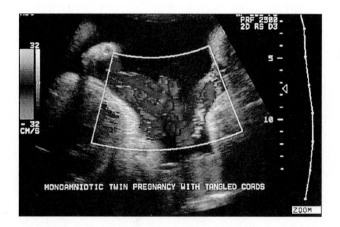

MONOAMNIOTIC TWIN PREGNANCY WITH TANGLED CORDS

5. This image of the umbilical cord demonstrates this abnormality.

mult. knots in the cord

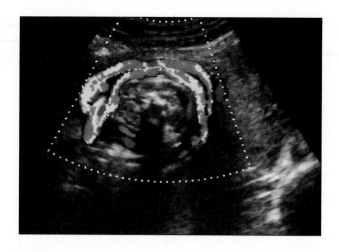

6. This is a transverse image at the level of the fetal neck. Color flow is shown as white. Describe your findings.

nuchal cord around fetal neck

53 Amniotic Fluid and Membranes: Polyhydramnios and Oligohydramnios

KEY TERMS

Exercise 1

Match the following terms with their definitions.

1. _____ amniotic bands

2. _____ amniotic cavity

3. _____ amniotic fluid

4. _____ amniotic fluid index

5. _____ chorion frondosum

6. _____ keratinization

7. _____ maximum or deep vertical pocket

8. _____ oligohydramnios

9. _____ placental insufficiency

10. _____ polyhydramnios

11. _____ subjective assessment of fluid

12. _____ uterine synechiae

13. _____ vernix caseosa

A. Too little amniotic fluid; associated with intrauterine growth restriction, renal anomalies, premature rupture of membranes, postdate pregnancy, and other factors

B. The process of keratin formation that takes place within the keratinocytes as they progress upward through the layers of the epidermis of skin to the surface stratum corneum

C. Sonographer surveys uterine cavity to determine visual assessment of amniotic fluid present

D. Multiple fibrous strands of amnion that develop in utero that may entangle fetal parts to cause amputations or malformations of the fetus

E. Too much amniotic fluid; associated with central nervous system disorder, gastrointestinal anomalies, fetal hydrops, skeletal anomalies, renal disorders, and other factors

F. The portion of the chorion that develops into the fetal portion of the placenta

G. Another method (used more often in multiple gestation pregnancy) to determine the amount of amniotic fluid; pocket less than 2 cm may indicate oligohydramnios; greater than 8 cm indicates polyhydramnios

H. Inability of placenta to adequately provide blood and/or nutrient supply to the fetus caused by underlying maternal disease, such as hypertension or diabetes, or extensive placental abruption

I. Forms early in gestation and surrounds the embryo; amniotic fluid fills the cavity to protect the embryo and fetus

J. Fatty material found on fetal skin and in amniotic fluid late in pregnancy

K. Scars within the uterus secondary to previous gynecologic surgery

L. Produced by the umbilical cord and membranes, the fetal lung, skin, and kidney

M. The uterus is divided into four quadrants; each quadrant is evaluated with the transducer perpendicular to the table in the deepest vertical pocket without fetal parts; the four quadrants are added together to determine the amniotic fluid index

Exercise 2

Fill in the blank(s) with the word(s) that best completes the statements about amniotic fluid.

1. _____ allows the fetus to move freely within the amniotic cavity while maintaining intrauterine temperature and protecting the developing fetus from injury.

2. The amnion can be visualized with endovaginal sonography in the early first trimester between 4 to 5 weeks of gestation as a thin membrane separating the _____ cavity (which contains the fetus) from the extraembryonic coelom and the secondary _____ sac.

3. Amniotic fluid is produced by the umbilical cord, the _____, _____, skin, and _____.

4. As the fetus and placenta mature, amniotic fluid production and consumption change to include movement of fluid across the _____ and fetal skin, fetal urine output and fetal swallowing, and gastrointestinal absorption.

5. Fetal skin is also permeable to water and some solutes to permit a direct exchange between the fetus and amniotic fluid until _____ occurs at 24 to 26 weeks.

6. Fetal production of urine and the ability to swallow begins between _____ weeks of gestation and becomes the major pathway for amniotic fluid production and consumption after this time period.

7. The fetus _____ amniotic fluid, which is absorbed by the digestive tract. The fetus also _____ urine, which is passed into the surrounding amniotic fluid.

8. Fetal urination into the amniotic sac accounts for nearly the total volume of amniotic fluid by the second half of pregnancy so that the quantity of fluid is directly related to _____ function.

9. Normal lung development depends critically on the _____ of amniotic fluid within the lungs.

10. Inadequate lung development may occur when severe _____ is present, placing the fetus at high risk for developing small or hypoplastic lungs.

11. Volume of amniotic fluid increases progressively until about 33 weeks of gestation, with the average increment per week of _____ mL from the 11th to the 15th week and _____ mL from the 15th to 28th week of gestation.

12. At 20 to 30 weeks of gestation, amniotic fluid may appear somewhat _____, although this typically represents a normal amniotic fluid variant.

13. At the end of pregnancy, the amniotic fluid is scanty, and _____ fluid pockets may be the only visible areas of fluid.

14. The small-for-age fetus has _____ amniotic fluid; the large-for-age fetus has _____ volume of fluid.

15. Amniotic fluid generally appears _____, although occasionally fluid particles (particulate matter) may be seen.

Exercise 3

Fill in the blank(s) with the word(s) that best completes the statements about the sonographic assessment of amniotic fluid.

1. As the sonographer initially scans "through" the entire uterus to determine the *visual "eyeball"* assessment of the

   fluid present, the lie of the fetus, and the position of the placenta, _____ is performed.

2. The uterine cavity is divided into four equal quadrants by two imaginary lines perpendicular to each other with the

   _____ method.

3. The largest vertical pocket of amniotic fluid, excluding fetal limbs or umbilical cord loops, is measured in the four

   quadrants and added together for the _____.

4. Subjective assessment of normal amniotic fluid correlates with AFI of 10 to 20 cm; borderline values of

   _____ cm indicate low fluid, and values of _____ cm indicate increased fluid.

5. The sonographer must be careful to hold the transducer _____ to the table (not the curved skin surface) when determining these pockets of fluid.

6. The _____ (i.e., fluid should measure greater than 1 cm "rule") assessment of amniotic fluid is done by identifying the largest pocket of amniotic fluid.

7. In twin pregnancies, the two-dimensional pocket measurement appears to be a better predictor of

   _____ than the AFI or the largest vertical pocket.

Exercise 4

Fill in the blank(s) with the word(s) that best completes the statements or provide a short answer about the abnormalities of amniotic fluid.

1. Hydramnios or _____ is defined as an amniotic fluid volume of greater than 2000 mL.

2. Polyhydramnios is often associated with _____ disorders and/or _____ problems.

3. This central nervous system disorder causes _____ swallowing.

4. With gastrointestinal abnormalities, often a _____ (atresia) of the esophagus, stomach, duodenum, and small bowel results in ineffective swallowing.

5. An overall reduction in the amount of amniotic fluid resulting in fetal crowding and decreased fetal movement is

   _____.

6. Oligohydramnios may be defined as a single pocket of fluid with a depth less than _____ cm or an

AFI of less than _____ cm.

7. Identify one of the five causes that may be attributed to the development of oligohydramnios.

_____

_____

_____

_____

8. The association between _____ and decreased amniotic fluid (oligohydramnios) is well recognized.

9. Evaluation of the _____ in the umbilical cord, the placenta, and the cerebral vascular system with color and Doppler techniques is critical to determine the presence or absence of intrauterine growth restriction.

10. Cord _____ by the fetus is another potential cause for fetal asphyxia leading to oligohydramnios.

Exercise 5
Fill in the blank(s) with the word(s) that best completes the statements about amniotic band syndrome.

1. A common, nonrecurrent cause of various fetal malformations involving the limbs, craniofacial region, and trunk

is the _____.

2. The site where the amniotic band cuts across the fetus is usually evident after _____.

3. Amniotic sheets are believed to be caused by uterine scars, or _____, from previous instrumentation of the uterus (usually curettage), cesarean section, or episodes of endometritis.

Exercise 6

Provide a short answer for each question after evaluating the images.

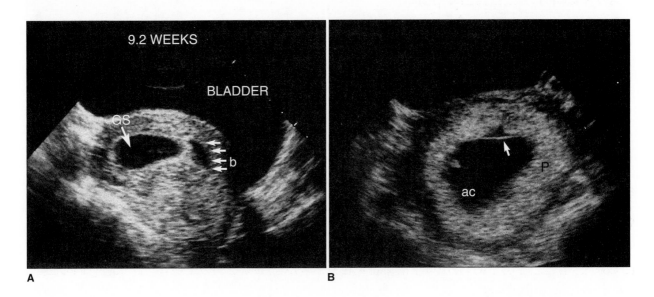

A   **B**

1. Identify the structure the arrow(s) are pointing to in image **A** and **B.**

_____

_____

_____

_____

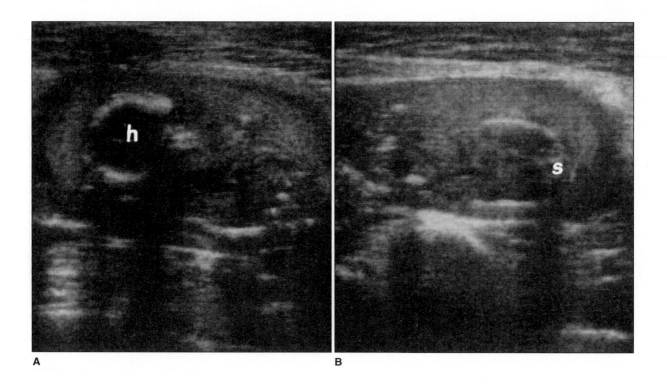

A   B

2. The patient stated she noted fluid leaking for the past 4 days. Describe the sonographic findings.

_____

_____

_____

_____

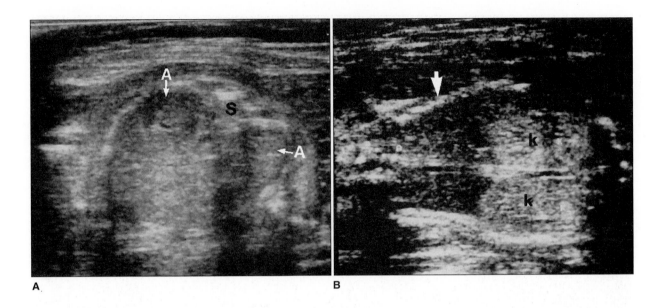

A.   B

3.   These two different fetuses both presented with oligohydramnios. The abnormalities for the fetus in image **A** and **B** are:

_____

_____

_____

_____

54 The Fetal Face and Neck

KEY TERMS

Exercise 1
Match the following terms with their definitions.

1. _____ anophthalmia

2. _____ arrhinia

3. _____ cephalocele

4. _____ craniosynostoses

5. _____ dacryocystocele

6. _____ exophthalmia

7. _____ fetal cystic hygroma

8. _____ fetal goiter (thyromegaly)

9. _____ holoprosencephaly

10. _____ hypertelorism

11. _____ microcephaly

12. _____ micrognathia

13. _____ nuchal lucency

14. _____ phenylketonuria (PKU)

15. _____ Treacher Collins syndrome

A. Malformation of the lymphatic system that leads to single or multiloculated lymph-filled cavities around the neck

B. Premature closure of the cranial sutures

C. Underdevelopment of the jaw and cheek bone and abnormal ears

D. Head smaller than the body

E. Cystic dilation of the lacrimal sac at the nasocanthal angle

F. Absent eyes

G. Small chin

H. Congenital defect caused by an extra chromosome, which causes a deficiency in the forebrain

I. Absence of the nose

J. Increased thickness in the nuchal fold area in the back of the neck associated with trisomy 21

K. Abnormal protrusion of the eyeball

L. Protrusion of the brain from the cranial cavity

M. Enlargement of the thyroid gland

N. Hereditary disease caused by failure to oxidize an amino acid (phenylalanine) to tyrosine because of a defective enzyme; if PKU is not treated early, mental retardation can develop

O. Eyes too far apart

Exercise 2
Match the following terms with their definitions.

1. _____ Beckwith-Wiedemann syndrome

2. _____ branchial cleft cyst

3. _____ epignathus

4. _____ hemifacial microsomia

5. _____ hypotelorism

A. Underdevelopment of the eyes, fingers, and mouth

B. A cylindrical protuberance of the face that in cyclopia or ethmocephaly represents the nose

C. Underdevelopment of the jaw that causes the ears to be located close together toward the front of the neck

D. A cystic defect that arises from the primitive branchial apparatus

E. Solid tumor

F. Eyes too close together

453

6. _____ macroglossia

7. _____ microphthalmia

8. _____ oculodentodigital dysplasia

9. _____ otocephaly

10. _____ Pierre Robin sequence

11. _____ proboscis

12. _____ strabismus

13. _____ teratoma

14. _____ trigonocephaly

G. Small eyes

H. Premature closure of the metopic suture

I. Abnormal smallness of one side of the face

J. Group of disorders having in common the coexistence of an omphalocele, macroglossia, and visceromegaly

K. Micrognathia and abnormal smallness of the tongue, usually with a cleft palate

L. Eye disorder in which optic axes cannot be directed to the same object

M. Teratoma located in the oropharynx

N. Hypertrophied tongue

ANATOMY

Exercise 3

Label the following illustrations.

1. Lateral view of the embryo at 28 days.

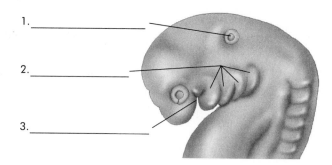

1. _____

2. _____

3. _____

2. Frontal view of the embryo at 24 days.

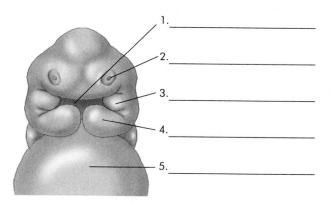

1. _____

2. _____

3. _____

4. _____

5. _____

3. Frontal view of the embryo at 33 days.

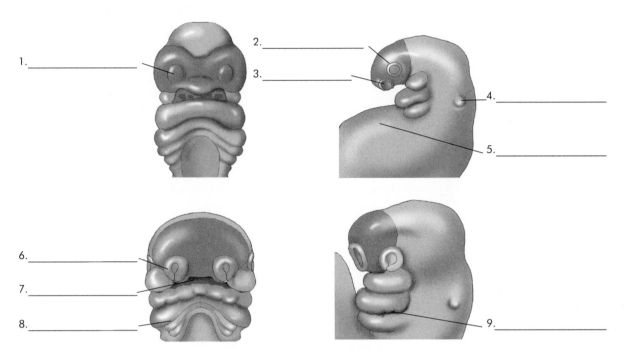

1. _____

2. _____

3. _____

4. _____

5. _____

6. _____

7. _____

8. _____

9. _____

Exercise 4

Fill in the blank(s) with the word(s) that best completes the statements about the embryology of the fetal face and neck.

1. The embryo in the 4th week has characteristic external features of the head and neck area in the form of a series

   of branchial arches, pouches, grooves, and membranes that are referred to as the _____ and bear a resemblance to gills.

2. There are _____ branchial arches; however, only the first four are visible externally.

3. The first branchial arch is also known as the _____ arch that forms the jaw, zygomatic bone, ear, and temporal bone.

4. The _____ crest cells develop the skeletal parts of the face, and the _____ of each arch develops the musculature of the face and neck.

5. The primitive mouth is an indentation on the surface of the _____ (referred to as the stomodeum).

6. The maxillary prominences grow _____ between the 5th and 8th weeks. This growth compresses the medial nasal prominences together toward the midline. The two medial nasal prominences and the two maxillary

   prominences lateral to them fuse together to form the _____ lip.

Exercise 5

Fill in the blank(s) with the word(s) that best completes the statements about the sonographic evaluation and abnormalities of the fetal face.

1. Fetal facial evaluation is not routinely included in a basic fetal scan; however, when there is a _____

   history of craniofacial malformation or when another _____ anomaly is found, the face should be screened for a coexisting facial malformation.

2. Many fetuses with a facial defect also have _____ abnormalities.

3. The fetal forehead (frontal bone) appears as a _____ surface with differentiation of the nose, lips, and chin seen inferiorly.

4. Anterior cephaloceles may arise from the frontal bone or midface; they may cause widely spaced orbits

   (_____).

5. Premature closure of any or all six or the cranial sutures or _____ causes the fetal cranium to become abnormally shaped.

6. Cloverleaf skull or _____ appears as an unusually misshapen skull with a cloverleaf appearance in the anterior view.

7. Cloverleaf skull has been associated with numerous skeletal dysplasias (most notably _____) and

   _____.

8. _____ (premature closure of the metopic suture) may cause the forehead to have an elongated (tall) appearance in the sagittal plane and appear triangular shaped in the axial plane.

9. _____ may be observed in a fetus with a lemon-shaped skull (from spina bifida) or with skeletal dysplasias.

10. An underdevelopment of the middle structures of the face is _____ or _____ hypoplasia with depressed or absent nasal bridge.

11. Midface hypoplasia may be seen in fetuses with chromosome anomalies, such as trisomy _____, craniosynostosis syndromes, such as Apert's syndrome, and with limb and skeletal abnormalities, such as achondroplasia, chondrodysplasia punctata, asphyxiating thoracic dysplasia, and others

12. A median-cleft face syndrome consisting of a range of midline facial defects involving the eyes, forehead, and

    nose is _____.

13. The optimum gestational age for the measurement of fetal NT is _____ weeks of gestation to

    _____ weeks _____ days of gestation.

14. The fetal crown-rump length should be within the range of _____ mm to _____ mm.

15. Tongue protrusion may suggest macroglossia (enlarged tongue), a condition found in _____ syndrome (congenital overgrowth of tissues).

456

16. Mandibular width is measured in an axial plane laterally from _____ to _____.

17. Mandibular length, or AP diameter, is assessed by measuring from the _____ of the mandible to the

    _____ of the lateral width line.

18. Micrognathia is associated with many conditions that can be subdivided into three groups of anomalies:

    _____ anomalies, _____ dysplasias, or primary _____ disorders.

19. The sonographer must document the presence of both eyes and assess the overall size of the eyes to exclude

    _____ (small eyes) and _____ (absent eyes).

20. A condition characterized by a decreased distance between the orbits is _____.

21. _____ is characterized by abnormally widely spaced orbits.

22. The contour of the nose, upper and lower lips, and chin is observed in a(n) _____ plane.

23. Evaluation of the nasal triad should assess: (1) _____, (2) _____, and

    (3) _____.

24. _____ lip with or without cleft palate represents the most common congenital anomaly of the face.

25. Defects range from clefting of the lip alone to involvement of the _____ palate, which may extend
    into the nose and in rare cases to the inferior border of the orbit.

26. Isolated cleft lip may occur as a unilateral or bilateral defect and when unilateral, commonly originates on the

    _____ side of the face.

27. In fetuses with epignathus, _____ may be impaired, resulting in hydramnios.

ABNORMALITIES

Exercise 6
Fill in the blank(s) with the word(s) that best completes the statements about the abnormalities of the neck.

1. The most common neck mass is _____ colli (lymphatic obstruction).

2. When a large neck tumor exists, delivery of the infant is complicated because the tumor may cause delivery

   _____ (inability to deliver the trunk once the head has been delivered) and obstruction of the airway,
   which may require an EXIT procedure at delivery.

3. A _____ observed prenatally suggests that the mother may have thyroid disease.

4. When cystic hygroma is found, there is a high risk for _____ syndrome (45, X).

5. A malformation of the lymphatic system that leads to single or multiloculated lymph-filled cavities around the neck

   results in _____.

6. Because of an accumulation of lymph in the fetal tissues, fetal _____ may result.

7. A fetal _____ usually appears as a symmetrical (bilobed), solid, homogeneous mass arising from the anterior fetal neck in the region of the fetal thyroid gland.

Exercise 7

Provide a short answer for each question after evaluating the images.

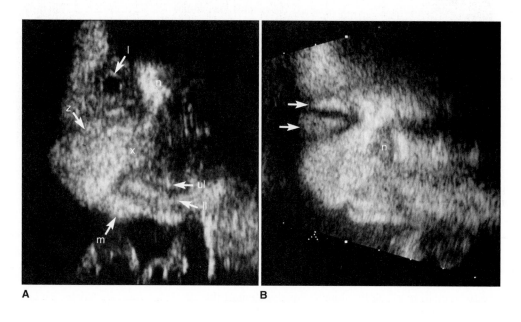

A   B

1. Identify what the arrows are pointing to in Figures **A** and **B.**

_____

_____

_____

_____

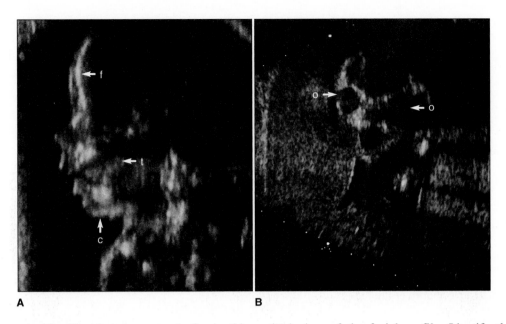

A

B

2. For image **A,** identify what the *t* stands for in this sagittal view of the facial profile. Identify the view that is demonstrated in **B.**

_____

_____

_____

_____

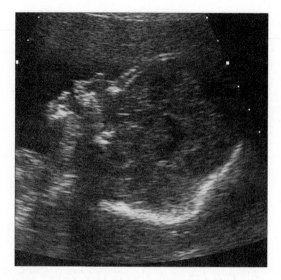

3. Describe this abnormality of the fetal skull.

_____

_____

_____

_____

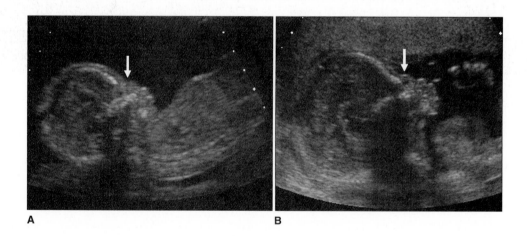

A   B

4. The arrow is pointing to this structure.

_____

_____

_____

_____

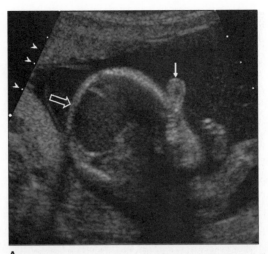

A

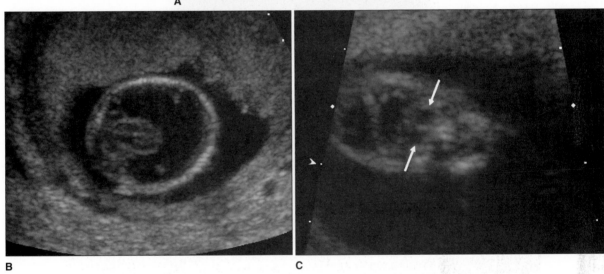

B   C

5. Describe the abnormality in this fetal head.

_____

_____

_____

_____

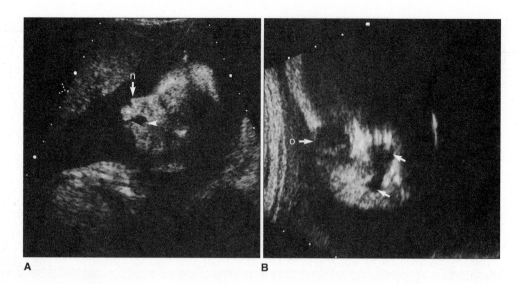

6. Describe the abnormality in this fetus.

_____

_____

_____

_____

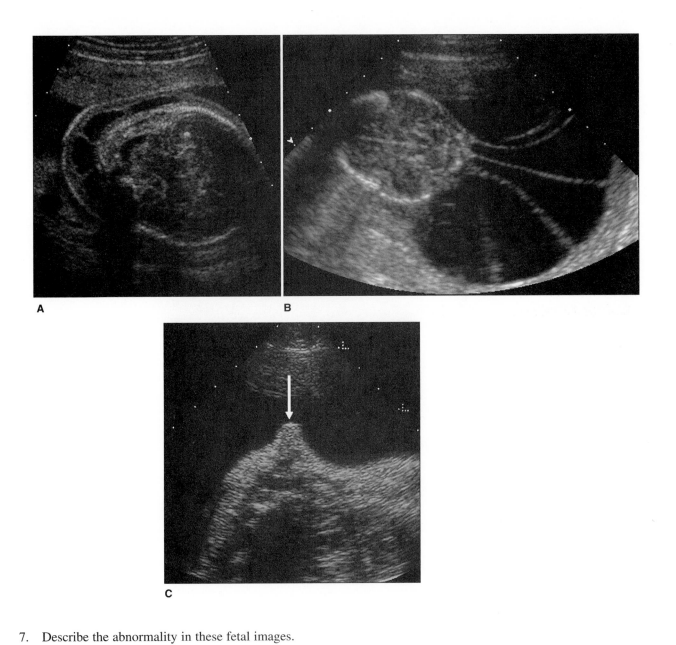

A

B

C

7. Describe the abnormality in these fetal images.

_____

_____

_____

_____

55 The Fetal Neural Axis

KEY TERMS

Exercise 1
Match the following terms with their definitions.

1. _____ acrania
2. _____ alobar holoprosencephaly
3. _____ anencephaly
4. _____ anomaly
5. _____ cebocephaly
6. _____ cyclopia
7. _____ cystic hygroma
8. _____ holoprosencephaly
9. _____ hydranencephaly
10. _____ hydrocephalus
11. _____ macrocephaly
12. _____ meningocele
13. _____ meningomyelocele
14. _____ spina bifida
15. _____ spina bifida occulta
16. _____ ventriculomegaly

A. Enlargement of the fetal cranium as a result of ventriculomegaly

B. Most severe form of holoprosencephaly characterized by a single common ventricle and malformed brain

C. An increase in size of the jugular lymphatic sacs because of abnormal development

D. Neural tube defect of the spine in which the dorsal vertebrae fail to fuse together, allowing the protrusion of meninges and/or spinal cord through the defect

E. Abnormal accumulation of cerebrospinal fluid within the cerebral ventricles resulting in dilation of the ventricles; compression of developing brain tissue and brain damage may result; commonly associated with additional fetal anomalies

F. An abnormality or congenital malformation

G. Congenital absence of the cerebral hemispheres because of an occlusion of the carotid arteries; midbrain structures are present, and fluid replaces cerebral tissue

H. Open spinal defect characterized by protrusion of meninges and spinal cord through the defect, usually within a meningeal sac

I. Ventriculomegaly in the neonate; abnormal accumulation of cerebrospinal fluid within the cerebral ventricles, resulting in compression and frequently destruction of brain tissue

J. Form of holoprosencephaly characterized by a common ventricle, hypotelorism, and a nose with a single nostril

K. Closed defect of the spine without protrusion of meninges or spinal cord

L. Neural tube defect characterized by the lack of development of the cerebral and cerebellar hemispheres and cranial vault; this abnormality is incompatible with life

M. Condition associated with anencephaly in which there is complete or partial absence of the cranial bones

N. Severe form of holoprosencephaly characterized by a common ventricle, fusion of the orbits with one or two eyes present, and a proboscis

O. Open spinal defect characterized by protrusion of the spinal meninges

P. A range of abnormalities from abnormal cleavage of the forebrain

465

Exercise 2

Fill in the blank(s) with the word(s) that best completes the statements or provide a short answer about the fetal neural axis.

1. The cephalic neural plate develops into the _____, and the caudal end forms the _____ cord.

2. The forebrain will continue to develop into the _____, the midbrain will become the

   _____, and the hindbrain will form the _____.

3. The failure of closure of the neural tube at the cranial end is _____.

4. List the sonographic features of anencephaly.

   _____

   _____

   _____

   _____

5. List the sonographic features of acrania.

   _____

   _____

   _____

   _____

6. A neural tube defect in which the meninges alone or meninges and brain herniate through a defect in the

   calvarium is a(n) _____.

7. The term used to describe herniation of the meninges and brain through the defect is _____.

8. Cranial _____ describes the herniation of only meninges.

9. Fetuses with myelomeningoceles often present with the cranial defects associated with the _____ malformation, which is identified in 90% of patients.

10. List the sonographic features of spina bifida.

    _____

    _____

    _____

    _____

11. Identify the sonographic features of DWM.

_____

_____

_____

_____

12. _____ holoprosencephaly is characterized by a monoventricle; by brain tissue that is small and may have a cup, ball, or pancake configuration; by fusion of the thalamus; and by absence of the interhemispheric fissure, cavum septi pellucidi, corpus callosum, optic tracts, and olfactory bulbs.

13. _____ holoprosencephaly presents with a single ventricular cavity with partial formation of the occipital horns, partial or complete fusion of the thalamus, a rudimentary flex and interhemispheric fissure, and absent corpus callosum, cavum septi pellucidi, and olfactory bulbs.

14. There is almost complete division of the ventricles with a corpus callosum that may be normal, hypoplastic, or absent, although the cavum septi pellucidi will still be absent in _____ holoprosencephaly.

15. A fibrous tract that connects the cerebral hemispheres and aids in learning and memory is the _____.

16. Identify the sonographic features of agenesis of the corpus callosum.

_____

_____

_____

_____

17. _____ results from an obstruction, atresia, or stenosis of the aqueduct of Sylvius causing ventriculomegaly.

18. Porencephaly or _____ cysts are cysts filled with cerebrospinal fluid.

19. A rare disorder characterized by clefts in the cerebral cortex is _____.

20. Enlargement of the ventricles occurs with _____ of cerebrospinal fluid flow.

21. Fetal ventriculomegaly typically progresses from the _____ horns into the temporal and then to the _____ ventricular horns.

22. A ventricle is considered dilated when its diameter exceeds _____ mm.

Provide a short answer for each question after evaluating the images.

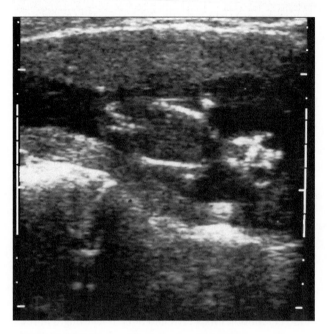

1. Mother presented with size greater than dates. Describe your findings.

_____

_____

_____

_____

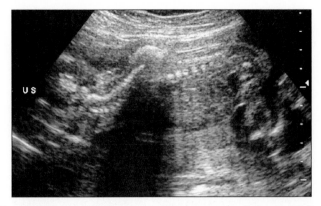

From Henningsen C: *Clinical guide to ultrasonography,* St Louis, Mosby, 2004.

2. The fetus is lying spine up. Describe the abnormality demonstrated.

_____

_____

_____

_____

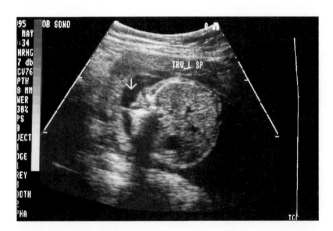

3. Describe the abnormality seen in this fetus.

_____

_____

_____

_____

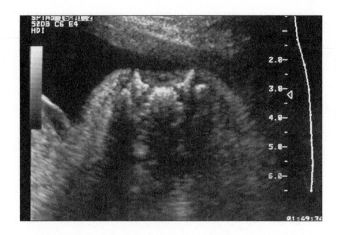

4. Describe this abnormality of the fetal spine.

_____

_____

_____

_____

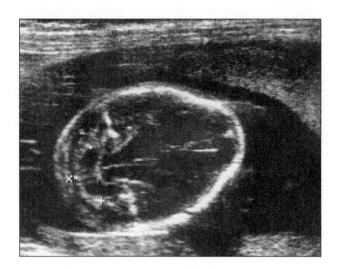

5. Describe this abnormality of the fetal head.

_____

_____

_____

_____

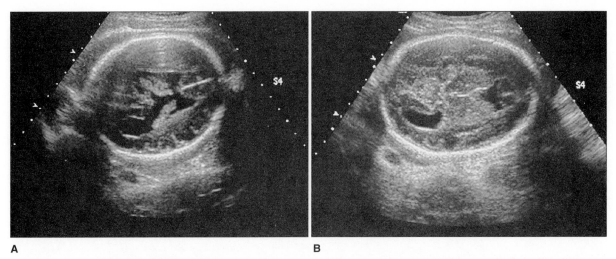

A   B

From Henningsen C: *Clinical guide to ultrasonography,* St Louis, Mosby, 2004.

6.   Describe this abnormality of the fetal head.

_____

_____

_____

_____

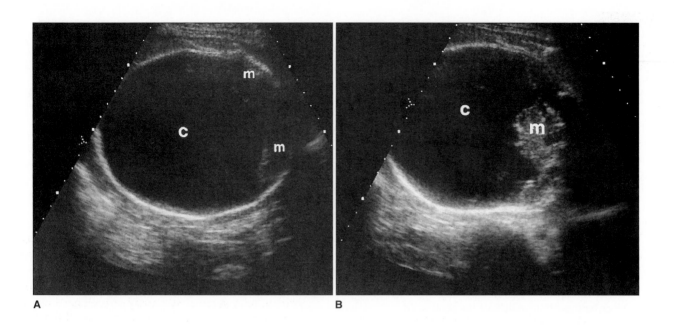

A   B

7. Describe this abnormality of the fetal head.

_____

_____

_____

_____

56 The Fetal Thorax

KEY TERMS

Exercise 1

Match the following fetal thorax terms with their definitions.

1. _____ asphyxiating thoracic dystrophy

2. _____ bronchogenic cyst

3. _____ congenital bronchial atresia

4. _____ congenital cystic adenomatoid malformation

5. _____ congenital diaphragmatic hernia

6. _____ foramen of Bochdalek

7. _____ foramen of Morgagni

8. _____ lymphangiectasia

9. _____ pleural effusion

10. _____ pulmonary hypoplasia

11. _____ pulmonary sequestration

A. Dilation of a lymph node

B. Abnormality in the formation of the bronchial tree with secondary overgrowth of mesenchymal tissue from arrested bronchial development

C. Small, underdeveloped lungs with resultant reduction in lung volume; secondary to prolonged oligohydramnios or as a consequence of a small thoracic cavity

D. Most common lung cyst detected prenatally

E. Type of diaphragmatic defect that occurs posterior and lateral in the diaphragm; usually found in the left side

F. Accumulation of fluid within the thoracic cavity

G. Pulmonary anomaly that results from the focal obliteration of a segment of the bronchial lumen

H. Extrapulmonary tissue present within the pleural lung sac or connected to the inferior border of the lung within its own pleural sac

I. Significantly narrow diameter of the chest in the fetus

J. Opening in the pleuroperitoneal membrane, which develops in the first trimester

K. Diaphragmatic hernia that occurs anterior and medial in the diaphragm that may communicate with the pericardial sac

Exercise 2

Fill in the blank(s) with the word(s) that best completes the statements about the embryology and sonographic characteristics of the thoracic cavity.

1. The lungs at birth are about half filled with _____ derived from the amniotic cavity, tracheal glands, and lungs.

2. The normal shape of the thoracic cavity is symmetrically _____ shaped, with the _____ forming the lateral margins, the _____ forming the upper margins, and the _____ forming the lower margin.

3. The thorax is normally slightly _____ than the abdominal cavity.

4. In the presence of oligohydramnios, resultant pulmonary _____ may be seen with a reduction in the overall thoracic size.

5. The location of the heart is important to document in a routine sonographic examination because the detection of abnormal position may indicate the presence of a chest _____, pleural _____, or cardiac _____.

6. The fetal lungs appear homogeneous on sonography with moderate _____.

7. Early in gestation, the lungs are similar to or slightly less echogenic than the _____, and as gestation progresses, there is a trend toward increased pulmonary echogenicity relative to the liver.

8. Fetal breathing becomes most prominent in the _____ and _____ trimesters.

9. Fetal breathing movements are documented to be present if characteristic seesaw movements of the fetal chest or abdomen are sustained for at least _____ seconds.

ABNORMALITIES

Exercise 3

Fill in the blank(s) with the word(s) that best completes the statements or provide a short answer about the abnormalities of the thoracic cavity.

1. Identify what a sonographer should evaluate when evaluating the fetus for a lung mass.

_____

_____

_____

_____

2. A decrease in the number of lung cells, airways, and alveoli, with a resulting decrease in organ size and weight causes pulmonary _____.

3. Pulmonary hypoplasia may occur when there is an extreme _____ in amniotic fluid volume.

4. The sonographer may be able to check for pulmonary hypoplasia by measuring the thoracic circumference at the level of the _____ heart view, excluding the skin and subcutaneous tissues.

5. _____ cysts occur as a result of abnormal budding of the foregut and lack any communication with the trachea or bronchial tree.

6. Accumulations of fluid within the pleural cavity that may appear as isolated lesions or secondary to multiple fetal anomalies are pleural effusions or _____.

7. In pulmonary _____, extrapulmonary tissue is present within the pleural lung sac (_____) or is connected to the inferior border of the lung within its own pleural sac (_____).

8. The arterial supply referred to in question 7 is usually from the _____, with venous drainage into the vena cava.

9. In reference to question 7, a(n) _____ solid mass resembling lung tissue is observed sonographically, usually in the lower lobe of the lung.

10. A multicystic mass within the lung consisting of primitive lung tissue and abnormal bronchial and bronchiolar-like structures is _____ malformation.

11. Congenital diaphragmatic hernia (CDH) is a herniation of the _____ viscera into the chest, which results from a congenital defect in the fetal diaphragm.

12. The most common type of diaphragmatic defect (more than 90% of defects) occurs posteriorly and laterally in the diaphragm (herniation through foramen of _____).

13. Diaphragmatic hernias may occur anteriorly and medially in the diaphragm through the foramen of _____ and may communicate with the pericardial sac.

14. Hydrops is usually not present with left-sided congenital diaphragmatic hernias unless associated fetal _____ are present.

15. On sonographic examination, a _____ congenital diaphragmatic hernia is usually found when the cardiac silhouette is displaced to the right, and an ectopic stomach is in the chest.

16. The sonographer will see the liver in the chest; collapsed bowel may be present; and the heart may be deviated far to the left in a _____-sided diaphragmatic hernia.

17. At birth the majority of infants with congenital diaphragmatic hernia have pulmonary _____ and secondary respiratory insufficiency.

18. The development of the _____ procedure has allowed such babies with severe diaphragmatic hernias a chance for survival immediately postdelivery.

Provide a short answer for each question after evaluating the images.

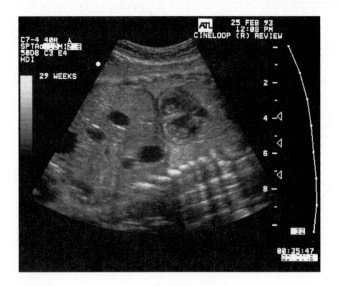

1. State whether the lungs are more or less echogenic than the liver.

_____

_____

_____

_____

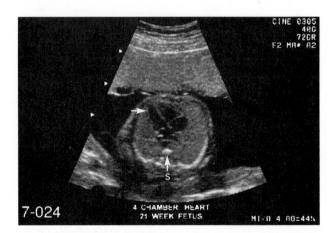

2. Describe where the apex of the fetal heart is in this image. State whether the fetal heart axis is normal in this image.

_____

_____

_____

_____

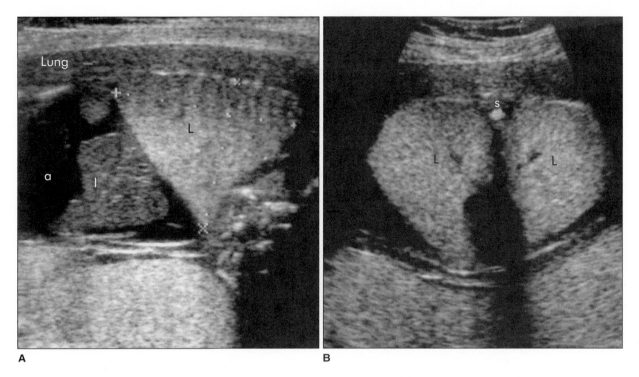

A **B**

3. Describe the abnormalities seen in these images.

_____

_____

_____

_____

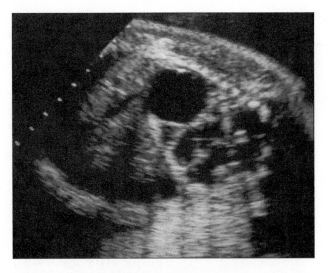

4. Describe which type of cystic adenomatoid malformation is shown in this fetal lung.

_____

_____

_____

_____

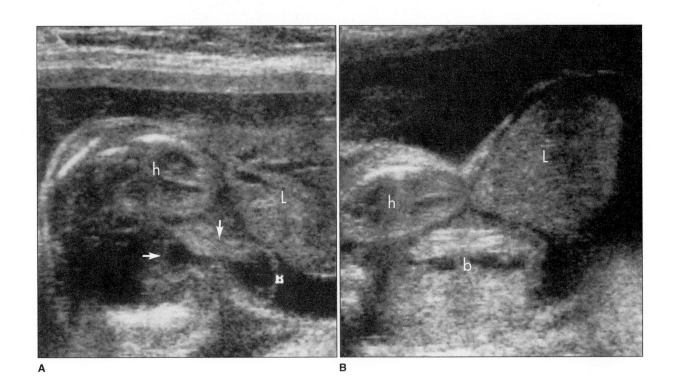

A   B

5. Describe the complication in this fetus with a known omphalocele.

_____

_____

_____

_____

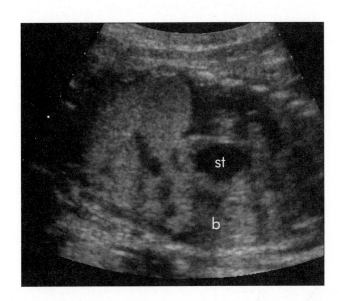

6. Describe the sonographic findings in this 25-week fetus.

_____

_____

_____

_____

57 The Fetal Anterior Abdominal Wall

KEY TERMS

Exercise 1
Match the following terms with their definitions.

1. _____ amniotic band syndrome

2. _____ Beckwith-Wiedemann syndrome

3. _____ cloacal exstrophy

4. _____ encephalocele

5. _____ exencephaly

6. _____ gastroschisis

7. _____ limb-body wall complex

8. _____ omphalocele

9. _____ pentalogy of Cantrell

10. _____ scoliosis

A. Opening in the layers of the abdominal wall with evisceration of the bowel

B. Rupture of the amnion that leads to entrapment or entanglement of the fetal parts by the "sticky" chorion

C. Develops when there is a midline defect of the abdominal muscles, fascia, and skin that results in herniation of intraabdominal structures into the base of the umbilical cord

D. Defect in the lower abdominal wall and anterior wall of the urinary bladder

E. Anomaly with large cranial defects, facial cleft, large body wall defects, and limb abnormalities

F. Abnormal curvature of the spine

G. Group of disorders having in common the coexistence of an omphalocele, macroglossia, and visceromegaly

H. Abnormal condition in which the brain is located outside the cranium

I. Rare anomaly with five defects: omphalocele, ectopic heart, lower sternum, anterior diaphragm, and diaphragmatic pericardium

J. Protrusion of the brain through a cranial fissure

Exercise 2

Fill in the blank(s) with the word(s) that best completes the statements about the fetal anterior abdominal wall.

1. The embryo is a flat disk consisting of three layers: _____, _____, and _____ that form by the end of the 5th week of development.

2. Umbilical hernia of the _____ occurs during the 8th week of development as the midgut extends to the extraembryonic coelom in the proximal portion of the umbilical cord.

3. The intestines return to the abdominal cavity by the _____ week of gestation.

4. The most common types of abdominal wall defects are _____, _____, and

   _____.

5. Abdominal wall defects cause _____ of the normal contour of the ventral or anterior surface of the fetal abdomen.

6. When bowel loops fail to return to the abdomen, a bowel-containing _____ occurs.

7. This omphalocele herniation is covered by a _____ that is composed of amnion and peritoneum.

8. Fetuses with an omphalocele that contains only bowel have a higher risk for _____ abnormalities and other anomalies.

9. _____ omphaloceles may contain bowel and demonstrate a relatively large abdominal wall defect in comparison with the abdominal diameter.

10. Gastroschisis is a periumbilical defect that nearly always is located to the _____ of the umbilicus.

11. _____ bowel is always found in the herniation.

12. _____ levels are significantly higher in gastroschisis compared with omphalocele because of the exposed bowel.

13. The edges of the bowel are irregular and free floating _____ a covering membrane, as is seen with omphalocele.

14. The rupture of the amnion, which leads to entrapment or entanglement of the fetal parts by the "sticky" chorion is

    the _____.

15. A rare group of disorders having in common the coexistence of an omphalocele, macroglossia, and visceromegaly

    is _____ syndrome.

16. A defect in the lower abdominal wall and anterior wall of the urinary bladder is a characteristic of bladder

    _____.

17. The _____ is rare and is the association of a cleft distal sternum, diaphragmatic defect, midline anterior ventral wall defect, defect of the apical pericardium with communication into the peritoneum, and an internal cardiac defect.

18. The exposed heart presents outside the chest wall through a cleft sternum in _____.

19. The anomaly that is associated with large cranial defects (exencephaly or encephalocele) is _____; facial cleft; body wall complex defects involving the thorax, abdomen, or both; and limb defects.

Exercise 3
Provide a short answer for each question after evaluating the images.

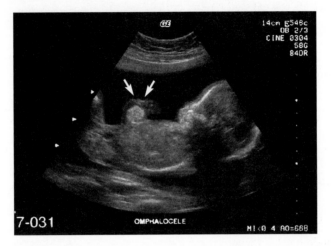

1. Name the structure that the arrows are pointing to in this 14-week fetus.

_____

_____

_____

_____

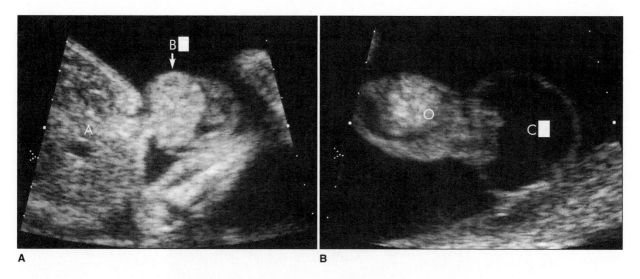

A

B

2. This is a fetus with trisomy 18. These abnormalities are seen.

_____

_____

_____

_____

_____

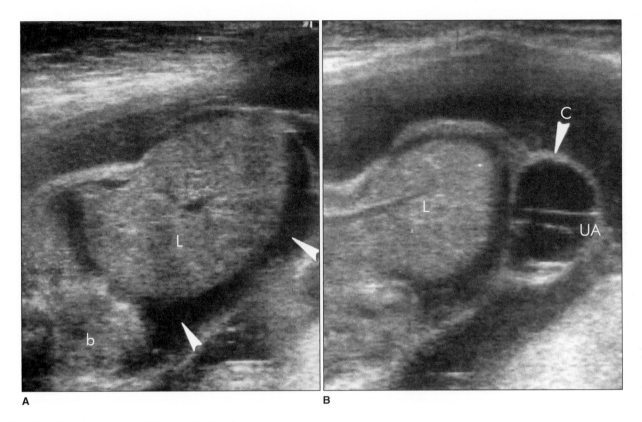

A   B

3. Describe the abnormality seen in this fetus.

_____

_____

_____

_____

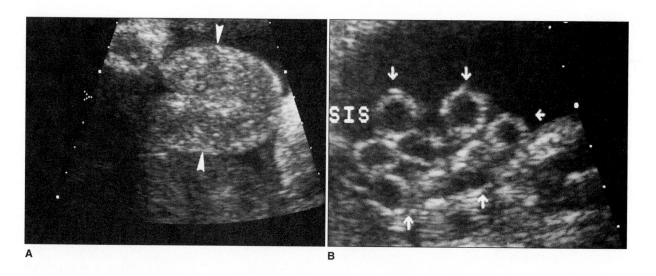

4. Describe the abnormality seen in this 34-week fetus.

_____

_____

_____

_____

58 The Fetal Abdomen

KEY TERMS

Exercise 1
Match the following embryology and sonographic evaluation terms with their definitions.

1. _____ duodenal stenosis

2. _____ esophageal atresia

3. _____ esophageal stenosis

4. _____ gastroschisis

5. _____ haustral folds

6. _____ hemopoiesis

7. _____ Meckel's diverticulum

8. _____ omphalocele

9. _____ peristalsis

A. Abnormality of the abdominal wall in which the bowel without a covering membrane protrudes outside of the wall

B. Abnormality of the abdominal wall in which bowel and liver, both covered by a membrane, protrude outside the wall

C. Congenital hypoplasia of the esophagus; usually associated with a tracheoesophageal fistula

D. Narrowing of the esophagus, usually in the distal third segment

E. Remnant of the proximal part of the yolk stalk

F. One of the sacculations of the colon caused by longitudinal bands that are shorter than the gut

G. Narrowing of the pyloric sphincter

H. Formation of blood

I. Movement of the bowel

Exercise 2
Match the following terms with their definitions.

1. _____ anorectal atresia

2. _____ asplenia

3. _____ choledochal cyst

4. _____ cholelithiasis

5. _____ cystic fibrosis

6. _____ duodenal atresia

7. _____ Hirschsprung's disease

8. _____ jejunoileal atresia

9. _____ meconium ileus

10. _____ partial situs inversus

A. Cystic growth of the common bile duct

B. Sonolucent band near the fetal anterior abdominal wall from the abdominal wall muscles in the fetus over 18 weeks

C. A congenital disorder in which there is abnormal innervation of the large intestine

D. Small-bowel disorder marked by the presence of thick echogenic meconium in the distal ileum

E. No development of splenic tissue

F. Complete blockage at the pyloric sphincter

G. Heart and abdominal organs are completely reversed

H. Gallstones

I. More than one spleen; associated with cardiac malformations

J. Vertebral defects, anal atresia, heart defects, tracheoesophageal fistula, renal and limb abnormalities

K. Blockage of the jejunum and ileal bowel segments that appears as multiple cystic structures within the fetal abdomen

11. _____ polysplenia

12. _____ pseudoascites

13. _____ situs inversus

14. _____ VACTERL

L. Mucus buildup within the lungs and other areas of the body

M. Complex disorder of the bowel and genitourinary tract

N. Condition in which only the heart or the abdominal organs are reversed

FETAL ABDOMEN

Exercise 3

Fill in the blank(s) with the word(s) that best completes the statements about the fetal gastrointestinal tract.

1. The derivatives of the _____ are the pharynx, lower respiratory system, esophagus, stomach, part of the duodenum, liver and biliary apparatus, and pancreas.

2. Amniotic fluid cannot pass to the intestines for absorption, and hydramnios results when _____ occurs.

3. The stomach appears as a fusiform dilatation of the caudal part of the _____.

4. The dorsal mesogastrium is carried to the left during rotation of the stomach and formation of a cavity known as

   the omental bursa or _____ of peritoneum.

5. The lesser sac communicates with the main peritoneal cavity or greater peritoneal sac through a small opening,

   called the _____.

6. The duodenum develops from the caudal part of the _____ and cranial part of the _____.

7. The junction of the two embryonic parts of the duodenum in the adult is just _____ to the entrance of the common bile duct.

8. Normally the duodenum is recanalized by the end of the 8th week. Partial or complete failure of this process

   results in either duodenal _____ (narrowing) or duodenal _____ (blockage).

9. The liver grows rapidly and intermingles with the vitelline and _____ veins, divides into

   _____ parts, and fills most of the abdominal cavity.

10. During the 6th week, _____ (blood formation) begins and accounts for the large size of the liver between the 7th and 9th weeks of development.

11. The derivatives of the _____ are the small intestines (including most of the duodenum), the cecum and vermiform appendix, the ascending colon, and most of the transverse colon. All of these structures are supplied by the superior mesenteric artery.

12. A remnant of the proximal part of the yolk stalk that fails to degenerate and disappear during the early fetal period

   is a _____.

Exercise 4

Fill in the blank(s) with the word(s) that best completes the statements about the stomach, small bowel, and colon.

1. The stomach should be identified as a _____ structure in the left upper quadrant inferior to the diaphragm.

2. If no fluid is apparent, the stomach should be reevaluated in _____ minutes to rule out the possibility of a central nervous system problem (swallowing disorders), obstruction, oligohydramnios, or atresia.

3. The abdominal circumference is measured at the level of the _____ sinus and the _____ portion of the left portal vein ("hockey stick" appearance on the sonogram).

4. The insertion of the umbilical cord must be imaged with _____ because it inserts both into the fetal abdomen and into the placenta.

5. The fetus is capable of _____ sufficient amounts of amniotic fluid to permit visualization of the stomach by 11 menstrual weeks.

6. After the 15th to 16th week, _____ begins to accumulate in the distal part of the small intestine as a combination of desquamated cells, bile pigments, and mucoproteins.

7. The region of the small bowel can be seen because it is slightly _____, compared with the liver, and may appear "masslike" in the central abdomen and pelvis.

8. After 27 weeks, _____ of normal small bowel is increasingly observed.

9. The _____ of the colon help to differentiate it from the small bowel.

10. The _____ does not have peristalsis like the small bowel does.

11. The meconium within the lumen of the colon appears _____ relative to the fetal liver and in comparison with the bowel wall.

12. The _____ lobe of the liver is larger than the _____ in utero secondary to the greater supply of oxygenated blood.

13. The normal gallbladder may be seen sonographically after _____ weeks of gestation.

Exercise 5

Fill in the blank(s) with the word(s) that best completes the statements about abnormalities of the fetal abdomen.

1. _____ may present as a total reversal of the thoracic and abdominal organs or as a partial reversal (mirror image of some organs).

2. The stomach may or may not be reversed in _____.

3. True ascites is identified within the peritoneal recesses, whereas _____ is always confined to an anterior or anterolateral aspect of the fetal abdomen.

4. A bowel obstruction results in _____ bowel dilatation that is characteristically recognized as one or more tubular structures within the fetal abdomen.

5. The most reliable criterion for diagnosing dilated bowel is the bowel _____, rather than the sonographic appearance.

6. A congenital blockage of the esophagus resulting from the faulty separation of the foregut into its respiratory and digestive components is _____.

7. In reference to the diagnosis in question 6, the sonographer may observe the _____ stomach and

   _____.

8. Blockage of the jejunum and ileal bowel segments (jejunoileal atresia or stenosis) appears as multiple cystic structures (more than two) _____ to the site of atresia within the fetal abdomen.

9. A small-bowel disorder marked by the presence of thick meconium in the distal ileum is _____.

10. _____ may present as part of the VACTERL association or in caudal regression.

11. Hyperechoic bowel is a _____ impression of unusually echogenic bowel, typically seen during the second trimester.

12. True ascites in the fetal abdomen is always _____; it usually outlines the falciform ligament and umbilical vein.

Exercise 6
Provide a short answer for each question after evaluating the images.

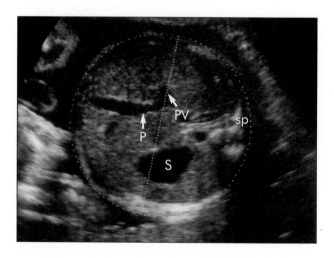

1. This image is representative of the level at which the abdominal circumference should be taken. Identify the following structures: *P, PV, S,* and *sp*.

_____

_____

_____

_____

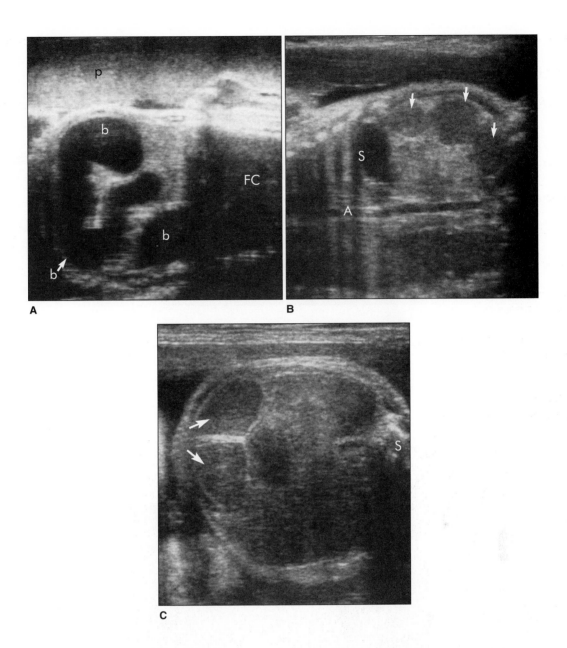

A

B

C

2. This fetus was known to have gastroschisis. Describe the further sonographic findings demonstrated in these images.

_____

_____

_____

_____

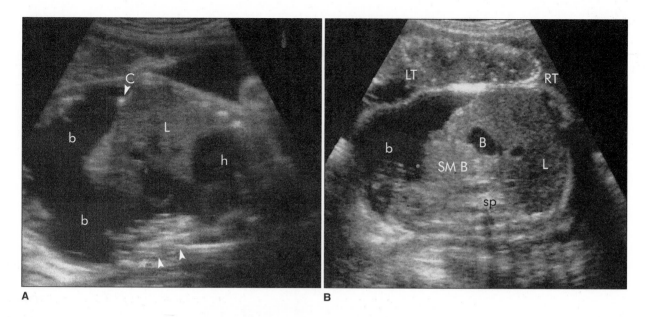

A   B

3. Describe the appearance of the fetal abdomen in these images.

_____

_____

_____

_____

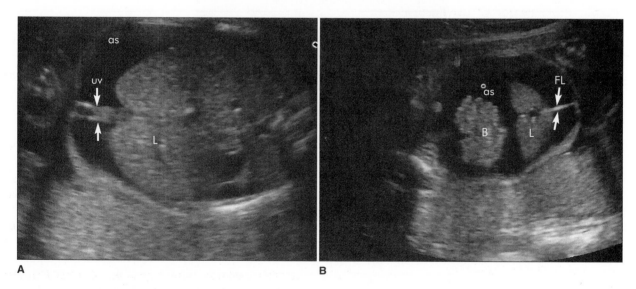

A   B

4. Describe the sonographic findings in these images of the fetal abdomen.

_____

_____

_____

_____

59 The Fetal Urogenital System

KEY TERMS

Exercise 1

Match the following urinary system and sonographic evaluation terms with their definitions.

1. _____ crossed renal ectopia

2. _____ horseshoe kidney

3. _____ hydroureters

4. _____ pelvic kidney

5. _____ posterior urethral valve

6. _____ renal agenesis

7. _____ urachal cyst

A. Renal system fails to develop

B. Dilated ureters

C. Occurs only in male fetuses; is manifested by the presence of a valve in the posterior urethra

D. Occurs when the kidney is located on the opposite side of its ureteral orifice

E. A small part of the lumen of the allantois that persists while the urachus forms

F. Forms when the inferior poles of the kidney fuse while they are in the pelvis

G. Occurs when the kidney does not migrate upward into the retroperitoneal space

Exercise 2

Match the following terms with their definitions.

1. _____ caliectasis

2. _____ fetal hydronephrosis

3. _____ infantile polycystic kidney disease

4. _____ megacystis

5. _____ megaureter

6. _____ multicystic dysplastic kidney disease

7. _____ Potter's syndrome

8. _____ prune-belly syndrome

9. _____ pyelectasis

10. _____ ureteropelvic junction

11. _____ ureterovesical junction

12. _____ urethral atresia

A. The level of the urethra where the urinary tract may become obstructed

B. Dilated renal pelvis measuring 5 to 9 mm in the anteroposterior direction

C. Dilated renal pelvis

D. Junction where the ureter enters the bladder

E. Multiple cysts replace normal renal tissue throughout the kidney; usually causes renal obstruction

F. Dilation of the fetal abdomen secondary to severe bilateral hydronephrosis and fetal ascites; fetus also has oligohydramnios and pulmonary hypoplasia

G. Autosomal recessive disease that affects the fetal kidneys and liver; the kidneys are enlarged and echogenic on ultrasound

H. This condition causes a massively distended bladder

I. Dilation of the lower end of the ureter; the common presentation of ureterovesical junction obstruction

J. Rounded calyces with renal pelvis dilation measuring greater than 10 mm in the anteroposterior direction

K. Junction of the ureter entering the renal pelvis; most common site of obstruction

L. Characterized by renal agenesis; oligohydramnios, pulmonary hypoplasia, abnormal facies, and malformed hands and feet

493

Exercise 3

Match the following terms with their definitions.

1. _____ bicornuate uterus

2. _____ cryptorchidism

3. _____ hermaphroditism

4. _____ hydrometrocolpos

5. _____ hypospadias

6. _____ ovarian cyst

7. _____ unicornuate uterus

8. _____ uterus didelphys

A. Collection of fluid in the vagina and uterus

B. May be found in the fetus; results from maternal hormone stimulation and is usually benign

C. Duplication of the uterus

D. Anomaly of the uterus in which only one horn and tube develop

E. Abnormal congenital opening of the male urethra on the undersurface of the penis

F. Failure of the testes to descend into the scrotum

G. Double uterus and double vagina

H. Condition in which both ovarian and testicular tissues are present

FETAL URINARY SYSTEM

Exercise 4

Fill in the blank(s) with the word(s) that best completes the statements about the fetal urinary system.

1. A complete ultrasound examination includes evaluation of both _____, documentation of the urinary

   _____, and assessment of _____.

2. The urinary system and the genital system develop from the intermediate _____ and the excretory ducts of both systems initially enter a common cavity called the cloaca.

3. The part of the urogenital ridge that gives rise to the urinary system is known as the nephrogenic cord or

   _____ ridge.

4. The part that gives rise to the genital system is known as the gonadal ridge or _____ ridge.

5. The permanent kidneys or _____ begin to develop early in the 5th week while the mesonephroi are still developing.

6. Urine formation begins toward the end of the first trimester, around the _____ week, and continues actively throughout fetal life.

7. Urine is excreted into the amniotic cavity and forms a _____ part of the amniotic fluid.

8. The kidneys do not need to function in utero because the _____ eliminates waste from the fetal blood.

9. The kidneys initially lie very close together in the _____; gradually, they migrate into the abdomen and become separated from one another.

10. In adolescent and adult patients, persistence of the fetal lobulation and groove may be seen on ultrasound as an

    _____ triangular notch along the anterior wall of the _____ kidney.

Exercise 5

Fill in the blank(s) with the word(s) that best completes the statements about the development of the fetal urinary system.

1. Complete absence of the kidneys is known as renal _____.

2. Division of the ureteric bud at an early stage results in a double or _____ kidney.

3. When the inferior poles of the kidney fuse while they are in the pelvis, a _____ kidney forms.

4. The fetal urinary bladder is derived from the hindgut derivative known as the _____ sinus.

5. _____ of the bladder occurs primarily in males and is characterized by the protrusion of the posterior wall of the urinary bladder, which contains the trigone of the bladder and the ureteric orifices.

6. Early in development the urinary bladder is continuous with the _____.

7. The allantois regresses to become a fibrous cord known as the _____.

8. If the lumen of the allantois persists while the urachus forms, a urachal _____ develops, which causes urine to drain from the bladder to the umbilicus.

9. If only a small part of the lumen of the allantois persists, it is called a _____.

Exercise 6

Fill in the blank(s) with the word(s) that best completes the statements about the sonographic evaluation of the urinary system.

1. The fetal kidneys and bladder may be seen on sonography by _____ weeks of gestation.

2. At this time period, the kidneys appear as bilateral _____ structures in the paravertebral regions.

3. By _____ weeks it is possible to distinguish the renal cortex from the medulla, outline the renal capsule clearly, and see a central echogenic area in the renal sinus region.

4. The upper limit of normal for the renal pelves is _____ mm up to 33 weeks gestation and

   _____ mm from 33 weeks gestation until term.

5. If the bladder appears too large, it should be evaluated again at the end of the study (assuming the examination

   takes at least _____ minutes) to see if normal emptying has occurred.

6. When obstruction occurs at the level of the urethra, the bladder wall becomes _____.

7. Dilation of the posterior _____ is highly suggestive for an obstructive process, such as posterior urethral valve syndrome, known as the "keyhole" sign on sonography because the dilated bladder has the shape of a key-hole superior to the obstructed urethra.

8. It is possible to have unilateral renal agenesis, but the contralateral kidney is usually quite _____ to compensate for this abnormality.

9. The _____ kidney shows a large central cyst with multiple small peripheral cysts to look like a pelviureteric junction obstruction; however, these cysts do not communicate with one another as is seen with hydronephrosis.

10. When the kidneys appear enlarged and echogenic, the sonographer should think of infantile _____ disease (with oligohydramnios) or occasionally adult polycystic disease (normal amniotic fluid volume).

11. Dilatation of the renal collecting system suggests either _____ or _____ .

12. Pelviureteric junction obstruction shows dilatation of the renal _____, whereas ureteric dilatation

    suggests either a _____ junction obstruction or reflux.

13. When the hydronephrosis is _____, then the possibility of bladder outlet obstruction should be considered.

Exercise 7

Fill in the blank(s) with the word(s) that best completes the statements about the pathophysiology of the fetal urinary system.

1. A critical marker in the assessment of renal function is _____ .

2. The fetal kidneys begin to excrete urine after the _____th week but do not become the major

   contributor of fetal urine (hence, amniotic fluid volume) until _____ weeks of pregnancy.

3. It usually takes at least _____ minutes to fill and empty the fetal bladder.

4. Renal agenesis and infantile polycystic kidney disease are fetal conditions _____ with life.

5. In renal agenesis, the _____ glands may be large and may mimic the kidneys.

6. _____ kidneys should be considered when the kidneys are not located in their normal retroperitoneal location.

7. _____ syndrome is characterized by renal agenesis, oligohydramnios, pulmonary hypoplasia, abnormal facies, and malformed hands and feet.

8. Infantile polycystic kidney disease (IPKD) is an autosomal-recessive disorder (25% chance of recurrence) that

   affects the fetal _____ and _____ .

9. In the most severe cases of IPKD, renal failure occurs with _____ and an _____ urinary bladder.

10. Multicystic dysplastic kidney disease is the most common form of renal _____ disease in childhood and represents one of the most common abdominal masses in the neonate.

11. Multicystic dysplastic kidney disease is composed of multiple, smooth-walled, nonfunctioning, _____ cysts of variable size and number.

12. In autosomal-dominant (adult) polycystic kidney disease, the fetal kidneys appear _____ and

    _____, and rarely, cysts may be observed prenatally.

13. In obstructive cystic dysplasia, renal dysplasia occurs secondary to _____ in the first or early second trimester of pregnancy.

14. The urinary tract may be obstructed at the junction of the ureter entering the renal pelvis (_____ junction) or at the junction of the ureter where it enters the bladder (_____ junction) or at the level of the urethra (_____).

15. If the obstruction is _____, a multicystic kidney may develop.

16. _____ obstruction produces hydronephrosis.

Exercise 8

Fill in the blank(s) with the word(s) that best completes the statements about the dilatation of the fetal urinary system.

1. Measurements of the renal pelvis have a wide discrepancy, varying between _____ and _____ mm in the second trimester and _____ and _____ mm in the third trimester.

2. Dilatation of the renal pelves should not be misinterpreted as an abnormal collection of urine within the renal pelves, _____ (5 to 9mm), or _____, rounded calyces with renal pelvis dilation (greater than 10 mm), which may lead to severe hydronephrosis.

3. Unilateral renal hydronephrosis commonly results from an obstruction at the junction of the renal pelvis and the ureter; this is called a _____ obstruction.

4. _____ junction obstruction commonly presents with dilatation of the lower end of the ureter (megaureter).

5. A dilatation of the intravesical (bladder) segment of the distal ureter is a _____ .

6. _____ outlet obstruction is produced by a membrane within the posterior urethra; the bladder wall is severely thickened with a dilated posterior urethra, the "_____ sign."

7. Sonographic findings in prune-belly syndrome include _____, mild to severe bilateral hydronephrosis, fetal _____, and hypoplastic lungs.

Exercise 9

Fill in the blank(s) with the word(s) that best completes the statements about fetal genital development.

1. The phallus elongates to form the penis; with sonography this finding is known as the "_____ sign."

2. Both the urethra and vagina open into the urogenital sinus, the vestibule of the vagina. The urogenital folds become the labia minora, the labioscrotal swellings become the labia majora, and the phallus becomes the clitoris; on sonography this is known as the "_____ sign."

3. Complete failure of the fusion will give rise to a duplication of the entire female genital tract, uterus _____ (double uterus and double vagina).

4. Duplication of the uterus or _____ uterus with one vagina may also occur.

5. If only one paramesonephric duct develops, a _____ uterus (single uterine tube and horn) is formed.

6. _____ occurs in the male fetus and is seen as an accumulation of serous fluid surrounding the testicle resulting from a communication with the peritoneal cavity.

7. Failure to completely descend results in undescended testes, or _____ .

8. The condition that occurs when errors are made determining male or female sexuality is _____ .

9. A collection of fluid in the vagina and uterus is _____ .

Exercise 10

Provide a short answer for each question after evaluating the images.

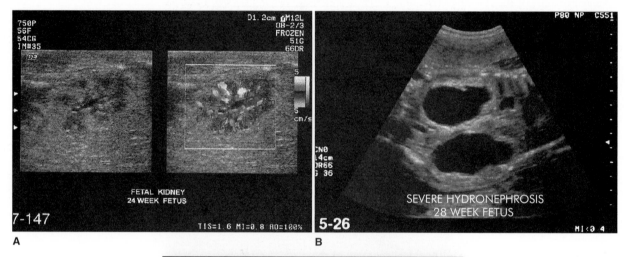

A   B

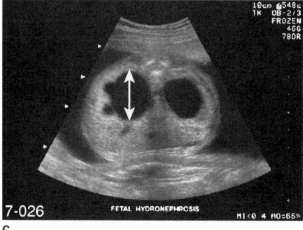

C

1. From these images of the fetal kidneys, describe how you can tell normal separation of the renal pelvis from severe hydronephrosis.

_____

_____

_____

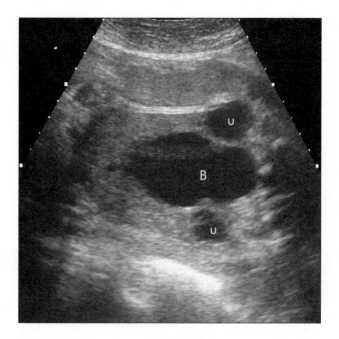

2. Describe the sonographic findings on this image with the possible cause.

_____

_____

_____

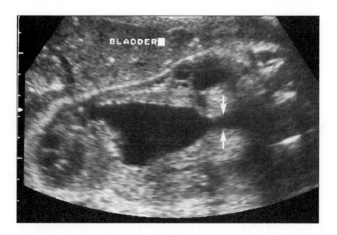

3. Name the sonographic term for this image.

_____

_____

_____

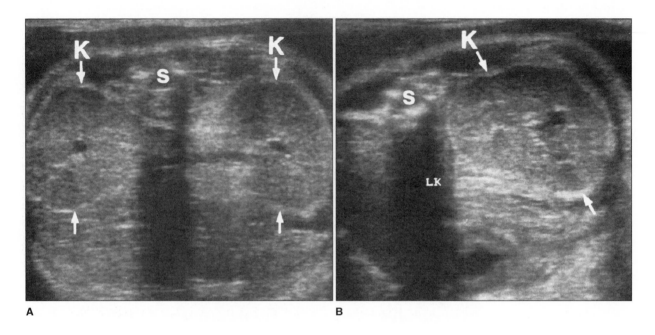

4. This fetus was known to have Beckwith-Wiedemann syndrome. Describe the sonographic findings in these images.

_____

_____

_____

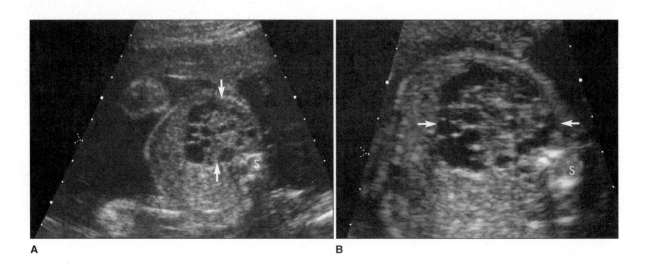

5. Describe the sonographic findings in this 25-weeks-of-gestation fetal abdomen.

_____

_____

_____

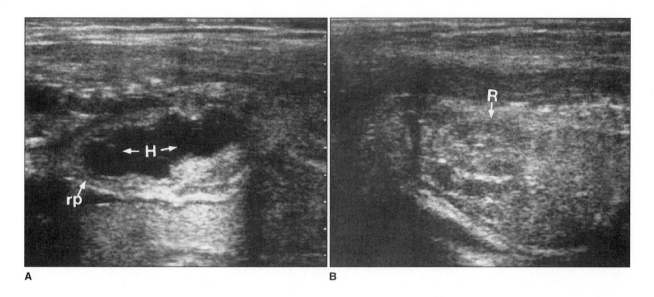

A   B

6. Discuss the sonographic findings in this fetal abdomen. Image **A** is left kidney; image **B** is right kidney.

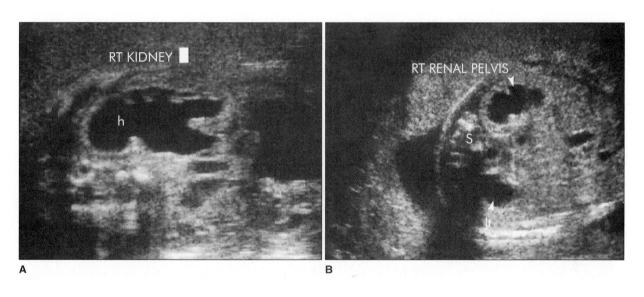

A   B

7. A 24-week fetus with oligohydramnios. Describe the sonographic findings.

60 The Fetal Skeleton

KEY TERMS

Exercise 1

Match the following fetal skeletal terms with their definitions.

1. _____ achondrogenesis

2. _____ achondroplasia

3. _____ craniosynostosis

4. _____ heterozygous achondroplasia

5. _____ homozygous achondroplasia

6. _____ hypophosphatasia

7. _____ osteogenesis imperfecta

8. _____ polydactyly

9. _____ thanatophoric dysplasia

A. Early ossification of the calvarium with destruction of the sutures; hypertelorism frequently found in association; sonographically the fetal cranium may appear brachycephalic

B. Congenital condition characterized by decreased mineralization of the bones resulting in "ribbonlike" and bowed limbs, underossified cranium, and compression of the chest; early death often occurs

C. A defect in the development of the cartilage at the epiphyseal centers of the long bones producing short, square bones

D. Anomalies of the hands or feet in which there is an addition of a digit; may be found in association with certain skeletal dysplasias

E. Lethal autosomal-recessive short-limb dwarfism marked by long bone and trunk shortening, decreased echogenicity of the bones and spine, and "flipperlike" appendages

F. Short-limb dwarfism affecting fetuses of achondroplastic parents

G. Lethal short-limb dwarfism characterized by a notable reduction in the length of the long bones, pear-shaped chest, soft tissue redundancy, and frequently cloverleaf skull deformity and ventriculomegaly

H. Short-limb dysplasia that manifests in the second trimester of pregnancy; conversion abnormality of cartilage to bone affecting the epiphyseal growth centers; extremities are notably shortened at birth, with a normal trunk and frequent enlargement of the head

I. Metabolic disorder affecting the fetal collagen system that leads to the varying forms of bone disease: intrauterine bone fractures, shortened long bones, poorly mineralized calvaria, and compression of the chest found in type II forms

Exercise 2

Fill in the blank(s) with the word(s) that best completes the statements or provide a short answer about the fetal musculoskeletal system.

1. The majority of the musculoskeletal system forms from the primitive _____ arising from mesenchymal cells that are the embryonic connective tissues.

2. The vertebral column and ribs arise from the _____, and the limbs arise from the lateral plate

   _____.

3. Initially the limbs have a paddle shape with a ridge of thickened _____, known as the apical ectodermal ridge, at the apex of each bud.

4. The fingers are distinctly evident by day 49, although they are still webbed, and by the _____ week of development the fingers are longer.

5. The development of the feet and toes is essentially complete by the _____ week, although the soles of the feet are still turned inward at this time.

6. The term used to describe abnormal growth and density of cartilage and bone is skeletal _____.

7. When skeletal dysplasia is suspected, the protocol of the obstetric ultrasound examination should be adjusted to include the following criteria:

   _____

   _____

   _____

   _____

Exercise 3

Fill in the blank(s) with the word(s) that best completes the statements or provide a short answer about the fetal skeleton.

1. Type I _____ is characterized by short, curved femurs and flat vertebral bodies.

2. Type II is characterized by straight, _____ femurs, flat vertebral bodies, and a _____ skull.

3. The most common nonlethal skeletal dysplasia is _____.

4. The sonographic features of achondroplasia may not be evident until after 22 weeks of gestation when biometry becomes abnormal. Ultrasound findings include the following:

   _____

   _____

   _____

   _____

5. Achondrogenesis is caused by cartilage abnormalities that result in abnormal _____ formation

   and _____.

6. Osteogenesis imperfecta is a rare disorder of collagen production leading to _____ bones;

   manifestations in the teeth, skin, and ligaments; and blue _____.

7. Type II is considered the most severe form of _____, having a lethal outcome.

8. A condition that presents with diffuse hypomineralization of the bone caused by an alkaline phosphatase defi-

   ciency is congenital _____.

9. Camptomelic (bent bone) dysplasia is a group of lethal skeletal dysplasias that are characterized by

   _____ of the long bones.

10. Short-rib polydactyly syndrome is a lethal skeletal dysplasia characterized by short ribs, short _____,
    and polydactyly.

11. Ellis-van Creveld syndrome may present with a _____ thorax, causing pulmonary hypoplasia, and

    heart defects, the most common of which is the _____.

12. An anomaly in which there is fusion of the lower extremities is _____.

13. For the VACTERL association to be considered, _____ features must be identified; a

    _____ umbilical artery may also be identified.

14. Amputation defects may be identified as total or partial absence and may be associated with _____
    syndrome.

15. Clubfoot, also known as _____, describes deformities of the foot and ankle.

16. _____ foot is characterized by a prominent heel and a convex sole.

Exercise 4

Provide a short answer for each question after evaluating the images.

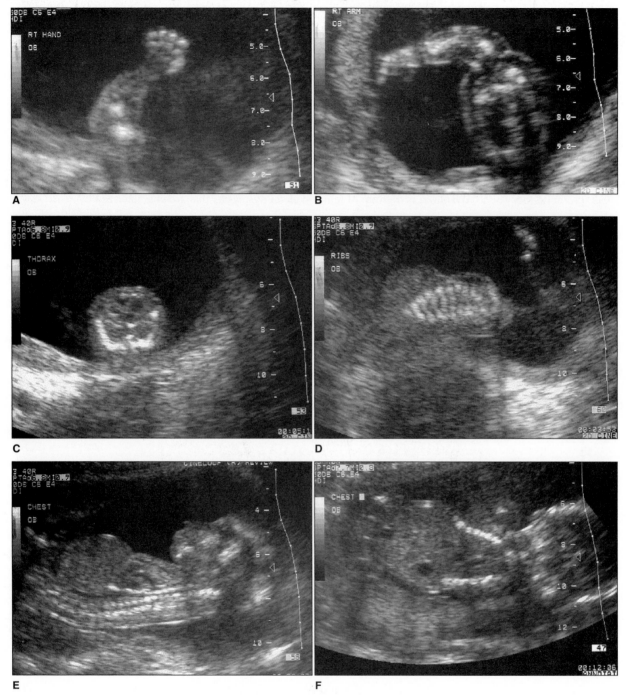

A

B

C

D

E

F

1. Discuss the sonographic findings in this fetus with a lethal skeletal dysplasia.

_____

_____

_____

_____

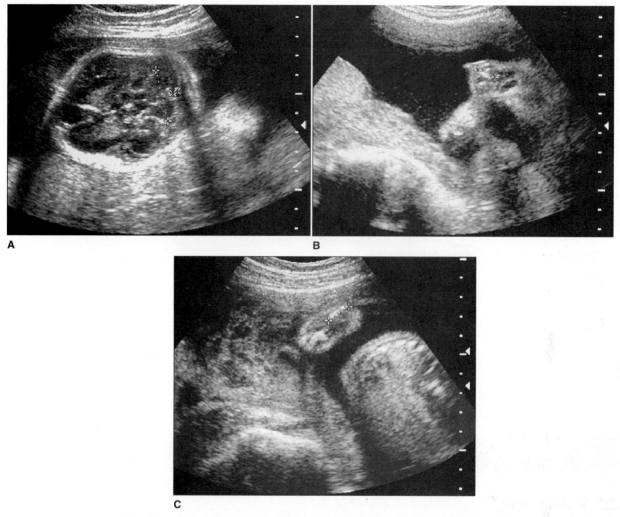

A

B

C

From Henningsen C: *Clinical guide to ultrasonography,* St Louis, Mosby, 2004.

2. Discuss the sonographic findings in this fetus with achondrogenesis.

_____

_____

_____

_____

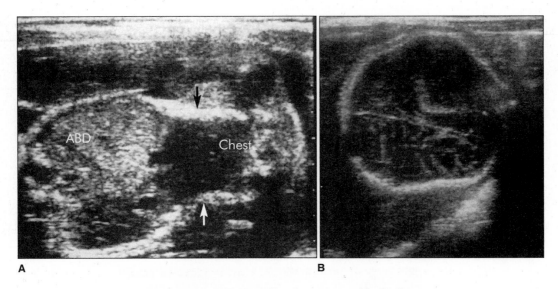

A   B

3. This fetus had osteogenesis imperfecta, type II. Describe the sonographic findings.

_____

_____

_____

_____

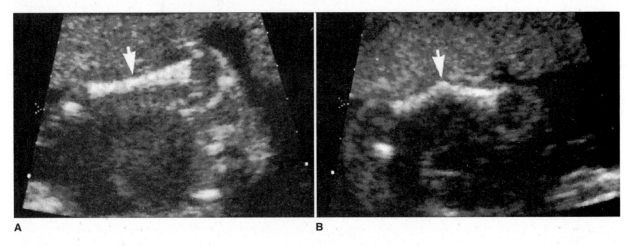

A   B

4. Images of both femurs in a 22-week fetus. Describe the sonographic findings.

_____

_____

_____

_____

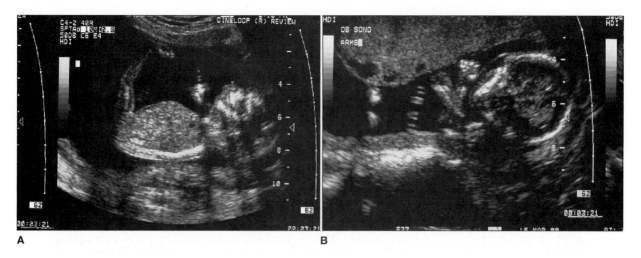

A   B

5. This 19-week fetus demonstrated findings of Pena-Shokeir syndrome. Describe the sonographic findings.

_____

_____

_____

_____

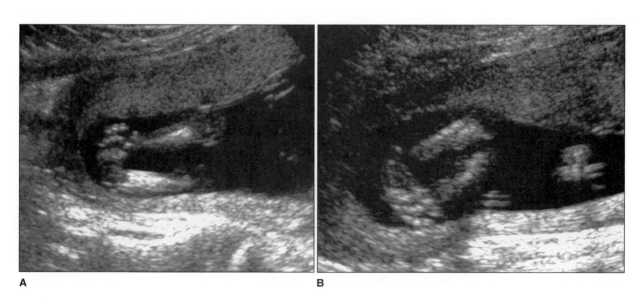

A   B

6. Images of the lower fetal extremity. Describe the sonographic findings in these images.

_____

_____

_____

_____

Image Analysis Exercises

Provide a short answer for each question after evaluating the images.

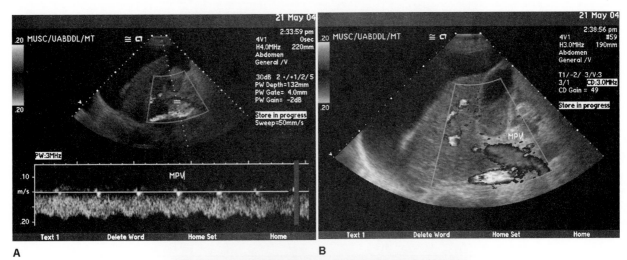

A

B

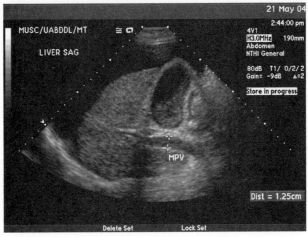

C

A 62-year-old male with abdominal distention and hepatomegaly by physical examination presented to the gastrologist for evaluation. Describe your ultrasound findings.

_____

_____

_____

_____

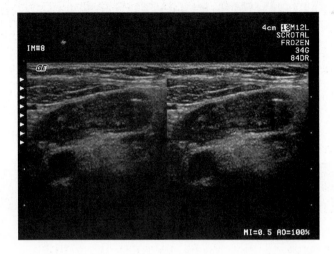

A 13-year-old female was evaluated for spiking fevers, nausea and vomiting, and flank pain. Describe the ultrasound findings.

_____

_____

_____

_____

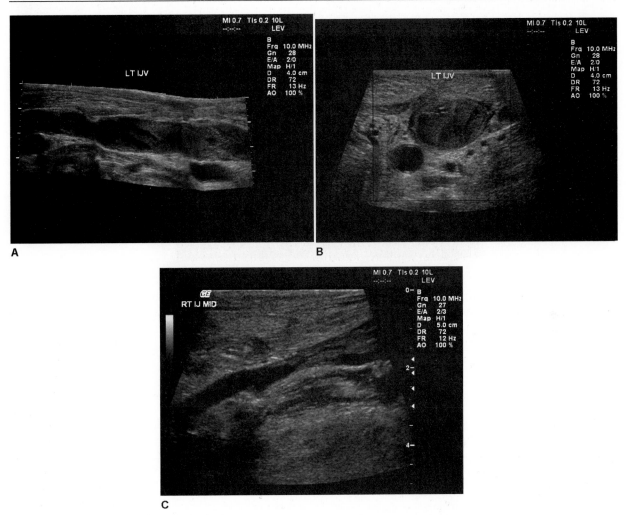

An 83-year-old male presented with right upper extremity swelling and a recent right IJ PermaCath placement. Describe your ultrasound findings.

_____

_____

_____

_____

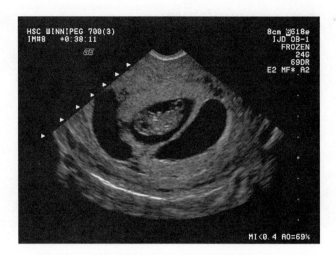

A 24-year-old female presents with several weeks of nausea. Describe your ultrasound findings of the uterus.

_____

_____

_____

_____

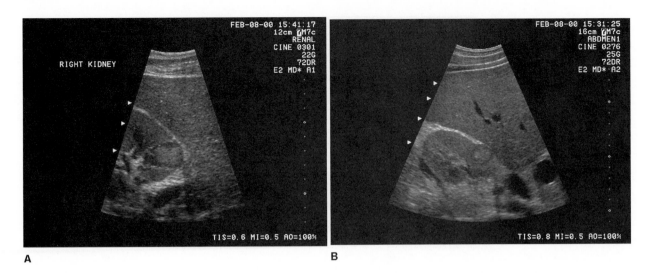

A 61-year-old male presented with right-sided pain and hematuria. The patient had a nuclear medicine scan earlier that showed a defect in the right upper pole. Describe the ultrasound findings.

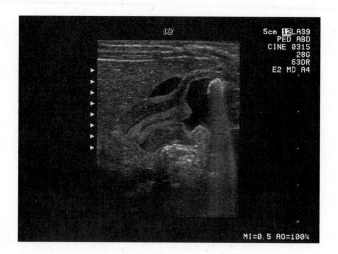

An 8-day-old neonate presented with a 4-day history of projectile vomiting suspicious for pyloric stenosis. Describe the ultrasound findings.

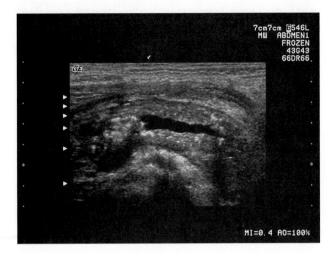

A 57-year-old female presents with a 1-week history of abdominal pain, tenderness, nausea, and vomiting. She smokes and drinks only at night. Lab values that are elevated include amylase, lipase, BUN, creatinine. Describe what you would look for and the ultrasound findings in this transverse image of the pancreas.

_____

_____

_____

_____

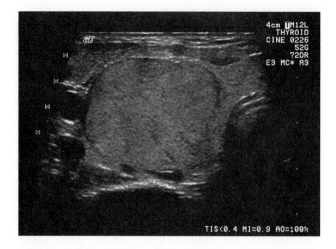

A middle-aged woman presented with the feeling of "fullness in her neck" for several months. Describe your ultrasound findings.

_____

_____

_____

_____

CASE 9

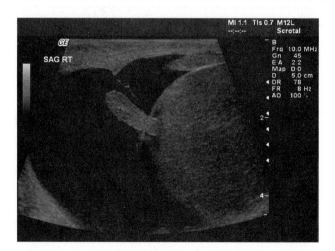

A young male presented with swelling, fever, and tenderness in the right testicle. Describe your ultrasound findings.

_____

_____

_____

_____

CASE 10

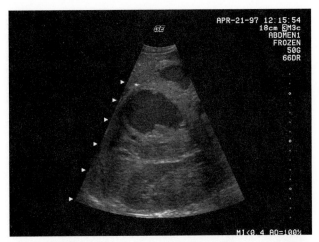

Ching-ling-Sung is a 75-year-old female with a history of acute onset of chronic right upper quadrant pain. There was a previous history of jaundice, hepatitis, and fever. Hepatomegaly was present on physical examination. Describe your findings of the pancreas.

_____

_____

_____

_____

CASE 11

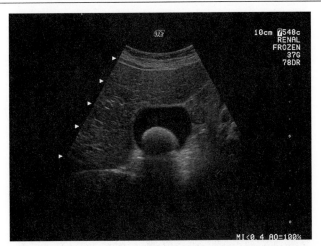

A 44-year-old obese, diabetic female with a history of alcohol abuse presents with right upper quadrant pain. Her liver function tests are mildly elevated, but otherwise her clinical information is unremarkable. Describe your diagnosis of the gallbladder.

_____

_____

_____

_____

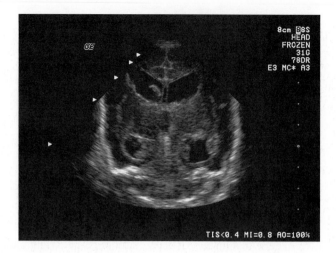

A premature infant with a difficult delivery was evaluated for neurologic changes and a drop in hematocrit. Describe your ultrasound findings.

_____

_____

_____

_____

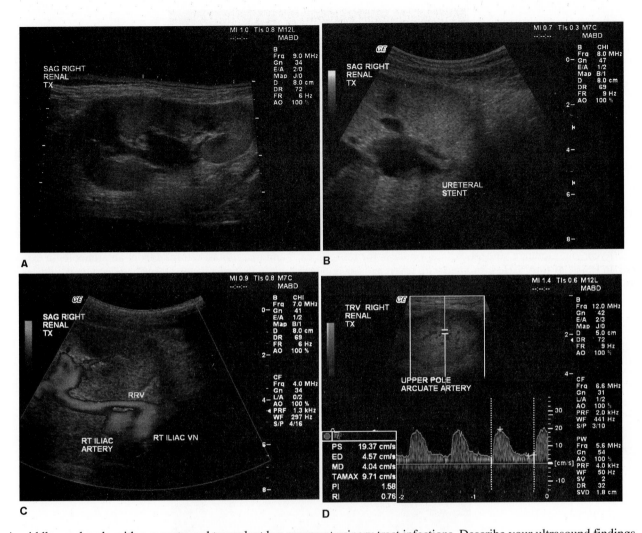

A middle-aged male with a recent renal transplant has recurrent urinary tract infections. Describe your ultrasound findings.

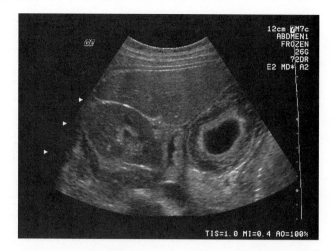

A 20-year-old graduate student, with a fondness for refried beans and margaritas, returned from an archeologic expedition in Baja California. He presented with fever, nausea, and vomiting for the past week. Describe what you would expect to find on the ultrasound and describe the ultrasound findings.

_____

_____

_____

_____

CASE 15

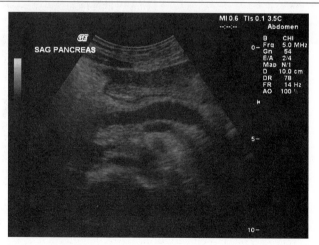

A 63-year-old female with a history of alcohol abuse, elevated LFTs, and intermittent abdominal pain came into the emergency room. Describe the sonographic findings.

_____

_____

_____

_____

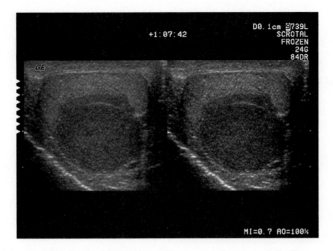

A young athlete presented with an enlarging testicle. Describe your ultrasound findings.

_____

_____

_____

_____

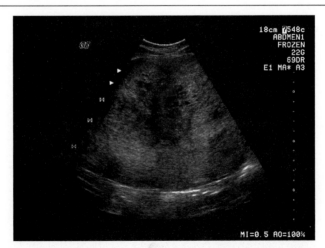

J.L. had lived as a ranch hand in Wyoming for 13 years on the Wrangle Peehs Ranch. He presented to the Mobile Medicine Man Clinic with right upper quadrant pain, abnormal liver function tests, and fever. Describe your ultrasound findings.

_____

_____

_____

_____

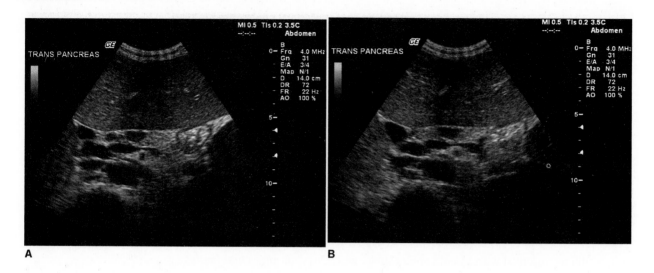

An elderly male has splenomegaly and myeloproliferative disorder. Describe your ultrasound findings.

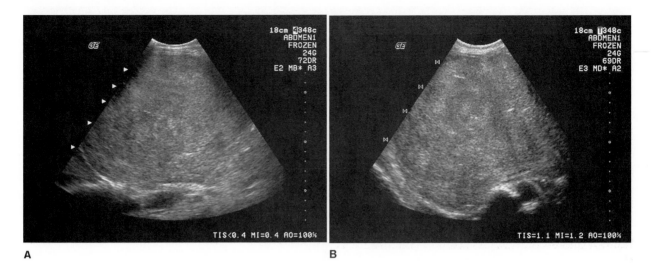

A 48-year-old male presents with abdominal pain, 30-lb weight loss, elevated liver function tests, and hepatomegaly on physical examination. He has a previous history of alcohol abuse, but has not had a drink in days. Describe your findings.

_____

_____

_____

_____

CASE 20

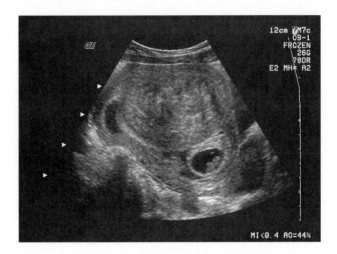

A young healthy woman with her first pregnancy is experiencing some pain and discomfort in her lower pelvic area. Describe your ultrasound findings.

_____

_____

_____

_____

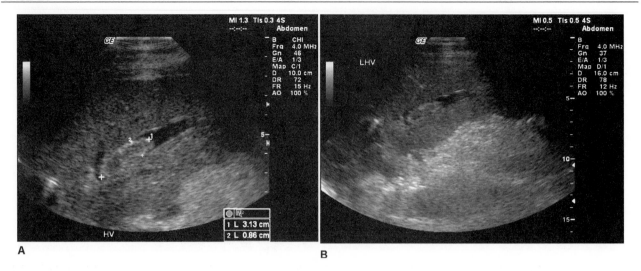

A middle-aged male has had a right hepatic lobectomy for hemangioma. Describe your ultrasound findings.

_____

_____

_____

_____

CASE 22

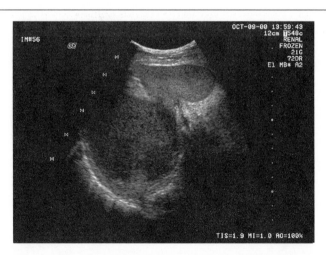

A 68-year-old male underwent exploratory laparotomy for retained common bile duct stones and resolving pseudocyst. Two weeks later, he presented with fever, sweats, and left upper quadrant pain. His bilirubin was normal, his alkaline phosphatase was mildly elevated, and there was leukocytosis with a left shift. Describe your findings.

_____

_____

_____

_____

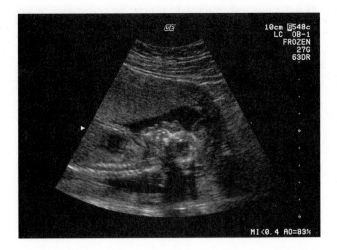

A second-trimester pregnancy was evaluated for decreased fetal movement and activity. Describe your ultrasound findings.

_____

_____

_____

_____

CASE 24

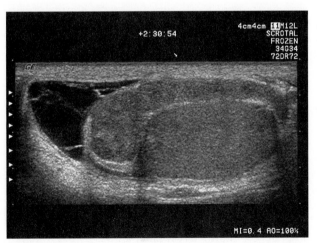

A young male presented with intense scrotal pain for 3 days. He developed a slight fever the night before the ultrasound examination. Describe your ultrasound findings.

_____

_____

_____

_____

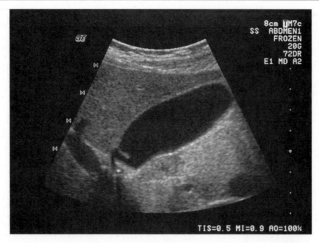

A 23-year-old pregnant woman presented to the ER with fever, increasing jaundice, and right upper quadrant pain. Describe your ultrasound findings.

_____

_____

_____

_____

CASE 26

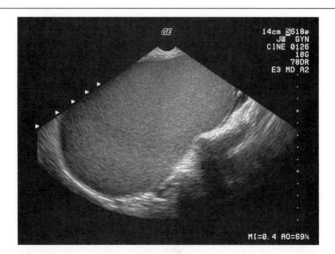

A 34-year-old female presented with ongoing pelvic pain and irregular menstrual periods. Describe your ultrasound findings of the right lower quadrant.

_____

_____

_____

_____

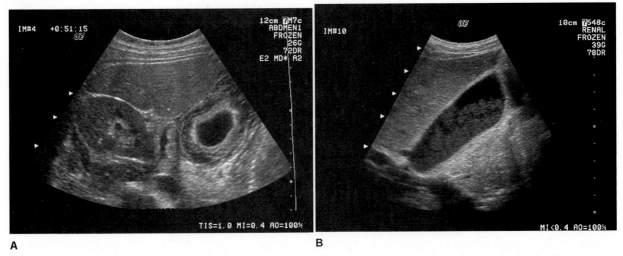

A   **B**

A 19-year-old female presented to the ER with a 3-day history of epigastric pain radiating to the back. She was nauseated for the past several days since returning from this great party at the beach house. Describe your ultrasound findings in these right upper quadrant images.

_____

_____

_____

_____

CASE 28

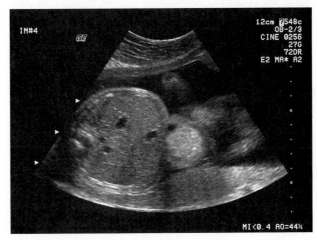

A second-trimester fetus presented with an abnormal abdominal mass on a routine ultrasound examination. Describe your ultrasound findings in this transverse image of the abdomen.

_____

_____

_____

_____

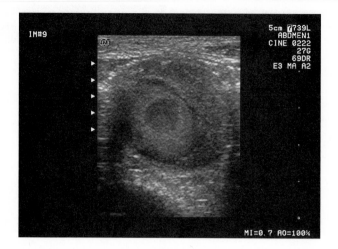

A 63-year-old female presented with a pulsatile mass in the abdominal aortic area. Describe your ultrasound findings.

_____

_____

_____

_____

CASE 30

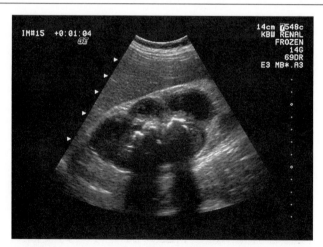

A patient with recurrent urinary tract infections is now running a fever. Describe your ultrasound findings in this sagittal image of the kidney.

_____

_____

_____

_____

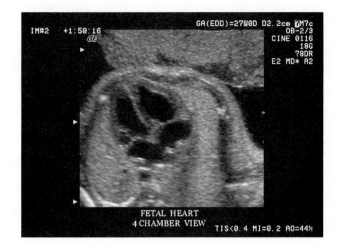

This second-trimester fetal heart shows the four-chamber view. Identify the chamber closest to the aorta.

_____

_____

_____

_____

CASE 32

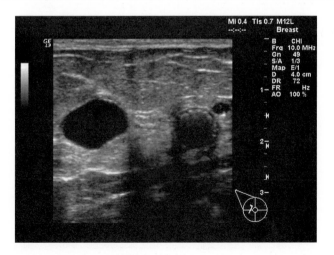

Name the criteria for a cystic mass in the breast.

_____

_____

_____

_____

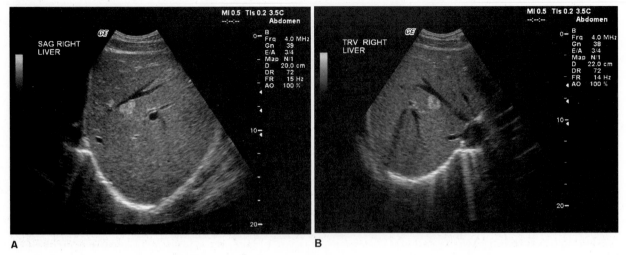

A 38-year-old male has staph bacteremia and hypotension. Describe your ultrasound findings.

_____

_____

_____

_____

CASE 34

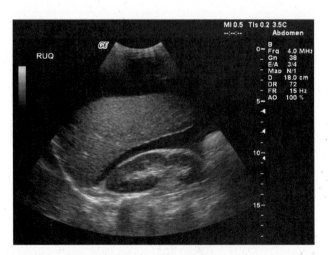

A 49-year-old male presented to his Minor Medical Clinic with a past history of six beers a day, one quart of J.D. on the weekends (only to relax), and increasing abdominal girth and increasing abdominal pain. List the lab values you think would be helpful in analyzing this case. Name your differential considerations. Describe what this image shows.

_____

_____

_____

_____

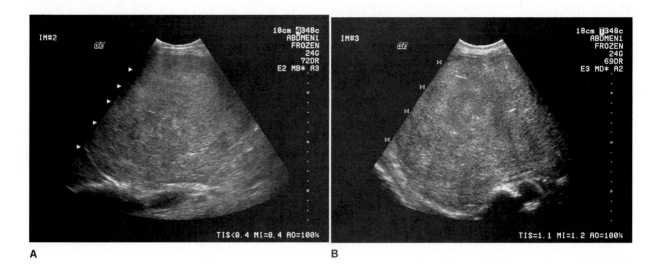

A

B

A 42-year-old female presents with a history of cirrhosis and hepatomegaly. Describe what you would look for and your findings.

_____

_____

_____

_____

CASE 36

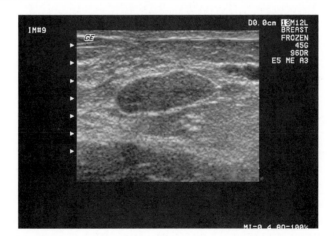

A 35-year-old female presented with a mass in the right breast. Describe your ultrasound findings.

_____

_____

_____

_____

General Ultrasound Review

Select the answer that best completes the following questions or statements.

1. Useful clinical history and clinical symptoms the sonographer should be aware of in a patient who presents with acute abdominal pain include all of the following except
   a. past history
   b. previous diagnostic examinations and pertinent laboratory findings
   c. age and present condition
   d. weight

2. The sonographer should use the following questions to help define the nature of the pain. (Identify the most specific questions.)
   a. Has the pain shifted?
   b. Locate the pain with your hand.
   c. Is there any radiation of the pain?
   d. Is the pain related to food ingestion?

3. All of the following questions relate to vomiting except
   a. Is it related to pain?
   b. How often does it occur?
   c. Is it related to inspiration?
   d. Is it associated with nausea?

4. When performing a pelvic exam, all of the following questions regarding menstruation should be answered except
   a. What was the date of the LMP?
   b. Was the LMP normal?
   c. How long have you been pregnant?
   d. Do you have pain associated with your period?

5. The following words relate to past history of the patient and include all of the following except
   a. apnea
   b. jaundice
   c. weight loss
   d. fatigue

6. Central upper abdominal pain would most likely be associated with which of the following diseases?
   a. Crohn's disease
   b. diverticulitis
   c. acute pancreatitis
   d. PID

7. Central pain with shock may be seen in all of the following conditions except
    a. cholelithiasis
    b. ectopic pregnancy
    c. internal hemorrhage
    d. dissecting aneurysm

8. An acute abdomen in a pregnant patient may represent any of the following conditions except
    a. degeneration of a fibroid
    b. hydatid disease
    c. ovarian torsion
    d. pelvic peritonitis

9. Patients who present with RUQ pain may have any of the following conditions except
    a. gallbladder disease
    b. hepatitis
    c. ectopic pregnancy
    d. renal stones

10. An abdominal trauma case may present with any of the following conditions except
    a. rupture of the liver, gallbladder, or spleen
    b. rupture of the liver, spleen, or kidney
    c. rupture of the bladder
    d. rupture of the intestine

11. Common clinical findings in patients with renal disease include any of the following except
    a. pain, frequency, retention
    b. hematuria
    c. flank pain
    d. pectoralis pain

12. The most specific lab value in detecting acute pancreatitis is
    a. serum amylase
    b. serum lipase
    c. BUN
    d. bilirubin

13. Clinical signs of urinary tract infection may include any or all of the following except
    a. fever
    b. tremors
    c. nausea
    d. flank pain

14. Alkaline phosphatase is markedly increased in patients with
    a. hepatocellular disease
    b. early obstruction
    c. hydatid disease
    d. polycystic disease

15. If there is an interruption of the IVC, what vascular structure will take over its "job"?
    a. SVC
    b. azygos
    c. lumbar
    d. iliac

16. The distribution to the liver, spleen, and stomach is via the
    a. portal vein
    b. celiac trunk vessels
    c. gastroduodenal artery
    d. superior mesenteric vein

17. The distribution of the proximal half of the colon and small intestine is via the
    a. splenic
    b. IMA
    c. SMA
    d. hepatic

18. A patient who presents with a clot in the main portal vein and hepatopetal flow in the collaterals most likely has
    a. hepatic vein thrombosis
    b. transformation of the portal vein
    c. renal vein thrombosis
    d. Budd-Chiari syndrome

19. When venous obstruction occurs within the liver or in extrahepatic portal veins, this condition exists.
    a. pulmonary hypertension
    b. portal hypertension
    c. superior mesenteric artery obstruction
    d. renal vein thrombosis

20. The most common collaterals in portal hypertension are
    a. left gastric and paraumbilical veins
    b. retroperitoneal and short gastric veins
    c. splenorenal and omental vein
    d. splenoperitoneal and retroperitoneal veins

21. The shunt that is performed via a transjugular approach is called
    a. PITS
    b. SIPS
    c. JITS
    d. TIPS

22. As portal venous flow to the liver decreases, hepatic arterial flow
    a. decreases
    b. increases
    c. stabilizes
    d. remains the same

23. Clinical symptoms of hepatic vein obstruction are characterized by all of the following except
    a. hepatomegaly
    b. shrunken liver
    c. ascites
    d. pain

24. Ultrasound excels over CT in its ability to image
    a. fascial planes and fat-containing structures
    b. ascites and intraperitoneal abscesses
    c. mesenteric infiltration
    d. omental seeding

25. The intraperitoneal fluid first accumulates in
    a. cul-de-sac or retrovesical fossa
    b. mesentery
    c. omental bursa
    d. pericolic ligaments

26. The location and distribution of intraperitoneal fluid are influenced by all of the following except
    a. patient position
    b. viscosity of the fluid
    c. respiration
    d. peritoneal adhesions

27. When ascites is found unexpectedly, the abdomen must be surveyed to detect all of the following except
    a. malignancy
    b. renal hypertension
    c. portal hypertension
    d. hepatic or portal vein thrombosis

28. Serous fluid is
    a. echogenic
    b. inhomogeneous
    c. anechoic
    d. complex

29. Peritoneal fluid that contains septations, low-level echoes, or debris suggests all of the following except
    a. portal vein thrombosis
    b. infection
    c. hemorrhage
    d. carcinomatosis

30. Which statement is false?
    a. Long-standing bland ascites may contain internal septations and be loculated.
    b. Uninfected ascites usually has no mass effect and passively conforms to intraperitoneal compartments.
    c. Abscesses never displace adjacent bowel or organs.
    d. Abscesses usually have significant mass effect.

31. Acute intraperitoneal hemorrhage is most often caused by all of the following except
    a. lymphadenopathy
    b. blunt trauma
    c. ruptured ectopic pregnancy
    d. interventional procedures

32. The _____ layer is a constant anatomic feature of the GI tract and serves as a useful landmark to identify a loop of bowel.
    a. muscularis propria
    b. submucosal layer
    c. muscularis mucosa
    d. adventitial surface

33. Neoplastic invasion of the bowel may cause a target or _____ appearance.
    a. sandwich sign
    b. comet tail
    c. pseudokidney
    d. mirror image

34. The landmarks the sonographer should use to image the appendix include all of the following except
    a. right colon
    b. cecum
    c. left colon
    d. psoas muscle

35. Complications of appendicitis may include all of the following except
    a. gangrenous infection
    b. periappendiceal abscess
    c. appendicolith
    d. cholecystitis

36. A mucocele is the result of
    a. acute appendicitis
    b. phlegmon
    c. chronic obstruction of the appendix
    d. intramural hemorrhage

37. Optimal color flow and spectral Doppler sonography of the liver requires
    a. high-frequency scanning
    b. low-frequency scanning
    c. high PRF
    d. increased scan angle

38. Flash artifact is associated with
    a. wraparound
    b. diaphragm interface
    c. color related to tissue motion
    d. decreased respiration

39. Thicker septations seen within a cyst are usually
    a. complicated cyst or neoplasm
    b. adenoma
    c. polycystic disease
    d. focal nodular hyperplasia

40. The most common benign hepatic neoplasm is
    a. adenoma
    b. hepatoma
    c. cavernous hemangioma
    d. angiomyolipoma

41. The most common liver metastases originate from all of the following except
    a. lung
    b. colon
    c. pancreas
    d. brain

42. The most common primary liver cancer in the United States is
    a. hemangioma
    b. hepatoblastoma
    c. liposarcoma
    d. hepatocellular carcinoma

43. The type of tumor that arises from the bile ducts to account for 10% of all primary liver cancers is
    a. cholangioma
    b. cholangiocarcinoma
    c. cholangiosarcoma
    d. cholangiolipoma

44. This type of abscess should be suspected when a patient presents from a high-risk population (recent immigrant from an endemic area, patients living in poor sanitary conditions, and HIV-positive patients).
    a. pyogenic
    b. echinococcal
    c. fungal microabscess
    d. amebic

45. The most common symptomatic liver tumor in children under 5 years is
    a. Wilms' tumor
    b. hepatoblastoma
    c. neuroblastoma
    d. nephroblastoma

46. In chronic viral hepatitis, hepatomegaly and inhomogeneous patchy or diffuse increased echogenicity are common and are related to the
    a. amount of fatty infiltration and fibrosis present
    b. amount of fibrosis present
    c. amount of portal hypertension present
    d. amount of vascular compression present

47. Fatty liver is a nonspecific response to liver injury and may occur in dysnutritional states including all of the following except
    a. obesity
    b. hyperlipidemia
    c. dehydration
    d. diabetes mellitus

48. Fatty infiltration is often patchy or focal. A less affected region of the liver is also called
    a. spared
    b. infiltrated
    c. hyperfused
    d. revascularized

49. In sonographic evaluation of patients with cirrhosis of the liver, all of the following should be considered except
    a. ratio of LLL to RLL
    b. nodularity of the liver surface
    c. attenuation of the ultrasound transmission
    d. increased size of the caudate lobe

50. The thyroid gland can be located at the level of the
    a. thyroid cartilage
    b. manubrium
    c. hyoid bone
    d. cricoid cartilage

51. Which of the following is typically the largest vascular structure located in the neck?
    a. common carotid artery
    b. internal jugular vein
    c. internal carotid artery
    d. external jugular vein

52. Which muscle divides the neck into anterior and posterior triangles?
    a. trapezius
    b. platysma
    c. longissimus dorsi
    d. sternocleidomastoid

53. The superior vena cava is formed by the junction of the
    a. internal jugular veins
    b. external jugular veins
    c. subclavian veins
    d. brachiocephalic veins

54. Which of the following makes up the apex of the heart?
    a. right atrium
    b. left atrium
    c. right ventricle
    d. left ventricle

55. Collateral circulation between the IVC and the SVC is supplied by the
    a. thoracic veins
    b. subclavian veins
    c. azygos veins
    d. intercostal veins

56. Which of the following is not considered a mediastinal structure?
    a. heart
    b. lungs
    c. trachea
    d. thymus gland

57. What vein passes anterior to the third part of the duodenum and posterior to the neck of the pancreas?
    a. portal
    b. splenic
    c. superior mesenteric
    d. inferior mesenteric

58. The gastroepiploic artery is a branch of the
    a. left gastric artery
    b. hepatic artery
    c. splenic artery
    d. pancreatic artery

59. The distribution of blood to the liver, spleen, and stomach is via the
    a. portal vein
    b. celiac trunk vessels
    c. gastroduodenal artery
    d. superior mesenteric vein

60. The distribution of the proximal half of the colon and small intestine is via the
    a. splenic
    b. IMA
    c. SMA
    d. hepatic

61. The most common cause for abdominal aneurysms is
    a. cystic medial necrosis
    b. syphilis
    c. atheroma
    d. arteriosclerosis

62. An aneurysm that is connected to the vascular lumen by a neck that varies in size is
    a. fusiform
    b. saccular
    c. berry
    d. cylindroid

63. The triphasic waveform seen in the hepatic veins reflects the contractility of the
    a. right atrium
    b. left atrium
    c. right ventricle
    d. left ventricle

64. Which structure is retroperitoneal?
    a. gallbladder
    b. spleen
    c. pancreas
    d. stomach

65. Which of the following arteries is NOT one of the branches of the celiac axis?
    a. hepatic artery
    b. splenic artery
    c. gastric artery
    d. cystic artery

66. Which part of the pancreas is located in the curve of the duodenum?
    a. head
    b. neck
    c. body
    d. tail

67. What is the smallest lobe of the liver?
    a. right
    b. left
    c. caudate
    d. Riedel's

68. What thin, tendinous structure connects the two rectus abdominis muscles at the midline?
    a. linea alba
    b. transversus abdominis
    c. internal oblique
    d. ligamentum teres

69. Morison's pouch is located in the
    a. subhepatic space
    b. subphrenic space
    c. paracolic gutter
    d. pararenal space

70. Which of the following does not unite to form the portal vein?
    a. superior mesenteric vein
    b. inferior mesenteric vein
    c. hepatic vein
    d. splenic vein

71. The peritoneum is divided into the _____ layer, which lines the abdominal walls, and the _____ layer, which covers the organs.
    a. parietal, visceral
    b. visceral, parietal
    c. serous, mucous
    d. outer, inner

72. The major renal calyces empty urine into the
    a. pyramids
    b. arteries
    c. papilla
    d. pelvis

73. What anatomic area would you examine to rule out a rectus sheath hematoma?
    a. posterior abdominal wall
    b. anterior chest wall
    c. lateral wall
    d. anterior abdominal wall

74. The interlobar arteries of the kidneys can be found
    a. at the base of the medullary pyramids
    b. branching at right angles from the arcuate arteries
    c. coursing toward the cortex along the lateral borders of the pyramids
    d. along the capsule of the kidney

75. The glomerulus is
    a. contained in the loop of Henle
    b. a network of capillaries encased in Bowman's capsule
    c. located in the renal papilla
    d. found in the renal pelvis

76. The apices of the renal pyramids project into the minor calyces as the
    a. convoluted tubules
    b. renal columns of Bertin
    c. renal papillae
    d. glomerulus

77. Which of the following statements is(are) true regarding the sonographic appearance of the neonatal kidney?
    a. The medullary pyramids are larger in relation to the cortex than in adult life.
    b. The kidneys are generally much more echogenic than the liver in the newborn and become increasingly less echogenic with age.
    c. In the normal newborn, the kidneys are often echogenic compared with the liver and spleen.
    d. The kidneys are generally smaller in relation to the other organs than they will appear in adult life.

78. The right adrenal gland is located
    a. anterior to the IVC, superior and medial to the upper pole of the right kidney, and posterior to the crus of the diaphragm
    b. posterior to the IVC, superior and lateral to the upper pole of the right kidney, and anterior to the crus of the diaphragm
    c. medial to the IVC, superior and medial to the upper pole of the right kidney, and posterior to the crus of the diaphragm
    d. posterior to the IVC, superior and medial to the upper pole of the right kidney, and anterior to the crus of the diaphragm

79. Arcuate arteries in the kidney are branches of the
    a. segmental arteries
    b. interlobar arteries
    c. renal arteries
    d. papillary arteries

80. The left renal vein courses
    a. posterior to the IVC
    b. anterior to the IVC
    c. anterior to the AO
    d. anterior to the SMA

81. The common bile duct can be seen at the _____ aspect of the pancreatic head.
    a. anterolateral
    b. superior
    c. anteromedial
    d. posteromedial

82. A choledochal cyst is an abnormality of the
    a. sphincter of Oddi
    b. gallbladder
    c. common bile duct
    d. pancreatic duct

83. The major renal calyces empty urine into the
    a. minor calyces and/or pyramids
    b. arteries
    c. papilla
    d. pelvis

84. Which of the following statements is TRUE regarding the common bile duct?
    a. It crosses the duodenum anteriorly before reaching the pancreas.
    b. It extends from the neck of the gallbladder to the duodenum.
    c. It is formed by the confluence of the cystic and common hepatic ducts.
    d. It courses posterior to the portal vein.

85. A thickened gallbladder wall may be encountered in all of the following states except?
    a. ascites
    b. acute cholecystitis
    c. hydrops
    d. cholangiocarcinoma

86. In a 50-year-old female, the intraluminal diameter of the normal distal common bile duct should not exceed
    a. 4 mm
    b. 5 mm
    c. 6 mm
    d. 7 mm

87. Which of the following statements is NOT true regarding the spleen?
    a. The stomach lies on the posterior border of the spleen.
    b. The spleen is positioned posteriorly in the left upper quadrant.
    c. The spleen is bordered posteriorly by the ribs and the left kidney.
    d. The splenic artery is a branch of the portal trunk.

88. Which of the following is NOT true regarding multicystic dysplastic kidney?
    a. The reniform contour of the kidney is maintained.
    b. The cysts are of variable size and have a random distribution.
    c. Contralateral disease occurs in approximately one third of patients.
    d. The normal central echo pattern of the renal pelvis is generally absent.

89. An 8-year-old boy presents with a recent sore throat, hematuria and proteinuria, urinary red cell casts, and a slightly elevated BUN. His history is very suggestive of acute poststreptococcal glomerulonephritis. Which of the following is false?
    a. The renal sonogram may demonstrate a diffuse increase in cortical echogenicity similar to that of the renal sinus.
    b. Acute glomerulonephritis is usually an incidental finding.
    c. The kidneys may be enlarged in acute glomerulonephritis.
    d. The disease may reverse or progress to end-stage renal disease.

90. Which of the following is NOT a true statement about renal allograft rejection?
    a. The allograft increases in size at a greater rate than that associated with compensatory hypertrophy.
    b. Shrinking and increased echogenicity of the renal medullary pyramids occurs.
    c. The size and echogenicity of the central renal sinus fat is diminished.
    d. The allograft may lose its elliptical configuration and become more globular in shape.

91. Which of the following is NOT a sign of renal transplant rejection?
    a. enlargement and decreased echogenicity of the pyramids
    b. hyperechoic cortex
    c. localized area of renal parenchyma presenting with an anechoic appearance
    d. hydronephrosis

92. Sonographic findings of acute cholecystitis include all of the following except
    a. positive Murphy's sign
    b. thickened gallbladder wall
    c. hydrops
    d. contracted gallbladder filled with stones

93. A tumor of the adrenal medulla that produces intermittent hypertension is
    a. neuroblastoma
    b. adenoma
    c. pheochromocytoma
    d. hyperplasia

94. A fluid collection that tends to occur 2 to 6 weeks posttransplantation and is associated with a chronic diminution in renal function rather than an acute decrease in urine output is the
    a. seroma
    b. abscess
    c. urinoma
    d. lymphocele

95. Which of the following describes the Doppler criteria used to diagnose acute vascular rejection of a renal allograft?

    a. In acute vascular rejection, the diastolic flow in the renal, arcuate, and interlobar arteries rises significantly in relation to the systolic value.

    b. In acute vascular rejection, the diastolic value in the renal artery decreases in relation to the systolic value in the interlobar and arcuate arteries.

    c. In acute vascular rejection, the systolic to diastolic ratio decreases in the arcuate, interlobar, and renal artery.

    d. In acute vascular rejection, the diastolic flow decreases, reverses, or becomes absent in the renal, arcuate, and interlobar arteries, increasing the systolic to diastolic ratio.

96. Which of the following would most likely cause anterior displacement of the superior mesenteric artery and vein?

    a. pancreatic neoplasm

    b. paraaortic lymphadenopathy

    c. cholelithiasis

    d. small-bowel obstruction

97. Courvoisier's gallbladder is associated with

    a. cholesterolosis

    b. multiple cholesterol polyps

    c. pancreatic head mass

    d. chronic cholecystitis

98. A form of infection seen in patients with obstruction secondary to longstanding calculi and chronic renal infections is

    a. acute lobar nephronia

    b. acute bacterial nephritis

    c. xanthogranulomatous pyelonephritis

    d. chronic atrophic pyelonephritis

99. A localized process in the kidney that forms a wedge-shaped phlegmonous lesion in which no true abscess exists is a

    a. renal carbuncle

    b. acute lobar nephronia

    c. xanthogranulomatous pyelonephritis

    d. chronic atrophic pyelonephritis

100. Empyema of the gallbladder refers to

    a. gas in the gallbladder wall

    b. pus-filled gallbladder

    c. distention of the gallbladder with mucus and stones

    d. calcified gallbladder

101. Which of the following is NOT a true statement regarding adult polycystic disease?

    a. It is a form of primary renal disease transmitted as an autosomal-dominant trait.

    b. Typically patients present with a large kidney, which contains multiple cysts of varying sizes, loss of the reniform contour, and no definable central echo complex.

    c. Associated cysts are always found in the liver and pancreas.

    d. Clinically patients present with deteriorating renal function.

102. The blood supply to the gallbladder is accomplished by the
    a. gastroduodenal artery
    b. right gastric artery
    c. portal vein
    d. cystic artery

103. Cholangitis refers to
    a. inflammation of a bile duct
    b. inflammation of the gallbladder
    c. inflammation of a choledochal cyst
    d. inflammation of the bladder

104. A high level of serum amylase may be a result of
    a. liver disease
    b. dilated intrahepatic ducts
    c. pancreatitis
    d. insulinoma

105. Which of the following is NOT a retroperitoneal structure?
    a. pancreas
    b. kidney
    c. adrenal
    d. liver

106. The PRIMARY hormones produced in the pancreas are
    a. glucagon and insulin
    b. collagen and fibrin
    c. lipase and cholase
    d. pancreatin and secretin

107. The membrane that lines the abdominal cavity is the
    a. retroperitoneum
    b. omentum
    c. mesentery
    d. peritoneum

108. Chronic pancreatitis is usually associated with all of the following sonographic patterns except
    a. hyperechoic, more echogenic than liver
    b. generalized decrease in size
    c. bright, discrete echoes from calcification, dilated pancreatic duct
    d. hypoechoic with diffuse swelling

109. The targetlike structure, anterior to the aorta, posterior to the left lobe of the liver, represents the normal
    a. appendix
    b. pylorus
    c. antrum
    d. esophagogastric junction

110. Which of the following statements about the right crus of the diaphragm is true?
    a. It is larger and longer than the left.
    b. It attaches the psoas muscle to the diaphragm.
    c. It is the frequent site of metastasis in lymphoma.
    d. It is shorter than the left.

111. Which of the following does not describe the pancreas?
    a. It lies within the peritoneal space.
    b. It is a retroperitoneal structure.
    c. It is nonencapsulated.
    d. It is a multilobulated gland.

112. Which of the following is the correct order of abdominal wall structures from the skin inward?
    a. linea alba, rectus muscle, subcutaneous fat
    b. subcutaneous fat, rectus sheath, rectus muscle, peritoneum
    c. peritoneum, linea alba, rectus sheath
    d. rectus muscle, peritoneum, linea alba

113. With aging, the pancreas becomes
    a. smaller and more echogenic
    b. larger and more echogenic
    c. smaller and less echogenic
    d. the same and less echogenic

114. The most common posthepatic transplant vascular complication is
    a. portal vein thrombosis
    b. hepatic artery thrombosis
    c. portal hypertension
    d. hepatic vein thrombosis

115. The most common abdominal organ transplant performed is
    a. pancreas
    b. liver
    c. renal
    d. heart

116. The aorta is named the "abdominal aorta" when it passes through the
    a. diaphragm
    b. Glisson's capsule
    c. spleen hiatus
    d. aortic arch

117. Atherosclerosis involves the accumulation of lipids in the
    a. intima only
    b. media only
    c. intima and media
    d. adventitia only

118. The most common type of aneurysm is
    a. saccular
    b. mycotic
    c. fusiform
    d. pseudoaneurysm

119. A complication of pancreatitis is
    a. formation of islet cell tumor
    b. formation of pseudocyst
    c. formation of cystadenoma
    d. pancreatic carcinoma

120. The most common cause of aortic aneurysm is
    a. infection
    b. atherosclerosis
    c. trauma
    d. congenital

121. The spleen is a peritoneal structure lying between
    a. the right hemidiaphragm and the stomach
    b. the left hemidiaphragm and the stomach
    c. the hepatic flexure of the colon and the left kidney
    d. spleen is not peritoneal

122. The most echogenic organ or structure listed below is the
    a. liver
    b. spleen
    c. renal sinus
    d. pancreas

123. The remnant of the fetal umbilical vein is the
    a. main lobar fissure
    b. ligamentum venosum
    c. falciform ligament
    d. ligamentum teres

124. Focal calcifications seen in the spleen as small, bright, echogenic foci with or without shadow are often the result of
    a. metastasis
    b. primary neoplasm
    c. previous granulomatous infections
    d. hydatid disease

125. Splenomegaly may be associated with diffuse splenic disease that includes all of the following except
    a. sickle cell
    b. hereditary spherocytosis
    c. polycythemia vera
    d. abscess

126. The pancreas is both an exocrine and endocrine gland. The endocrine function is to produce
    a. insulin
    b. lipase
    c. amylase
    d. trypsin

127. Mild to moderate splenomegaly is most often caused by all of the following except
    a. infection, portal hypertension, or AIDS
    b. metastatic disease
    c. trauma
    d. leukemia

128. A phlegmon of the pancreas represents
    a. an inflammatory process
    b. a malignant neoplasm
    c. a benign adenoma
    d. a functioning islet cell tumor

129. If a mass in the head of the pancreas is found, special attention should be directed to which of the following areas?
    a. the portal vein for portal hypertension
    b. the liver for fatty changes
    c. the spleen for splenomegaly
    d. the bile ducts for dilatation

130. When the gallbladder fundus is folded over on itself, it is called
    a. junctional fold
    b. Hartmann's pouch
    c. phrygian cap
    d. Morison's pouch

131. One sonographic method to distinguish dilated bile ducts is by demonstrating the
    a. double-barrel shotgun sign
    b. Mirizzi syndrome
    c. Courvoisier's sign
    d. stop sign

132. A congenital insertion of the CBD into the pancreatic duct causing a focal and abnormal dilatation of the CBD is called
    a. sclerosing cholangitis
    b. Courvoisier's gallbladder
    c. choledochal cyst
    d. biliary atresia

133. Adenomyomatosis of the gallbladder is
    a. proliferation and thickening of the epithelial layer with glandlike outpouchings in the wall
    b. an inflammation of the gallbladder wall
    c. strongly associated with a positive Murphy's sign
    d. always accompanied by dilated ducts

134. A 42-year-old female presents with right upper quadrant pain and nausea that comes and goes. Her sonogram reveals a normal-sized gallbladder with a slightly thick wall and contains a small, echogenic focus that casts an acoustic shadow. This most likely represents
    a. choledochal cyst
    b. cholangitis
    c. cholelithiasis with chronic cholecystitis
    d. choledocholithiasis with intermittent jaundice

135. Nonshadowing, nonmobile, echogenic foci attached to the gallbladder wall most likely represent
    a. calculi
    b. gravel
    c. sludge
    d. polyps

136. Thick, viscid bile ("sludge") within the gallbladder indicates
    a. obstruction of the intrahepatic ducts
    b. an incidental finding sometimes linked to gallbladder pathology
    c. the definite presence of calculi
    d. carcinoma of the gallbladder

137. All of the following describe the appearance of a gallbladder filled with stones is all of the following except
    a. WES triad
    b. double arc sign
    c. two parallel echogenic lines separated by a thin anechoic space with distal acoustic shadowing
    d. single echogenic line from the falciform ligament with posterior shadowing

138. The usual sonographic appearance of acute pancreatitis is
    a. hyperechoic and generalized decrease in size
    b. hypoechoic and generalized enlargement
    c. isoechoic and generalized increase in size
    d. isoechoic and increase in size

139. Focal gallbladder tenderness is referred to as
    a. Mirizzi syndrome
    b. Courvoisier's sign
    c. Klatskin's sign
    d. positive Murphy's sign

140. Perforation of the gallbladder is strongly associated with
    a. gangrenous cholecystitis
    b. acute cholecystitis
    c. chronic cholecystitis
    d. biliary atresia

141. In regards to bile duct dimensions after a cholecystectomy, the size of the CHD or CBD may be
    a. somewhat larger
    b. somewhat smaller
    c. slow to return to normal size for several months
    d. shortened

142. Jaundice is due to a buildup of _____ in the body.
    a. glycogen
    b. urea
    c. heparin
    d. bilirubin

143. One way to distinguish hepatic veins from portal veins is by
    a. size; the hepatic veins are much smaller than the portal veins
    b. tracing them to their points of origin
    c. the decrease in caliber as they approach the IVC
    d. visualizing the wall thickness of the vessels knowing that hepatic veins have thicker walls

144. A patent umbilical vein may be found in the
    a. ligamentum venosum
    b. main labor fissure
    c. ligamentum teres
    d. intersegmental fissure

145. The portal veins can be distinguished from the hepatic veins by their
    a. thicker wall and echogenic rim surrounding them
    b. thin wall and echo-poor rim surrounding them
    c. origin to the IVC
    d. close proximity to the periphery
    e. clusterlike appearance close to the hepatic periphery

146. The portal triad consists of
    a. portal vein, hepatic artery, bile duct
    b. left hepatic vein, middle hepatic vein, right hepatic vein
    c. common duct, cystic duct, pancreatic duct
    d. caudate lobe of liver, right lobe of liver, left lobe of liver
    e. hepatocellular carcinoma

147. A high level of serum lipase would be most associated with
    a. liver disease
    b. dilated intrahepatic ducts
    c. pancreatitis
    d. insulinoma

148. Which of the following is the most common site for pseudocyst formation?
    a. iliac fossa
    b. lesser sac
    c. Morison's pouch
    d. pouch of Douglas

149. The celiac axis gives rise to the following vessels except
    a. splenic artery
    b. hepatic artery
    c. superior mesenteric artery
    d. left gastric artery

150. A linear echodensity that connects the gallbladder to the main portal vein is the
    a. ligamentum teres
    b. main lobar fissure
    c. ligamentum venosum
    d. coronary ligament

151. Chronic pancreatitis is most often caused by
    a. cholelithiasis
    b. ETOH abuse
    c. trauma
    d. choledocholithiasis

152. The vessel that can be seen posterior to the IVC is the
    a. right renal artery
    b. splenic artery
    c. pancreaticoduodenal artery
    d. left renal vein

153. Which of the following vessels courses between the SMA and aorta?
    a. right renal vein
    b. right renal artery
    c. gastroduodenal artery
    d. left renal vein

154. Which of the following structures is seen in close relation to the anterolateral aspect of the head of the pancreas?
    a. common bile duct
    b. pancreaticoduodenal artery
    c. right gastric vein
    d. gastroduodenal artery

155. In the liver, the right and left hepatic ducts will join to form the
    a. cystic duct
    b. common bile duct
    c. valves of Heister
    d. common hepatic duct

156. Calcifications, pancreatic duct dilatation, and pseudocyst formation are most consistent with
    a. islet cell tumor
    b. acute and chronic pancreatitis
    c. cholelithiasis
    d. adenocarcinoma

157. Budd-Chiari syndrome may present sonographically as
    a. relative enlargement of the caudate lobe caused by hepatic vein thrombosis of the liver
    b. relative shrinkage of the caudate lobe caused by splenic vein thrombosis
    c. relative enlargement of the quadrate lobe caused by splenic vein thrombosis
    d. relative shrinkage of all of the lobes of the liver caused by IVC thrombosis

158. The liver is supplied with blood via the
    a. inferior vena cava and hepatic veins
    b. splenic artery and splenic vein
    c. abdominal aorta and iliac artery
    d. hepatic artery and portal vein

159. The normal echographic pattern of the liver is
    a. diffusely inhomogeneous throughout
    b. patchy areas of increased echogenicity
    c. decreased areas of echogenicity diffusely situated
    d. homogeneous throughout without interruption of the echo pattern

160. Lymphocele is a fluid collection caused by
    a. lymph duct obstruction secondary to inflammation
    b. agenesis of a lymphatic chain
    c. lymph-filled spaces secondary to surgery
    d. enlarged lymph nodes secondary to neoplasm

161. The segments of the right lobe of the liver are
    a. medial and lateral
    b. anterior and posterior
    c. cephalad and caudad
    d. caudad and quadrate

162. Loculations within ascites are most commonly the result of
    a. malignancy or inflammation
    b. benign conditions
    c. pedal edema
    d. pleural effusions

163. Riedel's lobe is a normal liver variant defined as a(an)
    a. elongated left lobe of the liver
    b. tonguelike extension of the caudate lobe of the liver
    c. tonguelike extension of the right lobe of the liver
    d. tonguelike extension of the quadrate lobe of the liver

164. Ascites is defined as accumulation of fluid in the
    a. abdominal wall
    b. peritoneal cavity
    c. retroperitoneal cavity
    d. any abdominal cavity

165. The visceral peritoneum refers to the surface that is in contact with the
    a. abdominal wall
    b. organs
    c. skin
    d. retroperitoneum

166. Ultrasound is capable of demonstrating the ligaments and fissures of the liver because
    a. they are hyperechoic
    b. collagen and fat are present within and around these structures
    c. they contain heparin, an echogenic substance
    d. they are perpendicular to the beam

167. Crohn's disease is an inflammatory bowel disease usually affecting the
    a. terminal ileum
    b. stomach
    c. pylorus
    d. esophagus

168. Compared with the adult adrenal gland, the neonatal adrenal gland
    a. appears larger and increased in medullary echogenicity
    b. appears smaller and hypoechoic
    c. appears no different
    d. cannot be seen

169. An echogenic linear echo located immediately anterior to the caudate lobe represents the
    a. main lobar fissure
    b. ligamentum venosum
    c. falciform ligament
    d. ligamentum teres

170. The segments of the left lobe of the liver are
    a. medial and lateral
    b. anterior and posterior
    c. cephalad and caudad
    d. caudate and quadrate

171. When longitudinal scans of the liver are performed with a subcostal approach, the patient is asked to take in a deep breath. This technique displaces the liver
    a. anteriorly
    b. posteriorly
    c. superiorly
    d. inferiorly
    e. medially

172. Sonographic visualization of the anterior wall of the appendix greater than _____ in an adult with RLQ pain is highly suggestive of acute appendicitis.
    a. 1.6 cm
    b. 16 mm
    c. 6 cm
    d. 6 mm

173. Portal vein obstruction may develop as an extension of
    a. hepatocellular carcinoma
    b. Budd-Chiari syndrome
    c. marked dilation of the interhepatic veins
    d. fatty liver infiltration

174. Portal vein gas is an important diagnosis in the infant associated with
    a. right renal cell carcinoma
    b. ascites
    c. abdominal tumor
    d. necrotizing enterocolitis

175. The reflection of the liver above the diaphragm is due to
    a. reverberation
    b. mirror-image artifact
    c. reflection
    d. ring-down artifact

176. Metastatic lesions in the liver may sonographically appear as all of the following except
    a. anechoic with decreased transmission
    b. hyperechoic with decreased transmission
    c. hypoechoic
    d. anechoic with good transmission

177. Glycogen storage disease is associated with
    a. adenomas
    b. angiomyolipomas
    c. lipomas
    d. pancreatitis

178. An amebic abscess of the liver is most frequently located
    a. superior to the liver
    b. in the right lobe of the liver
    c. in the caudate lobe of the liver
    d. inferior to the liver, posterior to the right kidney

179. Which of the following disorders may not produce a complex sonographic pattern?
    a. infected cyst
    b. hemorrhagic cyst
    c. hematoma
    d. congenital cyst

180. All of the following structures form neighboring structures for the thyroid gland except
    a. superficial and deep fascia
    b. parotid muscle
    c. strap muscles
    d. sternocleidomastoid muscle

181. Characteristic findings of a thyroid cyst include all of the following except
    a. cysts account for 20% of all cold thyroid nodules
    b. lesions are usually multiple
    c. the vast majority result from hemorrhage or degenerative changes in an adenoma
    d. incidence of carcinoma in cystic lesions less than 4 cm is less than 2%

182. Clinical signs of a thyroid goiter include
    a. lymph node enlargement
    b. rapidly enlarging mass
    c. fainting
    d. thyroid enlargement

183. Characteristics of thyroid carcinoma include all of the following except
    a. central sonolucent halo
    b. most common endocrine malignancy
    c. found in women more than 40 years of age
    d. rapid growth

184. The most descriptive sonographic finding in thyroid carcinoma is
    a. well-defined borders
    b. lesion is more hyperechoic than normal thyroid tissue
    c. solid complex mass with heterogeneous echo pattern and irregular margins
    d. normal size lymph nodes

185. The most common feature of a thyroid adenoma is
    a. diffuse echogenicity
    b. hemorrhage
    c. peripheral sonolucent halo
    d. inhomogeneity

186. The most common cause of hyperparathyroidism is
    a. thyroid adenoma
    b. parathyroid adenoma
    c. parathyroid cyst
    d. parathyroid hemorrhagic cyst

187. Fat, Cooper's ligaments, connective tissue, blood vessels, nerves, and lymphatics are found
    a. in the retromammary region
    b. in the parenchyma
    c. in the subcutaneous layer
    d. in the subareolar area

188. The most important signs to look for in determining a cystic lesion of the breast include all of the following except
    a. well-defined borders
    b. good through transmission
    c. anechoic
    d. disruption of architecture

189. The most common solid benign tumor of the breast is
    a. cystosarcoma phyllodes
    b. fibroadenoma
    c. papilloma
    d. lipoma

190. A cystic enlargement of a distal duct filled with milk is called a
   a. lactoadenoma
   b. lactoma
   c. galactocele
   d. lactiferoma

191. The most common malignant neoplasm of the breast in women is
   a. lymphoma
   b. adenocarcinoma
   c. mucinous carcinoma
   d. cystosarcoma phyllodes

192. A breast lesion that presents with well-defined borders, low-level internal echoes, and moderate through transmission most likely represents
   a. infected cyst
   b. simple cyst
   c. fibroadenoma
   d. cystosarcoma phyllodes

193. A linear stripe of variable thickness and echogenicity running through the testis in a craniocaudal direction represents the
   a. Cowper's fascia
   b. mediastinum testis
   c. epithelial fascia
   d. dartos muscle

194. The epididymis is located
   a. anterior and inferior to the testis
   b. anterior and superior to the testis
   c. posterior and inferior to the testis
   d. posterior and lateral to the testis

195. Which fact about undescended testes is false?
   a. The testis originates in the retroperitoneum at the level of the fetal kidney.
   b. All undescended testes are found in the inguinal canal.
   c. There is a 40% to 50% association with testicular malignancy.
   d. There is an increased incidence of infertility.

196. Common causes of a secondary hydrocele include all of the following except
   a. trauma
   b. undescended testes
   c. infection
   d. neoplasm

197. Which of the following statements is false regarding varicocele?
    a. Varicoceles refer to dilated, serpiginous, and elongated veins of the pampiniform plexus.
    b. They are more common on the right side.
    c. Primary varicoceles result from incompetent valves in the spermatic vein.
    d. Secondary varicoceles develop from compression of the spermatic vein.

198. A common problem that is viral in origin and affects some adolescent and middle-aged men is
    a. epididymal cyst
    b. epididymitis
    c. spermatocele
    d. testiculitis

199. An infection that has spread to the testicle is
    a. epididymitis
    b. hydrocele
    c. orchitis
    d. spermatocele

200. Sonographic patterns of testicular neoplasms include all of the following except
    a. focal and well-defined homogeneous hypoechoic region
    b. diffuse and ill-defined region of decreased echogenicity
    c. complex mass with internal anechoic and echogenic areas
    d. anechoic pattern with increased transmission

Pediatric Review

Select the answer that best completes the following questions or statements.

1. The neural plate develops at
   a. 4.5 menstrual weeks
   b. 6 menstrual weeks
   c. 9 menstrual weeks
   d. 12 menstrual weeks

2. The conus medullaris is located at approximately the level of
   a. T12-L1
   b. L1-L2
   c. L2-L3
   d. L3-L4

3. What are the common clinical findings in a patient with appendicitis?
   a. RLQ pain, fever, nausea and vomiting
   b. nausea and projectile vomiting
   c. right flank pain and bile stasis
   d. abdominal pain radiating to the right shoulder

4. Early in development, the brain segments into three primary vesicles:
   a. prosencephalon, forebrain, midbrain
   b. prosencephalon, mesencephalon, rhombencephalon
   c. hindbrain, midbrain, rhombencephalon
   d. forebrain, midbrain, prosencephalon

5. What are the outgrowths on either side of the diencephalon?
   a. choroid plexus
   b. cerebral hemispheres
   c. midbrain
   d. pons

6. What structure invaginates into the lateral ventricles?
   a. pia
   b. forebrain
   c. choroid plexus
   d. subarachnoid

7. Extrahepatic obstruction in the neonate includes all except
   a. choledochal cyst
   b. biliary atresia
   c. hepatitis
   d. spontaneous perforation of the bile ducts

8. Dysgenesis of the fourth ventricle results in
   a. corpus callosum malformation
   b. cystic dilatation of the lateral ventricle
   c. Dandy-Walker malformation
   d. hypospadias

9. Define the measurement used to determine if appendicitis is present.
   a. an outer diameter greater than 10 mm with compression
   b. an outer diameter less than 5 mm with compression
   c. an outer diameter greater than 12 mm without compression
   d. an outer diameter greater than 6 mm with compression

10. What structure forms between the corpus callosum and fornices?
    a. septum pellucidum
    b. Dandy-Walker
    c. 4th ventricle
    d. sylvian fissure

11. The normal size of the lateral ventricle as measured in the axial plane should be less than
    a. 4 mm
    b. 10 mm
    c. 8 mm
    d. 6 mm

12. The cisterna magna gradually decreases with gestational age.
    a. True
    b. False

13. What two pitfalls should be avoided in determining lateral ventricular size?
    a. developing fetal cortical mantle
    b. choroid plexus
    c. echogenic subarachnoid space
    d. echogenic white matter

14. Approximately 30% of fetuses identified with hydrocephalus are associated with
    a. calcified cortex
    b. spina bifida
    c. subarachnoid hemorrhage
    d. agenesis of the corpus callosum

15. Which statement is false regarding the choroid plexus?
    a. It fills the lateral ventricle from side to side during the second trimester.
    b. With the development of hydrocephalus, the choroid plexus in the far ventricle separates from the medial wall of the lateral ventricle.
    c. The texture of the choroid plexus is heterogeneous.
    d. The choroid plexus in the near ventricle separates from the lateral wall of the lateral ventricle.

16. The most characteristic finding of absence of the corpus callosum is
    a. complete or partial agenesis of the cerebellar vermis
    b. dilatation and superior displacement of the third ventricle
    c. enlargement of the fourth ventricle
    d. hydrocephalus

17. What is the term used for any cavitation or CSF-filled cyst in the brain?
    a. hydranencephaly
    b. schizencephaly
    c. porencephaly
    d. encephalocele

18. What bony parts contribute to the formation of the vertebral arch?
    a. two pedicles, two laminae, one spinous process, two transverse processes, two superior and two inferior articular processes
    b. one pedicle, two laminae, one spinous process, two transverse processes, two superior and two inferior articular processes
    c. one pedicle, two laminae, one spinous process, one transverse process, two superior and two inferior articular processes
    d. two pedicles, two laminae, two spinous processes, two transverse processes, one superior and one inferior articular process

19. A vein of Galen aneurysm is best imaged with color Doppler as
    a. disturbed flow within the structure
    b. disturbed flow surrounding the structure
    c. disturbed flow posterior to the structure
    d. absence of flow within the structure

20. Describe intussusception in the infant.
    a. occurs when bowel prolapses into more distal bowel and is propelled in an antegrade fashion
    b. occurs when one segment of bowel twists around another
    c. occurs in the presence of appendicitis
    d. occurs in utero only

21. What percentage of premature infants may have intracranial hemorrhage?
    a. 30
    b. 40
    c. 80
    d. 90

22. What clinical criterion is used to determine whether an infant has pyloric stenosis?
    a. jaundice
    b. frequent urination
    c. hypoemesis
    d. projectile vomiting

23. What soft tissue structure is seen to form a bridge of gray matter across the third ventricle when it is abnormal?

 a. mass intermedia

 b. thalamus

 c. hypothalamus

 d. cerebral peduncle

24. The lateral ventricles drain into the third ventricle via what structure?

 a. aqueduct of Sylvius

 b. medulla oblongata

 c. cerebellar vermis

 d. foramen of Monro

25. Define the measurements used to evaluate a patient with pyloric stenosis.

 a. length greater than 16 mm, thickness greater than 4 mm

 b. length less than 16 mm, thickness greater than 4 mm

 c. length greater than 12 mm, thickness greater than 2 mm

 d. length greater than 13 mm, thickness greater than 6 mm

26. What connects the third and fourth ventricles?

 a. cerebral aqueduct

 b. aqueduct of Sylvius

 c. foramen of Monro

 d. foramen of nucleus

27. What anatomic landmark within the brain is used to find the middle cerebral arteries?

 a. vein of Galen

 b. aqueduct of Monro

 c. caudate nucleus

 d. sylvian fissure

28. What are the most common age and gender for pyloric stenosis to occur?

 a. female, age birth to 3 months

 b. female, age 1 to 5 months

 c. male, age 3 to 6 weeks

 d. male, age 1 to 3 months

29. Name the four segments of the lateral ventricles.

 a. frontal horn, body, occipital and temporal horns

 b. anterior, medial, lateral, posterior

 c. anterior, body, frontal, temporal horn

 d. anterior, body, occipital, frontal horn

30. What is the "pseudokidney" or "sandwich" sign?

 a. the sign of a pelvic kidney

 b. sonographic finding in a patient with appendicitis

 c. sonographic finding in a patient with intussusception

 d. hydroureter with a pelvic kidney

31. Name the fontanelle through which the neonatal brain may be scanned in the coronal plane.
    a. posterior fontanelle
    b. occipital fontanelle
    c. temporal fontanelle
    d. anterior fontanelle

32. The layer of meninges closely adhering to the brain tissue is the
    a. dura mater
    b. pia mater
    c. arachnoid
    d. choroid plexus

33. A subependymal hemorrhage is found at what site?
    a. supraependymal germinal matrix
    b. subependymal choroid plexus
    c. subarachnoid plexus
    d. thalamic-caudate groove

34. In the pediatric ultrasound examination of the abdomen, all of the following are true except
    a. the right hepatic lobe should not extend more than 1 cm below the xyphoid process
    b. the common bile duct should measure less than 2 mm in infants up to 1 year of age
    c. the length of the gallbladder should not exceed the length of the kidney
    d. the texture of the pancreas is hypoechoic when compared with the liver

35. Where is the most common site for a choroid plexus hemorrhage?
    a. anterior horn
    b. occipital horn
    c. lateral horn
    d. temporal horn

36. Where does the germinal matrix lie?
    a. between the midbrain and the forebrain
    b. superior to the caudate nucleus in the floor of the lateral ventricle
    c. lateral to the cerebral peduncles
    d. inferior to the cisterna magna

37. Define acute periventricular leukomalacia.
    a. hemorrhagic germinal matrix with cavitation
    b. echogenic formations in the epidural cavity
    c. increased echogenicity in the subarachnoid space
    d. multiple foci or coagulation necrosis in periventricular white matter

38. Name the two complications seen in patients with periventricular leukomalacia.
    a. anomalous myelination of the immature brain
    b. hydrocephalus
    c. agenesis of the corpus callosum
    d. abnormal neurologic development

39. Which is the best definition for hydrocephalus?
    a. marked separation of the anterior horns and bodies of the lateral ventricles
    b. enlargement of the ventricular system
    c. decreased production of cerebrospinal fluid
    d. displacement of the inferior part of the cerebellum through the foramen magnum

40. Which statement is false regarding ventriculitis?
    a. common complication of purulent meningitis in newborns
    b. caused by hematogenous spread of the infection to the choroid plexus
    c. ventricular shunt decreases the risk
    d. leads to compartmentalization of the ventricular cavities

41. The hip bones are the fusion of all the following except
    a. ilium
    b. femur
    c. ischium
    d. pubis

42. Agenesis of the corpus callosum may indicate what malformation?
    a. Dandy-Walker malformation
    b. Arnold-Chiari malformation
    c. vein of Galen malformation
    d. choroid plexus cyst

43. When the hip is laterally and posteriorly displaced to the extent that the femoral head has no contact with the acetabulum and the normal "U" configuration cannot be obtained on ultrasound, this condition is
    a. frank dislocation
    b. dysplasia
    c. subluxation
    d. normal

44. The _____ nerve is the largest nerve in the body.
    a. cranial
    b. diaphragmatic
    c. sciatic
    d. optic

45. The passage of cerebrospinal fluid between the third and lateral ventricles is accomplished via the
    a. foramen of Magendie
    b. aqueduct of Sylvius
    c. foramen of Luschka
    d. foramen of Monro

46. What is the function of the hippocampus?
    a. taste
    b. smell
    c. memory
    d. motor control

47. Cerebrospinal fluid circulates between the
    a. pia mater and arachnoid
    b. dura mater and arachnoid
    c. pia mater and cerebral cortex
    d. dura mater and periosteum

48. The upper and lower vertebral notches of adjacent vertebrae meet to form the
    a. transverse foramina
    b. central canal
    c. intervertebral foramina
    d. apophyseal joints

49. The most inferior portion of the spinal cord, located at approximately the level of the first or second lumbar vertebra, is called the
    a. cauda equina
    b. filum terminale
    c. sacral plexus
    d. conus medullaris

50. The "ball on a spoon" refers to
    a. ilium and gluteus minimus
    b. femoral head and acetabulum
    c. ischium and pubis
    d. pectineus and iliacus

Cardiovascular Anatomy Review

Select the answer that best completes the following questions or statements.

1. The tricuspid valve opens when
   a. the right ventricular pressure drops below the right atrial pressure
   b. the papillary muscle contracts
   c. the velocity of blood flow in the right ventricle exceeds the velocity of flow in the right atrium
   d. the pulmonic valve opens

2. Blood normally flows from the right ventricle to the
   a. pulmonary artery
   b. aorta
   c. right atrium
   d. pulmonary vein

3. Which of the following statements regarding cardiac anatomy is false?
   a. The heart tends to assume a more vertical position in tall, thin people and a more horizontal position in short, heavy people.
   b. The ligamentum arteriosum runs from the left pulmonary artery to the descending aorta.
   c. The coronary arteries arise from the sinuses within the cusps of the aortic valve.
   d. The left ventricle constitutes most of the ventral surface of the heart.

4. The most posterior chamber to the left of the sternum is the
   a. right atrium
   b. left atrium
   c. right ventricle
   d. left ventricle

5. The medial wall of the right atrium contains the
   a. interventricular septum
   b. interatrial septum
   c. right upper pulmonary vein
   d. right lower pulmonary vein

6. The inferior vena cava is guarded by a fold of tissue called the _____ valve, whereas the coronary

   sinus is guarded by the _____ valve.
   a. eustachian, coronary
   b. thebesian, eustachian
   c. eustachian, thebesian
   d. eustachian, atrial

7. The interventricular septum is divided primarily into two major sections: membranous and muscular; which of the terms below would be identified with the muscular septum?
    a. inflow
    b. outflow
    c. infundibular
    d. trabecular

8. The wall of the aorta bulges slightly at each semilunar cusp to form
    a. coronary arteries
    b. sinus of Valsalva
    c. chordae tendineae
    d. Arantius nodule

9. The _____ valve lies behind the right half of the sternum opposite the 4th ICS.
    a. mitral
    b. aortic
    c. tricuspid
    d. pulmonic

10. The pulmonary artery may be distinguished from the aorta by all except that
    a. it runs upward and to the left, anterior to the aorta
    b. the cusps are thinner than the aorta
    c. it bifurcates into right and left branches
    d. it runs upward and to the right, posterior to the aorta

11. The point at which the ductus joins the aorta is near the
    a. left common carotid artery
    b. left subclavian artery
    c. brachiocephalic artery
    d. crux of the heart

12. Most coronary venous drainage is into the
    a. coronary veins
    b. coronary sinus
    c. thebesian veins
    d. atrial sinus

13. Atrial contraction follows the _____ on the ECG.
    a. T wave
    b. P wave
    c. QRS
    d. ST segment

14. The brightest returning echo signal on the echocardiogram is from the
    a. anterior wall of the heart
    b. anterior leaflet of the mitral valve
    c. aortic semilunar cusps
    d. pericardium

15. To image the aortic root with semilunar cusps, the sonographer should angle the transducer
    a. toward the right shoulder
    b. toward the left shoulder
    c. inferior toward the left hip
    d. toward the 4th left ICS

16. The coronary sinus is often identified as a
    a. vertical tubular structure posterior to the heart
    b. oblique tubular structure posterior and lateral to the heart
    c. vertical tubular structure lateral to the heart
    d. horizontal tubular structure posterior to the atria of the heart

17. The Doppler shift would best be explained in the following way:
    a. If the source is moving toward the listener, it is "catching up" with the wave it just generated; the wavelength becomes shorter, and the listener hears a higher frequency.
    b. If the source is moving away, the wavelength becomes longer, and the listener hears a higher frequency.
    c. If the source is moving toward the listener, the wavelength becomes longer, and the listener hears a higher frequency.
    d. The difference between the frequency generated by the source and that observed by the listener is the Doppler shift.

18. The inflammatory process of the cardiac muscle is known as
    a. endocarditis
    b. pericarditis
    c. epicarditis
    d. myocarditis

19. The term dyspnea refers to the condition of
    a. difficulty in digesting food
    b. difficulty in breathing
    c. rapid breathing
    d. deep breathing

20. The amplitude of aortic root motion has been used to assess
    a. the vigor of left ventricular contraction
    b. the degree of aortic stenosis
    c. the degree of aortic insufficiency
    d. the size of the left atrium

21. The best window to image the area of the fossa ovalis is the
    a. apical
    b. subcostal four chamber
    c. parasternal long axis
    d. subcostal short axis

22. Atrial septal defects are classified on the basis of their position in the septum and their embryologic origin. The most common is
    a. ostium primum defect
    b. ostium secundum defect
    c. sinus venosus defect
    d. primum secundum defect

23. The structure that plays a significant role in the development of the septum primum, atrioventricular valves, and membranous septum is the
   a. endocardial cushion
   b. ventral septal endocardium
   c. atrial septal endocardium
   d. endocardial fibroelastocushion

24. The heart is lined by a serous membrane called the
   a. pericardium
   b. endocardium
   c. myocardium
   d. epicardium

25. The middle muscular layer of the heart is the
   a. pericardium
   b. endocardium
   c. myocardium
   d. epicardium

26. The _____ is located between the pericardium and the heart wall and is most prominent around the inflow and outflow of the heart.
   a. epicardium
   b. visceral pericardium
   c. pericardial fat
   d. endocardium

27. Risk factors identified for stroke include all except
   a. age
   b. sex
   c. hypertension
   d. pregnancy

28. The warning signs of stroke include all except
   a. symptoms of weakness or numbness
   b. sudden confusion, trouble speaking or understanding
   c. hypotension
   d. trouble with seeing or walking

29. An ischemic neurologic deficit that lasts less than 24 hours is known as
   a. CVA
   b. TIA
   c. RIND
   d. BEND

30. Blood supply to the brain is provided by the _____ arteries.
   a. internal and external
   b. carotid and vertebral
   c. ophthalmic and posterior communicating
   d. middle cerebral and anterior cerebral

31. Symptoms of lower extremity occlusive arterial disease are
    a. claudication and rest pain
    b. shoulder pain
    c. thoracic pain
    d. lower abdominal pain

32. Characteristics of a normal Doppler arterial waveform include all except
    a. triphasic
    b. high velocity forward flow during systole
    c. low velocity forward flow during systole
    d. short flow reversal in early diastole

33. A potentially lethal complication of acute DVT is
    a. pulmonary embolism
    b. claudication
    c. abscess
    d. fistula

34. Dilated, elongated, tortuous superficial veins are
    a. perforating veins
    b. varicose veins
    c. abscessed veins
    d. tortellini veins

Obstetrics and Gynecology Review

Select the answer that best completes the following questions or statements.

1. The physiologic status of prepuberty is
   a. menarche
   b. menopause
   c. premenarche
   d. postmenarche

2. The bladder is considered adequately filled when
   a. it extends past the endometrial canal
   b. it extends past the uterine fundus
   c. it fills the true pelvic cavity
   d. it covers the fimbria

3. A routine image protocol of the pelvis consists of longitudinal and transverse scans of
   a. uterus, cervix, adnexa
   b. cervix, right adnexa, left adnexa, uterus, rectouterine recess
   c. endometrial canal, cervix, adnexa
   d. cervix, uterus, fallopian tubes

4. If pelvic pathology is present, what other areas should be examined?
   a. renal
   b. subphrenic
   c. Morison's pouch, subphrenic, renal
   d. Morison's pouch, renal, pouch of Douglas

5. To image the cervix on the EDV exam, the transducer should be
   a. inserted deep and angled anteriorly
   b. withdrawn and angled posteriorly
   c. withdrawn and angled anteriorly
   d. inserted deep and angled posteriorly

6. To image the fundus of the anteverted uterus on the EDV exam, the transducer should be
   a. inserted deep and angled anteriorly
   b. withdrawn and angled posteriorly
   c. withdrawn slightly and angled anteriorly
   d. inserted deep and angled posteriorly

7. What muscle group is inserted on the pubic ramus and is called paired parasagittal straps in the abdominal wall?
   a. piriformis
   b. coccygeus
   c. obturator fascia
   d. rectus abdominis

8. What muscles may be identified in the true pelvis in the transverse plane with cephalic angulation of the transducer at the pubis?
   a. piriformis
   b. coccygeus
   c. obturator internus
   d. rectus abdominis

9. This muscle is best imaged in a transverse plane with caudal angulation at the most superior aspect of the bladder.
   a. levator ani
   b. rectus abdominis
   c. coccygeus
   d. piriformis

10. What muscle group may be seen in the false pelvis along the lateral side walls of the pelvis?
    a. obturator internus
    b. iliopsoas
    c. rectus sheath
    d. psoas major

11. The müllerian duct is important to the development of the
    a. fallopian tube
    b. ovary
    c. female internal reproductive organs
    d. uterine canal

12. Bilateral support for the uterus is provided by the
    a. broad ligament
    b. round ligament
    c. uterosacral ligaments
    d. endometrial ligament

13. The ligament that occupies space between the layers of another ligament and occurs in front of and below the fallopian tube is
    a. broad ligament
    b. uterosacral ligament
    c. round ligament
    d. tubal ligament

14. The texture of the myometrium of the uterus may be described as
    a. heterogeneous
    b. homogeneous with smooth borders
    c. heterogeneous with smooth borders
    d. homogeneous with irregular borders

15. The vessels seen in the periphery of the uterus are called the
    a. arcuate
    b. uterine
    c. ovarian
    d. tubal

16. The best way to measure the cervical-fundal length of the uterus is
    a. TA, longitudinal
    b. EDV, sagittal
    c. EDV, coronal
    d. TA, transverse

17. The normal length of the young adult uterus should measure
    a. 3 to 5 cm
    b. 2 to 3 cm
    c. 5 to 6 cm
    d. 6 to 9 cm

18. The endometrium changes during the menstrual cycle. When the three-line sign appears, this is the
    a. secretory phase
    b. early proliferative phase
    c. midproliferative phase
    d. late proliferative phase

19. The endometrial thickness is measured
    a. from inner to inner border
    b. from the anterior to posterior layers
    c. from outer to outer layer including fluid
    d. from inner to inner on TA only

20. The normal measurement of the endometrium should be _____ in a menstrual woman.
    a. 10 to 12 mm
    b. 1 to 2 mm
    c. 4 to 6 mm
    d. 4 to 12 mm

21. The structure that lies above the uteroovarian ligaments, the round ligaments, and tuboovarian vessels is the
    a. ovary
    b. fallopian tube
    c. broad ligament
    d. uterine artery

22. The ovary produces two hormones; estrogen is secreted by the _____, whereas progesterone is

    secreted by the _____.
    a. follicles, corpus luteum
    b. secretory, proliferative
    c. follicles, corpuscle
    d. corpus luteum, nabothian

23. The release of an egg from the ruptured mature follicle is
    a. menstruation
    b. corpus luteum
    c. ovulation
    d. follicle-stimulating hormone (FSH)

24. The ovary is located lateral to the _____ and anteromedial to the _____.
    a. round ligament, broad ligament
    b. uterus, internal iliac vessels
    c. external iliac vessels, piriformis
    d. obturator internus, internal iliac vessels

25. The posterior component of the pelvic cavity is occupied by all of the following except the
    a. rectum
    b. cervix
    c. colon
    d. ileum

26. Which statement is false regarding the ureter?
    a. It crosses the pelvic inlet anterior to the bifurcation of the common iliac artery.
    b. It runs in front of the internal iliac artery and posterior to the ovary.
    c. It runs forward and lateral under the base of the broad ligament.
    d. It runs forward and lateral to the vagina to enter the bladder.

27. The uterus is supported by the
    a. levator ani muscles and pelvic fascia
    b. obturator internus muscles
    c. iliacus muscles
    d. piriformis muscles

28. The ligaments of the uterus include
    a. broad, suspensory, round, ovarian
    b. broad, round, ovarian
    c. broad, fundal, round
    d. broad, fundal, piriformis

29. The texture of the ovary is
    a. less echogenic than the uterus
    b. more echogenic than the uterus
    c. more hypoechoic than the uterus
    d. less hypoechoic than the uterus

30. The failure of fusion that has two vaginas, two cervices, two uterine bodies is
    a. bicornuate uterus
    b. didelphys uterus
    c. bicornis unicollis uterus
    d. arcuatus uterus

31. The transvaginal technique is contraindicated in all of the following except
    a. premenarche patients
    b. obese patients
    c. sexually inactive patients
    d. patient's refusal or intolerance of the exam

32. The Doppler indices used to evaluate the pelvic vessels include all of the following except
    a. A/B ratio
    b. Pourcelot resistive index
    c. Bernoulli's equation
    d. pulsatility index

33. The uterine vessels are found in the
    a. obturator internus
    b. broad ligaments
    c. piriformis
    d. aorta

34. The ovarian arteries and veins are found in the
    a. broad ligaments
    b. suspensory ligaments
    c. round ligaments
    d. oval ligaments

35. The three divisions of the fallopian tube are
    a. intramural, isthmus, ampullary
    b. intramural, ampullary, follicular
    c. isthmus, ampullary, follicular
    d. follicular, fimbriae, luteal

36. When only the body and fundus of the uterus are flexed posteriorly, it is
    a. anteflexed
    b. anteverted
    c. retroflexed
    d. retroverted

37. The end of the fallopian tube that is open to the peritoneal cavity is called the
    a. isthmus
    b. frondosum
    c. ampulla
    d. fimbria

38. Hydrometra would appear sonographically as
    a. a sonolucent tubular structure in the adnexa
    b. an echogenic thickening of the endometrium
    c. a sonolucent fluid collection in the uterine canal
    d. a sonolucent fluid collection in the uterus, cervix, and vagina

39. The human chorionic gonadotropin (hCG) levels in gestational trophoblastic disease
    a. decrease in time
    b. increase at a markedly higher rate than in a normal pregnancy
    c. increase at a subnormal rate
    d. remain at an even level throughout the course of the disease

40. The hormone responsible for estrogen stimulation is
    a. FSH
    b. luteinizing hormone (LH)
    c. cortisone
    d. progesterone

41. Polycystic ovaries usually have cysts that are
    a. around the periphery of the ovary
    b. throughout the ovary
    c. large and septated
    d. infected

42. Sonographic evaluation of the pelvis in the patient with a suspected mass has several objectives. Which of the following is NOT one?
    a. Confirm the presence of a mass.
    b. Determine its origin.
    c. Provide a pathologic diagnosis.
    d. Characterize its internal echoarchitecture.

43. Which of the following is usually a preponderantly cystic mass?
    a. hydrosalpinx
    b. teratoma
    c. ovarian abscess
    d. mucinous cystadenoma

44. Teratomas are
    a. complex masses
    b. cystic masses
    c. always malignant
    d. lethal

45. The most common site of an ectopic pregnancy is
    a. the isthmus of the fallopian tube
    b. the abdomen
    c. the ovary
    d. the ampullary portion of the fallopian tube

46. A fluid collection in the endometrium that simulates the gestational sac of an early pregnancy is called
    a. decidual reaction
    b. endometritis
    c. pseudogestational sac
    d. hydrometra

47. Which of the following is NOT an adnexal structure?
    a. ovarian ligaments
    b. ovaries
    c. uterus
    d. broad ligaments

48. A dermoid is
    a. a large cystic mass with prominent septations
    b. a benign teratoma in which ectodermal elements are preponderant
    c. the most common large cystic mass, which may contain a lattice of internal thin-walled septations
    d. the largest of the functional cysts, associated with trophoblastic disease

49. The total sum of the measurement of the largest pocket of amniotic fluid in four quadrants is called the
    a. amniotic fluid volume
    b. amniotic fluid index
    c. amniotic pocket volume
    d. amniotic quadrant volume

50. A parovarian cyst is a
    a. large cystic mass with prominent septations
    b. benign teratoma in which ectodermal elements are preponderant
    c. the largest of the functional cysts, associated with trophoblastic disease
    d. cyst that arises from the broad ligament

51. Theca lutein cysts are
    a. large cystic masses with prominent septations
    b. benign teratomas in which ectodermal elements are preponderant
    c. the most common large cystic masses, which may contain a lattice of internal thin-walled septations
    d. the largest of the functional cysts, associated with trophoblastic disease or hyperstimulation of the hCG

52. Biparietal diameter can be used for fetal dating as early as
    a. 6 weeks
    b. 8 weeks
    c. 10 weeks
    d. 12 weeks

53. BPD measurement should be taken from the following borders:
    a. outer to outer
    b. outer to inner
    c. inner to inner
    d. inner to outer

54. A brachycephalic head means that the head is
    a. round
    b. elongated
    c. abnormal
    d. small

55. The crown-rump length (CRL) measurement is the longest length of the embryo
    a. excluding the limbs
    b. including the limbs
    c. including the yolk sac
    d. including the femur

56. An intrauterine growth-restricted fetus is one who
    a. is always born with genetic defects
    b. has an abnormal heart rate
    c. is RH sensitive
    d. is born at or below the 10th percentile of weight for gestational age

57. The abdominal circumference should be taken at the level of
    a. the fetal stomach and the portal vein
    b. the fetal heart and ribs
    c. the fetal kidneys
    d. the umbilical cord insertion site

58. A(an) _____ is formed when an oocyte unites with a sperm cell.
    a. oocyte
    b. zygote
    c. corpus albicans
    d. morula

59. When the uterus empties itself of all products of conception, it is referred to as a(an)
    a. blighted ovum
    b. complete abortion
    c. impending abortion
    d. missed abortion

60. What is the approximate hCG level when a gestational sac is first observed (transabdominally)?
    a. 800 mIU/ml
    b. 1200 mIU/ml
    c. 1800 mIU/ml
    d. 2100 mIU/ml

61. All of the following statements regarding hydatidiform mole are true except
    a. a previous mole results in an increased risk for recurrence
    b. it is associated with markedly elevated hCG levels
    c. the sonographic appearance is similar to a degenerating myoma
    d. although considered "tumors" of trophoblastic tissue, they are incapable of metastasizing

62. Causes of polyhydramnios include all of the following except
    a. congenital abnormalities
    b. heart failure
    c. gastrointestinal anomalies
    d. amniotic bands

63. Higher than normal levels of hCG are seen in which of the following conditions?
    a. multiple gestation
    b. corpus luteum cyst
    c. ectopic pregnancy
    d. anembryonic gestation

64. Postmenopausal ovaries are difficult to recognize sonographically for all of the following reasons except
    a. They are no longer responsive to pituitary gonadotropins.
    b. They are smaller than premenopausal ovaries.
    c. The parenchymal tissue becomes hypoechoic as a result of atrophy.
    d. The blood supply to the ovaries is diminished.

65. Fusion of the amnion and chorion normally occurs between
    a. 3 and 5 weeks
    b. 5 and 8 weeks
    c. 8 and 10 weeks
    d. 14 and 16 weeks

66. In the 8th to 9th week of gestation, the fetal heart rate on a transvaginal sonogram should measure
    a. 90 beats per minute
    b. 120 beats per minute
    c. 160 beats per minute
    d. 200 beats per minute

67. The most inaccurate measurement for fetal growth assessment is
    a. femur length
    b. biparietal diameter
    c. abdominal circumference
    d. head circumference

68. The fetal renal pelvis should be followed in utero if the measurement exceeds
    a. 1 to 2 mm
    b. 2 to 3 mm
    c. 4 to 5 mm
    d. 5 to 10 mm

69. If you are scanning a first-trimester pregnancy, documentation should be made of
    a. BPD
    b. crown-rump length
    c. head circumference
    d. abdominal circumference

70. To determine situs solitus, the following structures should be identified except
    a. stomach on left
    b. aorta on left, IVC right and anterior
    c. aorta on left, IVC right and posterior
    d. apex to left

71. A solid mass may exhibit all of the following except
    a. distal acoustic shadows
    b. distal acoustic enhancement
    c. irregular, poorly defined walls
    d. a heterogeneous interior

72. What type of cyst is commonly associated with pregnancy?
    a. a theca lutein cyst
    b. a parovarian cyst
    c. a corpus luteum cyst
    d. a follicular cyst

73. If an anterior abdominal wall mass is seen just to the right of the umbilical cord, the most likely diagnosis is
    a. gastroschisis
    b. omphalocele
    c. hernia
    d. limb body wall defect

74. Trophoblastic disease, which extends outside the uterus and spreads to the lungs or brain, is called
    a. choriocarcinoma
    b. hydatidiform mole
    c. endometrioma
    d. lung-gestational molar

75. In what anatomic site does fertilization of the ovum usually occur?
    a. the vagina
    b. the uterine cavity
    c. the ovary
    d. the fallopian tube

76. A 22-year-old gravid patient presents with oligohydramnios. Which of the following would be least likely?
    a. anencephaly
    b. postterm pregnancy
    c. renal agenesis
    d. premature rupture of the membranes

77. A patient is GPA 8,2,6. How many abortions has she had?
    a. four
    b. seven
    c. one
    d. six

78. A near-term gravid patient lying face up for more than 15 minutes will sometimes become ill with fainting and nausea. She is probably experiencing
    a. supine hypotensive syndrome
    b. supine hypertensive syndrome
    c. morning sickness
    d. hyperemesis gravidarum

79. The separation of the chorionic and amniotic membranes is normal
    a. after 24 weeks of gestation
    b. before 24 weeks of gestation
    c. after 16 weeks of gestation
    d. before 16 weeks of gestation

80. Which of the following is the appropriate description of gastroschisis?
   a. normal insertion of the umbilical cord, with herniation of the bowel occurring most often on the right side of the umbilicus
   b. herniation of the thoracic and abdominal contents, including the bowel and liver or spleen, with herniation at the base of the umbilical cord
   c. herniation of the umbilical cord
   d. herniation of bowel to the left of the umbilicus, containing spleen covered by peritoneum

81. A leiomyoma that deforms the endometrial cavity and may cause irregular or heavy menstrual bleeding is known as a
   a. pedunculated fibroid
   b. subserosal fibroid
   c. submucosal fibroid
   d. intramural fibroid

82. Calcifications of fibroids may be secondary to all of the following except
   a. diabetes mellitus
   b. hypertension
   c. hypotension
   d. chronic renal failure

83. If the endometrium measures more than 14 mm without hormone replacement therapy, the sonographer should think of
   a. endometrial hyperplasia
   b. adenomyosis
   c. endometritis
   d. endometrioma

84. Clear evidence for endometrial carcinoma is
   a. light bleeding during the secretory phase
   b. myometrial invasion
   c. calcification of the arcuate arteries
   d. gestational trophoblastic disease

85. The most common cause of tubal obstruction is
   a. endometrioma
   b. hydrometrocolpos
   c. adenomyosis
   d. pelvic inflammatory disease

86. The function of the ovary is to
   a. produce testosterone
   b. produce follicles
   c. mature oocytes until ovulation
   d. manufacture corpus luteum

87. The normal follicle may enlarge to _____ before ovulation.
   a. 8 cm
   b. 24 mm
   c. 39 mm
   d. 78 mm

88. Increased levels of hCG may cause
    a. hemorrhagic cysts to develop
    b. teratomas
    c. theca lutein cysts
    d. polycystic ovaries

89. Cysts less than _____ are not likely to be malignant.
    a. 2 cm
    b. 3 cm
    c. 4 cm
    d. 5 cm

90. Another name for a chocolate cyst is
    a. dermoid tumor
    b. endometrioma
    c. hemorrhagic cyst
    d. adenoma

91. Cysts with thick septations and solid elements are most likely
    a. filled with blood
    b. filled with fluid
    c. malignant
    d. benign

92. The most common mass in young girls is
    a. polycystic ovaries
    b. teratoma
    c. pelvic inflammatory disease
    d. Brenner tumor

93. Which statement is false regarding torsion of the ovary?
    a. The ovary becomes edematous, measuring more than 4 cm.
    b. Fluid is often found in the pelvis.
    c. Doppler shows increased blood surrounding the periphery of the ovary.
    d. The ovary is usually hypoechoic.

94. All of the following causes may mimic a pelvic mass except
    a. pelvic kidney
    b. omental cysts
    c. retroflexed ureter
    d. diverticular abscess

95. In an early gestation, the gestational sac
    a. represents the fluid-filled amniotic cavity
    b. surrounds the decidua capsularis and decidua parietalis
    c. can be visualized transvaginally by 4 weeks and transabdominally by 6 weeks
    d. cannot be correlated with hCG

96. The placenta develops from
    a. the portion of the trophoblast attached to the myometrium, the decidua basalis
    b. the portion of the trophoblast attached to the decidua capsularis
    c. the amnion before fusion with the chorionic cavity
    d. the double decidual sac

97. The echogenic secondary yolk sac is
    a. the first structure to be seen within the gestational sac
    b. not visualized in an ectopic gestation
    c. seen transabdominally at ±4 weeks after the LMP
    d. is usually between 5 to 7 mm in diameter

98. During the first trimester, the developing embryo grows approximately _____ every day
    a. 2 to 3 mm
    b. 4 to 5 mm
    c. 1 to 2 mm
    d. 2 to 3 mm

99. On transvaginal imaging, by the end of the first trimester, the choroid plexus
    a. is not present and cannot be imaged
    b. can be imaged as a hyperechoic structure in the lateral ventricle
    c. can be imaged as a hypoechoic structure in the lateral ventricle
    d. is seen as a linear echogenic structure in the gestational sac

100. A corpus luteum of pregnancy
    a. is a functional cyst of the ovary
    b. precedes the formation of a follicular cyst
    c. becomes a corpus luteum cyst only if fertilization does not take place
    d. is found with a hydatidiform mole

101. On sonography the sonographer finds the cul-de-sac to contain a small amount of clear fluid. This is MOST likely to be evidence of
    a. a normal situation
    b. an ectopic pregnancy
    c. pelvic inflammatory disease
    d. vesicouterine reflux

102. A patient with a positive serum hCG test presents with some bleeding. The LMP indicates 5 to 6 weeks - of gestation. Sonography does not reveal a fetal pole. The MOST likely diagnosis is a(n)
    a. hydatidiform mole
    b. complete spontaneous abortion
    c. ectopic pregnancy
    d. normal intrauterine gestation, but too early to detect the fetal pole

103. In a patient with a complete spontaneous abortion, the MOST likely finding is a(n)
    a. empty gestational sac with no evidence of decidua
    b. embryo with no evidence of a heartbeat
    c. complex mass in the cul-de-sac
    d. empty uterus with a decidual reaction

104. A patient presents with a closed cervical os and a distorted gestational sac in the lower uterine segment. This MOST likely represents a(n)

a. blighted ovum

b. complete spontaneous abortion

c. threatened abortion

d. inevitable abortion

105. With respect to ectopic pregnancies, which of the following is TRUE?

a. An adnexal mass can usually be palpated.

b. Implantation in the interstitial portion of the tube is a common occurrence.

c. Cornual ectopic pregnancies may have dangerous prognoses.

d. Ectopic pregnancies cannot be carried past the first trimester.

106. A succenturiate placenta is a(an)

a. early matured placenta

b. small placenta

c. accessory lobe of the placenta

d. benign tumor of the placenta

107. If a sonographer is unable to demonstrate the fetal urinary bladder, it is important to rescan the area in approximately

a. 5 to 10 minutes

b. 15 to 45 minutes

c. 2 hours

d. 24 hours

108. The normal fetal heart rate in the second and third trimester generally ranges between

a. 100 to 120 beats per minute

b. 120 to 140 beats per minute

c. 120 to 160 beats per minute

d. 160 to 200 beats per minute

109. The fetal umbilical cord contains

a. two arteries and one vein

b. two arteries and two veins

c. one artery and one vein

d. one artery and two veins

110. Measurement of the cerebellum is BEST made at the level of the

a. thalamus, hippocampus, midbrain, cavum septi pellucidi

b. vermis, midbrain, cisterna magna

c. sphenoid, temporal bone, pituitary stalk

d. foramen magnum, pons, fourth ventricle

111. When measuring the ventricular system of the fetal head, the MOST accurate level to use is the

a. frontal horn

b. lateral ventricle parallel to the falx

c. lateral ventricular atrium

d. cisterna magna

112. A percentage of fetal blood from the IVC is shunted from the
    a. left atrium to right atrium
    b. right atrium to left atrium
    c. ductus venosus to left atrium
    d. right atrium to the ductus arteriosus

113. Visualization of a four-chambered heart within the fetal thorax enables determination of all of the following except
    a. position of the heart and size of the chambers
    b. mobility of the atrioventricular valves
    c. mobility of the semilunar valves
    d. visualization of the ventricular inflow tract

114. With respect to ultrasound of the fetal thorax, which of the following is TRUE?
    a. The diaphragm presents as a linear echoic band.
    b. Increased thickness of skin at the ventral aspect of the thorax usually indicates pathology.
    c. The long axis of the fetal heart is usually perpendicular to the long axis of the body.
    d. Visualization of fluid in the pleural space is normal.

115. An embryo presents with an outpouching from the anterior abdominal wall into the base of the umbilical cord. This is MOST likely to be
    a. gastroschisis
    b. omphalocele
    c. normal herniation of the fetal gut
    d. umbilical hernia

116. Which of the following statements is TRUE with regard to fetal bowel?
    a. Peristalsis can be seen in the small bowel, but not in the large bowel.
    b. Peristalsis can be seen in the large bowel, but not in the small bowel.
    c. The presence of echogenic meconium in the large bowel is normal early in the second trimester.
    d. The presence of echogenic meconium may be distinguished from an amniotic bleed.

117. Which of the following statements is TRUE regarding the fetal bladder?
    a. If the bladder appears distended, pathology is always indicated.
    b. The fetus voids approximately once per hour.
    c. If the bladder is not seen, pathology is indicated.
    d. The sonographer should wait 10 minutes to rescan the fetal bladder.

118. Deoxygenated fetal blood enters the placenta through the
    a. umbilical vein
    b. umbilical artery
    c. spiral artery
    d. uterine artery

119. The most common tumor of the placenta is the
    a. choriocarcinoma
    b. subplacental hematoma
    c. chorioangioma
    d. placenta percreta

120. A single umbilical artery may indicate anomalies of all of the following systems except
    a. cardiovascular
    b. hepatobiliary
    c. central nervous
    d. genitourinary

121. Placenta previa is MOST likely to present in association with which of the following?
    a. increased maternal age, increased parity, or previous abortion
    b. second-trimester bleeding
    c. a distance from presenting part to maternal sacrum less than 1.5 cm
    d. a placenta extending to and covering the fundus

122. Regarding BPD measurement as a predictor of gestational age, which of the following is TRUE?
    a. BPD is more accurate than femur length in the late third trimester.
    b. BPD is more accurate than femur length in the second trimester.
    c. BPD is routinely measured at the level of the ventricles.
    d. BPD is more accurate than HC in the second trimester.

123. The largest transverse section of the abdomen is MOST likely found at the location of the
    a. umbilicus and stomach
    b. confluence of the umbilical and portal veins and stomach
    c. stomach and middle portal vein
    d. fetal kidneys

124. IUGR is BEST defined as a fetus that is
    a. below the 10th percentile in weight
    b. usually associated with maternal hypertension
    c. at high risk of perinatal morbidity
    d. usually associated with systemic disease

125. When two ova are fertilized, this is BEST described as
    a. monozygotic twinning
    b. dizygotic twinning
    c. monochorionic and monoamniotic twinning
    d. monochorionic and diamniotic twinning

126. Which of the following complication is NOT associated with multiple gestations?
    a. IUGR of one or both twins
    b. increased incidence of preeclampsia
    c. increased third-trimester bleeding
    d. postterm labor

127. In a twin pregnancy, visualization of a septum greater than 1 mm in width is MOST likely to represent which type of twinning?
    a. dichorionic
    b. monochorionic
    c. diamniotic
    d. monoamniotic

128. Which of the following is LEAST LIKELY to be found in the fetus of a diabetic mother?
    a. IUGR
    b. microsomia
    c. skeletal and CNS anomalies
    d. cardiac anomalies

129. The presence of hypertension in the second or third trimester is NOT likely to increase the risk of
    a. fetal hydrops
    b. IUGR
    c. placental abruption
    d. toxemia

130. With the PUBS procedure, it is BEST to involve percutaneous sampling of the
    a. umbilical vein near the cord insertion at the placenta
    b. umbilical vein near the cord insertion at the umbilicus
    c. umbilical artery near the cord insertion at the placenta
    d. umbilical vessels within the placenta

131. Which of the following is MOST likely to cause postpartum hemorrhage?
    a. obesity
    b. increased age or parity
    c. prolonged labor
    d. delayed uterine involution

132. Prolonged severe oligohydramnios is MOST likely to lead to which of the following conditions?
    a. femur dysplasia
    b. pulmonary hypoplasia
    c. postterm pregnancy
    d. single umbilical artery

133. The Spalding sign is most often associated with
    a. fetal hydrops
    b. IUGR
    c. fetal demise
    d. pleural effusion

134. The term "fetus papyraceus" refers to a condition wherein the fetus
    a. is reabsorbed, leaving no detectable sign
    b. lacks normal bone structure
    c. lacks red blood cells, rendering it white as paper
    d. dies, but persists as a flattened structure with bones

135. A malformation which is characterized by the fourth ventricle defect of a retrocerebellar cyst communicating with the fourth ventricle is
    a. choroid plexus cyst
    b. Dandy-Walker malformation
    c. hydranencephaly
    d. holoprosencephaly

136. The MOST accurate method for evaluating hydrocephalus is to measure the diameter of the
    a. atrium of the lateral ventricle through the choroid plexus
    b. superior lateral ventricle from the falx to the lateral margin of the ventricle
    c. fourth ventricle at the level of the cerebellum
    d. frontal horns at the level of the thalami

137. A complex mass appearing on either side of the fetal neck is MOST likely to be a
    a. meningomyelocele
    b. cephalocele
    c. teratoma
    d. choroid plexus cyst

138. A spinal defect containing meninges and neural tissue is MOST likely to be a
    a. cephalocele
    b. spina bifida
    c. meningocele
    d. meningomyelocele

139. The "lemon sign and banana sign" are MOST usually associated with
    a. Arnold-Chiari malformation
    b. Dandy-Walker malformation
    c. duodenal atresia
    d. renal agenesis

140. Sonographic visualization of a fluid-filled mass behind the left atrium and ventricle in the lower thorax MOST likely represents
    a. cystic adenomatoid formation
    b. congenital diaphragmatic hernia
    c. pleural effusion
    d. pericardial effusion

141. Oligohydramnios after week 16 of gestation is MOST likely to indicate which of the following?
    a. unilateral renal agenesis
    b. bilateral renal agenesis
    c. dominant polycystic renal disease
    d. unilateral multicystic renal disease

142. Which of the following is NOT likely to be seen as a fluid-filled mass in the RUQ?
    a. congenital duplication cyst
    b. choledochal cyst
    c. urachal cyst
    d. ascites

143. A fetus with findings of a narrow bell-shaped thorax, curved and shortened long bones, and a cloverleaf skull is MOST likely to have
    a. osteogenesis imperfecta
    b. achondroplasia
    c. VACTERL syndrome
    d. thanatophoric dysplasia

144. Failure of the atrioventricular valves to separate into mitral and tricuspid valves is part of
    a. tetralogy of Fallot
    b. atrioventricular canal defect
    c. hypoplastic heart syndrome
    d. Ebstein's anomaly

145. Sonographic findings of oligohydramnios, absent kidneys, IUGR, and pulmonary hypoplasia are MOST consistent with
    a. Meckel-Gruber syndrome
    b. Potter's syndrome
    c. amniotic band syndrome
    d. limb body wall syndrome

146. Uterine contractions throughout pregnancy may be confused with
    a. leiomyoma
    b. Braxton Hicks
    c. Breus' mole
    d. hemangioma

147. Ovarian hyperstimulation syndrome may be associated with
    a. polycystic ovaries
    b. theca lutein cysts
    c. corpus luteum cysts
    d. mesenteric cysts

148. An allantoic duct cyst is MOST likely to be associated with which of the following intrauterine structures?
    a. gallbladder
    b. cystic duct
    c. umbilical cord
    d. hepatic vein

149. When placental tissue is seen to extend beyond the external uterine wall into the bladder, this condition is
    a. placenta previa
    b. placenta percreta
    c. placenta increta
    d. placenta accreta

150. What usually happens to the hCG levels in 48 hours in the presence of an ectopic pregnancy?
    a. hCG levels drop.
    b. hCG levels rise at a subnormal rate.
    c. hCG levels double.
    d. hCG levels rise at a markedly high rate.

151. A fluid collection in the endometrium that simulates the gestational sac of an early pregnancy is called
    a. decidual reaction
    b. endometritis
    c. pseudogestational sac
    d. hydrometra

152. In a nonstimulated cycle, the maximum normal size of the dominant follicle before ovulation is
    a. 5 mm
    b. 15 mm
    c. 25 mm
    d. 35 mm

153. Ovarian hyperstimulation syndrome typically occurs
    a. after the patient has received hCG and may be pregnant
    b. before the patient has received hCG
    c. after failed induction of ovulation
    d. after the patient has received intrauterine artificial insemination

154. The cervical os is usually about _____ cm long.
    a. 1 to 2
    b. 3 to 4
    c. 5 to 7
    d. 6 to 8

155. The cephalic index is defined as the ratio of the biparietal diameter to
    a. femur length
    b. occipitofrontal diameter
    c. abdominal circumference
    d. binocular distances

156. The date of the last menstrual period indicates
    a. the date when fertilization occurred
    b. the date when menstrual bleeding ended
    c. the date when ovulation occurred
    d. the date when menstrual bleeding began

157. Which of the following is not a sonographic finding of a hydatidiform mole?
    a. theca lutein cysts
    b. grapelike clusters throughout the uterus
    c. homogeneous uterine texture
    d. low impedance, high-flow Doppler pattern

158. How early can the site of the placenta be identified on sonography?
    a. 8 weeks
    b. 14 weeks
    c. 16 weeks
    d. 20 weeks

159. Amniotic band syndrome is
    a. adhesions of torn amniotic membranes wrapped around fetal parts and producing congenital amputations
    b. complications of placental abruption
    c. a syndrome that occurs after the fetus swallows too much fluid
    d. a and c

160. A 30-year-old gravid patient, 32 weeks by dates, now presents with painless vaginal bleeding that has lasted for 5 days. The first condition to rule out by sonography is
    a. an ectopic pregnancy
    b. placenta previa
    c. an ovarian cyst
    d. hydatidiform mole

161. The kidneys should be scanned transversely at a level
    a. superior to the hepatic veins
    b. inferior to the bladder
    c. superior to the falciform ligament
    d. inferior to the stomach

162. Ovulation occurs
    a. always after intercourse
    b. approximately on the 7th day of the menstrual cycle
    c. around the 14th day of the menstrual cycle
    d. approximately on the 2nd day of the menstrual cycle

163. The most common cause of painless vaginal bleeding in the second and third trimesters of pregnancy is
    a. trauma
    b. ectopic pregnancy
    c. placental abruption
    d. placenta previa

164. A growth-restricted fetus will show a Doppler pattern in the umbilical cord that is
    a. high resistance
    b. low resistance
    c. normal
    d. indicative increased diastolic flow

165. The amount of amniotic fluid present increases the most during the
    a. embryonic period
    b. third trimester
    c. second trimester
    d. first trimester

166. What references should be used to document the biparietal diameter?
    a. thalamus, cavum septi pellucidi, falx
    b. thalamus, peduncles
    c. peduncles, cerebellum
    d. falx, cavum septi pellucidi, fourth ventricle

167. The age of conceptus from fertilization is called
    a. menstrual age
    b. embryonic period
    c. conceptional age
    d. zygotic period

168. The term that describes the transformed endometrial lining of the uterus during pregnancy is
    a. chorion
    b. decidua
    c. chorion laeve
    d. decidua basalis

169. The thin decidua overlying the portion of the gestational sac facing the endometrial cavity is
    a. decidua capsularis
    b. decidua
    c. decidua basalis
    d. decidua vera

170. The formula used to calculate gestational age from CRL is
    a. GA = CRL + 6.5
    b. GA = CRL + 2.3
    c. GA = CRL + 5.6
    d. GA = CRL + 4.2

171. What occurs when there is death of the embryo or fetus, but the gestational parts remain in utero?
    a. incomplete or missed abortion
    b. spontaneous abortion
    c. blighted ovum
    d. ectopic pregnancy

172. Oligohydramnios means the AFI
    a. is less than 12 cm
    b. is more than 9 cm
    c. is less than 8 cm
    d. is less than 5 cm

173. A bicornuate uterus may be identified by
    a. two cervices
    b. two vaginas
    c. two cornua
    d. two urethras

174. In a four-chamber view of the heart, the right side may be differentiated from the left by
    a. flap of the foramen ovale opening to the right
    b. foramen ovale, moderator band, apical position of tricuspid valve
    c. thebesian valve, eustachian valve, papillary muscles
    d. lack of trabeculations at the apex of the ventricle

175. The renal pyramids appear as _____ areas throughout the renal medulla.
    a. hyperechoic
    b. anechoic
    c. hypoechoic
    d. echogenic

176. A diabetic mother may have an increased incidence of delivering a fetus with
    a. neural tube or cardiac defect
    b. Potter's syndrome
    c. trisomy 18
    d. cystic hygroma

177. Hydrops fetalis is characterized by
    a. cystic masses within the lungs
    b. edema, ascites, pleural or pericardial effusion
    c. dilated ventricles
    d. pericardial effusion

178. When measuring AFI, the sonographer should use color to
    a. separate umbilical cord and uterine wall from fluid
    b. make sure the placenta does not have a tear
    c. look for a rupture in the membrane
    d. record cardiac activity

179. Evaluation of a(n) _____ would be required if intrauterine growth restriction in all its forms were to be detected.
    a. weight chart
    b. head circumference chart
    c. growth profile
    d. abdominal circumference

180. The biophysical profile should document all of the following except
    a. fetal breathing
    b. gross fetal movements
    c. AFI
    d. fetal position

181. What broad muscle covers the anterior surface of the iliac fossa?
    a. piriformis
    b. iliacus
    c. obturator internus
    d. psoas

182. The broad ligament encloses all of the following except
    a. ovaries
    b. uterus
    c. uterine tubes
    d. bladder

183. The thickened fold of mesentery that supports and stabilizes the position of each ovary is the
    a. ligamentum teres
    b. fibrous ligament
    c. broad ligament
    d. round ligament

184. The pouch located between the uterus and rectum is
    a. rectouterine
    b. rectovesicular
    c. Morison's
    d. uterine

185. The muscle that originates from the ilium and sacrum and passes through the great sciatic notch to insert on the greater trochanter is the
    a. obturator internus
    b. obturator externus
    c. piriformis
    d. coccygeus

Answers

CHAPTER 1

Exercise 1

1. I	7. U	13. F	19. P
2. B	8. K	14. V	20. G
3. L	9. W	15. J	21. E
4. Q	10. H	16. T	22. R
5. O	11. C	17. A	23. M
6. D	12. N	18. S	

Exercise 2

1. G	4. I	7. K	10. J
2. C	5. E	8. A	11. D
3. B	6. H	9. F	

Exercise 3

1. H	6. K	11. L	16. O
2. M	7. F	12. I	17. J
3. D	8. N	13. A	18. B
4. R	9. Q	14. P	19. S
5. C	10. E	15. G	

Exercise 4

1. generating, propagating, receiving

2. 20 kilohertz

3. Dussick, R. H. Bolt and H. T. Ballantyne, Fry, Holmes, Edler, Hertz, Howry, Wild, Ludwig, Rushmer, Franklin, Baker, Donald

4. diagnostic medical ultrasonography, sonography, ultrasound, and ultrasonography

5. echocardiography

6. sonographer

7. intellectual curiosity (keep abreast of developments in the field), perseverance to obtain high-quality images (ability to recognize artifact from structural anatomy), ability to conceptualize two-dimensional images into a three-dimensional format (very important), quick-thinking and analytic capabilities (always analyzing the image quality while keeping the clinical situation in mind), technical aptitude (very important), good physical health (continuous scanning may cause strain on back, shoulder, arm), independence and self-direction (must be able to analyze the patient, the history, the clinical findings, and tailor the examination to answer the clinical question), emotional stability to deal with patients in times of crisis (ability to understand the patient's concerns without losing objectivity), communication skills with peers, clinicians, and patients (ability to openly communicate ultrasound findings to physicians and the ability to be tactful with the patient by not revealing findings during the examination), and dedication

Exercise 5

1. L	4. D	7. I	10. E
2. C	5. A	8. B	11. K
3. F	6. G	9. H	12. J

Exercise 6

1. smooth, well-defined, and irregular
2. homogeneous and heterogeneous
3. increased, unchanged, and decreased
4. anechoic, hypoechoic, isoechoic, hyperechoic, and echogenic
5. smooth, well-defined borders, anechoic, increased through transmission
6. irregular borders, internal echoes, decreased through transmission
7. characteristics of both cystic and solid

Exercise 7

1. compression, rarefaction
2. electrical, mechanical
3. wave
4. frequency
5. longitudinal
6. wavelength
7. shorter
8. decreases
9. power
10. intensity
11. doubles
12. Curie
13. poor
14. faster
15. 1540
16. velocity of sound
17. perpendicular, angle of incidence
18. attenuation
19. axial
20. lateral
21. beam width
22. spatial
23. exam, size of patient, and amount of fatty or muscular tissue present
24. pulse repetition frequency
25. high
26. amplitude modulation
27. brightness modulation
28. gray scale
29. motion mode
30. real-time
31. twice
32. aliasing

Exercise 8

1. artifactual noise, absence of focusing, grating lobes, and side lobes
2. noise and banding
3. breathing
4. shadowing, reverberation, mirror image, enhancement, slice thickness, and comet effect

CHAPTER 2

Exercise 1

1. E	4. A	7. D	10. B
2. I	5. K	8. J	11. H
3. G	6. F	9. L	12. C

Exercise 2

1. F	5. H	9. E	13. A
2. J	6. N	10. C	14. G
3. D	7. B	11. M	
4. L	8. K	12. I	

Exercise 3

1. objective
2. Introduce yourself to patient and explain what you will be doing, reassure the patient everything will be kept confidential, be sure patient understands English and can hear well, and use a medical language patient can understand.
3. 96.7, 100.5
4. pulse
5. 60,100
6. 16, 20
7. systolic
8. diastolic

9. observe the abdomen for symmetry, note the patient's abdominal shape and contour, umbilicus should be midline and inverted, skin of abdomen smooth and uniform in color, presence or absence of dilated veins, and presence or absence of surgical scars

10. abdominal pain, diarrhea, hematochezia, and nausea and vomiting

11. concentration, memory loss, or disorientation

12. dysuria, urinary incontinence

Exercise 4

1. B	4. D	7. I
2. E	5. A	8. C
3. G	6. F	9. H

CHAPTER 3

Exercise 1

1. F	3. A	5. D
2. C	4. E	6. B

Exercise 2

1. J	5. G	9. N	13. L
2. D	6. C	10. E	14. M
3. K	7. B	11. P	15. I
4. A	8. H	12. F	16. O

Exercise 3

1. B	6. M	11. S	16. P
2. G	7. D	12. C	17. O
3. L	8. H	13. N	18. K
4. A	9. R	14. I	19. Q
5. E	10. J	15. F	

Exercise 4

System	Components	Functions
1. Muscular	Skeletal, cardiac, smooth muscle	Moves parts of skeleton, provides locomotion; pumps blood; aids movement of internal materials; produces body heat
2. Endocrine	Pituitary, adrenal, thyroid, pancreas, parathyroid, ovaries, testes, pineal, and thymus gland	Regulates body chemistry and many body functions
3. Circulatory	Heart, blood vessels, blood; lymph and lymph structures	Moves the blood through the vessels and transports substances throughout the body
4. Digestive	Mouth, tongue, teeth, salivary glands, pharynx, esophagus, stomach, liver, gallbladder, pancreas, and small and large intestines	Receives, breaks down, and absorbs food and eliminates unabsorbed material from the body
5. Urinary	Kidney, bladder, ureters	Excretes waste from the blood; maintains water and electrolyte balance; and stores and transports urine
6. Reproductive	Testes, scrotum, spermatic cord, vas deferens, ejaculatory duct, penis, epididymis, prostate, uterus, ovaries, fallopian tubes, vagina, breast	Allows reproduction; provides for continuation of the species

Exercise 5

1. anterior *or* ventral
2. proximal
3. superior
4. superficial
5. posterior *or* dorsal
6. distal
7. inferior
8. deep
9. medial
10. cephalic
11. lateral
12. caudal

Exercise 6

1. O
2. D
3. L
4. B
5. G
6. A
7. I
8. F
9. C
10. J
11. H
12. E
13. M
14. K
15. N

Exercise 7

1. dorsal cavity, ventral cavity
2. cranial cavity
3. ventral cavity, thoracic cavity, abdominal cavity
4. diaphragm
5. pleural sacs
6. pericardial sac

Exercise 8

1. diaphragm, abdominal wall, pelvis
2. hypochondrium, epigastrium, epigastrium, left hypochondrium
3. right
4. anterior, left
5. right
6. diaphragm
7. right
8. medial arcuate ligament
9. linea alba
10. rectus abdominis
11. pelvis major *or* false pelvis
12. pelvis minor *or* true pelvis
13. part of the large intestine, rectum, urinary bladder, and reproductive organs
14. vesicouterine
15. rectouterine
16. fallopian
17. coccygeus, levator ani
18. psoas, iliopsoas
19. piriformis
20. parietal, visceral
21. greater
22. lesser
23. epiploic foramen
24. peritoneum
25. falciform
26. ligamentum teres
27. gastrosplenic

Exercise 9

1. subphrenic
2. Morison's pouch
3. peritoneal recesses
4. right
5. hernia

Exercise 10

1. kidneys, ureters, adrenal glands, pancreas, aorta, inferior vena cava, bladder, uterus, prostate gland, ascending and descending colon, and most of the duodenum
2. anterior pararenal space
3. posterior pararenal space
4. perirenal

Exercise 11

1. gross anatomy, histology, embryology, pathology
2. cell
3. tissue
4. muscle, nervous, connective, epithelial
5. organs
6. body systems
7. metabolism
8. body temperature, blood pressure, pulse, breathing

Exercise 12

1. See Figure 3-1 in the textbook for the answers.
2. See Figure 3-2 in the textbook for the answers.
3. See Figure 3-3 in the textbook for the answers.
4. See Figure 3-4 in the textbook for the answers.
5. See Figure 3-6 in the textbook for the answers.
6. See Figure 3-11 in the textbook for the answers.
7. See Figure 3-12 in the textbook for the answers.
8. See Figure 3-15 in the textbook for the answers.
9. See Figure 3-16 in the textbook for the answers.
10. See Figure 3-19 in the textbook for the answers.
11. See Figure 3-20 in the textbook for the answers.

CHAPTER 4

Exercise 1

1. I	4. H	7. F	10. D
2. E	5. A	8. L	11. G
3. C	6. J	9. B	12. K

Exercise 2

1. E	4. J	7. D	10. K
2. A	5. B	8. I	11. C
3. H	6. F	9. G	

Exercise 3

1. H	5. D	8. I	11. E
2. M	6. A	9. L	12. J
3. C	7. F	10. B	13. G
4. K			

Exercise 4

1. left
2. left, right
3. scanning table
4. rib
5. 6 to 8
6. liver and porta hepatis, vascular structures, biliary system, pancreas, kidneys, spleen, and paraaortic area
7. above the baseline, below the baseline
8. systolic
9. hepatic veins

Exercise 5

1. See Figure 4-1 in the textbook for the answers.
2. See Figure 4-8 in the textbook for the answers.
3. See Figure 4-9 in the textbook for the answers.
4. See Figure 4-10 in the textbook for the answers.
5. See Figure 4-11 in the textbook for the answers.
6. See Figure 4-12 in the textbook for the answers.
7. See Figure 4-13 in the textbook for the answers.
8. See Figure 4-14 in the textbook for the answers.
9. See Figure 4-16 in the textbook for the answers.
10. See Figure 4-21 in the textbook for the answers.
11. See Figure 4-22 in the textbook for the answers.
12. See Figure 4-23 in the textbook for the answers.
13. See Figure 4-24 in the textbook for the answers.
14. See Figure 4-25 in the textbook for the answers.
15. See Figure 4-26 in the textbook for the answers.
16. See Figure 4-29 in the textbook for the answers.
17. See Figure 4-31 in the textbook for the answers.
18. See Figure 4-32 in the textbook for the answers.
19. See Figure 4-33 in the textbook for the answers.

CHAPTER 5

Exercise 1

1. A	3. E	5. D
2. F	4. B	6. C

Exercise 2

1. H	5. A	9. B	13. K
2. D	6. G	10. N	14. F
3. M	7. L	11. E	
4. I	8. J	12. C	

Exercise 3

1. A	4. I	7. G
2. F	5. B	8. E
3. C	6. D	9. H

Exercise 4

1. G	5. F	9. E	13. H
2. D	6. I	10. C	14. N
3. M	7. L	11. K	
4. A	8. B	12. J	

Exercise 5

1. E	5. F
2. B	6. D
3. A	7. G
4. C	

Exercise 6

1. See Figure 5-4 in the textbook for the answers.
2. See Figure 5-6 in the textbook for the answers.
3. See Figure 5-10 in the textbook for the answers.
4. See Figure 5-18 in the textbook for the answers.
5. See Figure 5-27 in the textbook for the answers.

Exercise 7

1. left ventricular
2. superior mesenteric vein
3. right hepatic artery
4. retroperitoneal, left
5. celiac
6. left renal vein
7. 2 to 3 cm, 1.0 to 1.5 cm
8. superior mesenteric artery
9. smaller
10. right renal artery
11. gastroduodenal artery
12. brachiocephalic, left common carotid, left subclavian arteries
13. portal vein
14. splenic
15. popliteal artery
16. hepatic veins

Exercise 8

1. root of the aorta, ascending aorta, descending aorta, abdominal aorta, and bifurcation of the aorta into iliac arteries.

2. The arteries are hollow elastic tubes that carry blood away from the heart. They are enclosed within a sheath that includes a vein and nerve. The smaller arteries contain less elastic tissue and more smooth muscles than the larger arteries. The elasticity of the larger arteries is important in maintaining a steady blood flow. The veins are hollow collapsible tubes with a diminished tunica media that carry blood toward the heart. The veins appear collapsed because they have little elastic tissue or muscle within their walls. Veins have a larger total diameter than the arteries, and they move blood more slowly.

3. the celiac trunk, the superior and inferior mesenteric arteries, and the renal arteries.

4. along with the heart and lymphatics, to transport gases, nutrient materials, and other essential substances to the tissues and subsequently transport waste products from the cells to the appropriate sites for excretion.

5. The veins contain special valves that prevent backflow and permit blood to flow only in one direction, toward the heart. Numerous valves are found within the extremities, especially the lower extremities, because flow must work against gravity. Venous return is also aided by muscle contraction, overflow from capillary beds, gravity, and suction from negative thoracic pressure.

6. Sagittal scans should be made beginning in the midline with a slight angulation of the transducer to the left, from the xiphoid to well below the level of bifurcation. In the normal individual, the luminal dimension of the aorta gradually tapers as it proceeds distally in the abdomen. A low-to-medium gain should be used to demonstrate the walls of the aorta without "noisy" artifactual internal echoes. These weak echoes may result from increased gain, reverberation from the anterior abdominal wall fat or musculature, or poor lateral resolution. These factors result in echoes being recorded at the same level as those from soft tissues that surround the vessel lumen, particularly if the vessels are smaller in diameter than the transducer. Try to use different techniques of breath holding to eliminate these artifactual echoes. Sometimes increased gentle pressure may help displace the bowel gas or compress the fatty tissue so the transducer will be closer to the abdominal aorta. If the abdomen is very concave, the patient may be instructed to "extend his abdomen" ("push the abdomen muscle out") so as to provide a better scanning plane.

Exercise 9

1. Doppler ultrasound frequently is used to differentiate vessels from nonvascular structures. For example, to distinguish the common bile duct from the hepatic artery, look for absence of flow in the common duct; to distinguish the hepatic artery from the splenic artery, look for direction of flow; to differentiate aneurysm from pancreatic pseudocyst, look for slow flow in the aneurysm; to differentiate dilated intrahepatic bile ducts and prominent hepatic artery, again look for absence of flow in the bile duct.

2. pseudoaneurysm

3. The patient should be instructed to hold his or her breath; this causes the patient to perform a slight Valsalva maneuver toward the end of inspiration, which dilates the inferior vena cava. The inferior vena cava may expand to 3 to 4 cm in diameter with this maneuver.

4. diastolic

Exercise 10

1. arteriosclerosis, atherosclerosis

2. intense back pain, hematocrit

3. outer, outer

4. anterior, anterolateral

5. pseudoaneurysm

6. A dissection may be detected by ultrasound and usually displays one or more clinical signs and symptoms. The typical patient is 40 to 60 years old and hypertensive; males are predominate over females. The patient is usually known to have an aneurysm, and sudden, excruciating chest pain radiating to the back may develop because of a dissection. The sonographer should look for a dissection "flap" or recent channel with or without frank aneurysmal dilation. The dissection of blood is along the laminar planes of the aortic media with formation of a blood-filled channel within the aortic wall.

7. The Type I dissection begins at the root of the aorta and may extend the entire length of the arch, descending to the aorta

7. Blood is carried away from the heart by the arteries and returned from the tissues to the heart by the veins. Arteries divide into progressively smaller branches, the smallest of which are the arterioles. These lead into the capillaries, which are minute vessels that branch and form a network where the exchange of materials between blood and tissue fluid takes place. After the blood passes through the capillaries, it is collected in the small veins, or venules. These small vessels unite to form larger vessels that eventually return the blood to the heart for recirculation.

8. The capillaries are minute, hair-size vessels connecting the arterial and venous systems. Their walls have only one layer. The cells and tissues of the body receive their nutrients from the fluids passing through the capillary walls; at the same time, waste products from the cells pass into the capillaries. Arteries do not always end in capillary beds; some end in anastomoses, which are end-to-end grafts between different vessels that equalize pressure over vessel length and also provide alternative flow channels.

5. external

6. The pulsatile aorta is easily differentiated from the inferior vena cava as the IVC travels in a horizontal course with its proximal portion curving slightly anterior as it pierces the diaphragm to empty into the right atrial cavity. On the contrary, the aorta follows the curvature of the spine with its distal portion lying more posterior before bifurcating into the iliac vessels.

7. plug flow

8. parallel

9. systolic, diastolic

10. low

11. increases

12. continuous

13. periportal

14. umbilical

and into the abdominal aorta. This is the most dangerous, especially if the dissection spirals around the aorta, cutting off the blood supply to the coronaries, carotid, brachiocephalic, and subclavian vessels. Dissection of the aorta (Type II) may be secondary to cystic medial necrosis (weakening of the arterial wall), to the inherited disease Marfan syndrome (individuals with this disorder are extremely tall, lanky, and double jointed; a progressive stretching disorder exists in all arterial vessels, especially in the aorta, causing abnormal dilation, weakened walls, and eventual dissection, rupture, or both), or to hypertension. Color flow Doppler may be used to detect flow into the false channel. The third type of dissection (Type III) begins at the lower end of the descending aorta and extends into the abdominal aorta. This may be critical if the dissection spirals around to impede the flow of blood into the renal vessels.

8. Masses that can simulate a pulsatile abdominal mass are retroperitoneal tumors, fibroid uterus, and para-aortic nodes.

Because the mass is adjacent to the aorta, the pulsations are transmitted from the aorta to the mass. After an abdominal aneurysm, the most common cause for a pulsatile abdominal mass is enlarged retroperitoneal lymph nodes.

9. collapse

Exercise 11

1. According to Figure 5-39 in the textbook, this is a large abdominal aortic aneurysm with thrombus along the anterior and posterior borders. The lumen of the vessel is anechoic.

10. Complete thrombosis of the inferior vena cava is life threatening. Patients present with leg edema, low back pain, pelvic pain, gastrointestinal complaints, and renal and liver abnormalities.

11. lower

2. Based on Figure 5-46 in the textbook, if the inferior vena cava measures greater than 2.4 cm and does not show collapse with expiration, it is enlarged.

3. The arrows in Figure 5-47, *A* in the textbook; the arrows are pointing to the thrombus.

CHAPTER 6

Exercise 1

1. C	5. M	9. B	13. E
2. A	6. D	10. F	14. L
3. N	7. H	11. J	
4. G	8. I	12. K	

Exercise 2

1. H	5. J	9. L	13. K
2. B	6. I	10. G	
3. D	7. F	11. M	
4. A	8. E	12. C	

Exercise 3

1. B	5. D
2. H	6. E
3. F	7. C
4. A	8. G

Exercise 4

1. See Figure 6-2 in the textbook for the answers.
2. See Figure 6-3 in the textbook for the answers.
3. See Figure 6-4 in the textbook for the answers.
4. See Figure 6-5 in the textbook for the answers.

Exercise 5

1. Riedel's lobe
2. Glisson's capsule
3. main lobar fissure
4. falciform ligament
5. ligamentum teres
6. ligamentum venosum
7. right, middle, left
8. metabolism
9. digestion
10. bilirubin
11. storage
12. detoxification
13. hepatocellular, obstructive
14. carbohydrates, fats, amino acids
15. glucose
16. lipoproteins
17. edema
18. enzymes
19. AST, ALT
20. alkaline phosphatase
21. bilirubin
22. jaundice

Exercise 6

1. The liver occupies almost all of the right hypochondrium, the greater part of the epigastrium, and the left hypochondrium as far as the mammillary line. The contour and shape of the liver vary according to patient habitus and lie. Its shape is also influenced by the lateral segment of the left lobe and the length of the right lobe of the liver. The liver lies inferior to the diaphragm. The ribs cover the greater part of the right lobe. (Usually a small part of the right lobe is in contact with the abdominal wall.) In the epigastric region, the liver extends several centimeters below the xiphoid process. Most of the left lobe is covered by the rib cage.

2. The right lobe of the liver is the largest of the liver's three lobes. It exceeds the left lobe by a ratio of 6:1. It occupies the right hypochondrium and is bordered on its upper surface by the falciform ligament, on its posterior surface by the left sagittal fossa, and in front by the umbilical notch. Its inferior and posterior surfaces are marked by three fossae: the porta hepatis, the gallbladder fossa, and the inferior vena cava fossa.

3. The left lobe of the liver lies in the epigastric and left hypochondriac regions. Its upper surface is convex and molded onto the diaphragm. Its undersurface includes the gastric impression and omental tuberosity. The medial segment of the left lobe is oblong and situated on the posteroinferior surface of the left lobe. In front it is bounded by the anterior margin of the liver, behind by the porta hepatis, on the right by the fossa for the gallbladder, and on the left by the fossa for the umbilical vein. The size of the left lobe of the liver varies considerably; the more prominent left lobe will allow the sonographer to image the pancreas and vascular structures anterior to the spine.

4. Glisson's capsule, main lobar fissure, falciform ligament, ligamentum teres, and ligamentum venosum

5. The best way to distinguish the hepatic from the portal vessels is to trace their points of entry to the liver. The hepatic vessels flow into the inferior vena cava, whereas the splenic vein and superior mesenteric vein join together to form the portal venous system. Real-time sector scanning allows the sonographer to make this assessment within a few seconds. Hepatic veins course between the hepatic lobes and segments. Hepatic veins are larger as they drain into the inferior vena cava before entering the right atrium; the portal veins are larger at their origin as they emanate from the porta hepatis. Portal veins have more echogenic borders than the hepatic veins because they have a thicker collagenous sheath.

6. AST (SGOT), ALT (SGPT), lactic acid dehydrogenase, alkaline phosphatase, bilirubin, prothrombin time, and albumin and globulins

Exercise 7

1. The normal, basically homogeneous parenchyma of the liver, allows imaging of the neighboring anatomic structures in the upper abdomen. Echo amplitude, attenuation, and transmission and parenchymal textures may be physically assessed with proper evaluation of the hepatic structures.

2. hepatic veins, portal veins, hepatic, hepatic

3. hepatopetal, hepatofugal

4. anterior, medial

5. The easiest way to do this is to hold the transducer over a deep segment of the right lobe of the liver. The far time-gain control pods should gradually be increased with a smooth motion of the index finger until the posterior aspect of the liver is well seen. The near-field time-gain controls should be adjusted (usually decreased) to image the anterior wall and musculature, the anterior hepatic capsule, and the near field of the hepatic parenchyma.

6. near field

7. sector or annular

Exercise 8

1. size, configuration, homogeneity, and contour

2. hepatocytes

3. cell

4. lipid accumulation

5. Moderate-to-severe fatty infiltration shows increased echogenicity on ultrasound. Enlargement of the lobe affected by fatty infiltration is evident. The portal vein structures may be difficult to visualize because of the increased attenuation of the ultrasound. The increased attenuation also causes a decrease in penetration of the sound beam, which may be a clue for the sonographer to think of fatty liver disease. Fatty infiltration is not always uniform and may demonstrate areas of focal sparing (hypoechoic masslike areas). Most common areas of focal sparing are located anterior to the gallbladder and portal vein and the posterior portion of the left lobe of the liver.

6. gallbladder, left lobe

7. coarse, decreased

8. degenerates, fat

9. The diagnosis of cirrhosis by ultrasound may be difficult. Specific findings may include coarsening of the liver parenchyma secondary to fibrosis and nodularity. Increased attenuation may be present with decreased vascular markings. Hepatosplenomegaly may be present with ascites surrounding the liver. The caudate lobe and left lateral lobe may be hypertrophied with the caudate to right lobe ratio exceeding 0.65. In addition, there may be atrophy of the right and left medial lobes of the liver. Chronic cirrhosis may show nodularity of the liver edge, especially if ascites is present. The hepatic fissures may be accentuated. The isoechoic regenerating nodules may be seen throughout the liver parenchyma. Portal hypertension may be present with or without abnormal Doppler flow patterns. Patients who have cirrhosis have an increased incidence of hepatoma tumors within the liver parenchyma.

10. hepatic adenomas, hyperplasia

11. cysts, abscess, hematoma, primary tumor, and metastases

12. The sonographer should be able to differentiate whether the mass is extrahepatic or intrahepatic. Intrahepatic masses may cause the following findings on ultrasound: displacement of the hepatic vascular radicles, external bulging of the liver capsule, or a posterior shift of the inferior vena cava. An extrahepatic mass may show internal invagination or discontinuity of the liver capsule, formation of a triangular fat wedge, anteromedial shift of the inferior vena cava, or anterior displacement of the right kidney.

13. fever, white cell elevation, and right upper quadrant pain

14. neoplasm

15. hemangioma

16. cirrhosis, hepatitis B

17. solitary massive tumor, multiple nodules throughout the liver, or diffuse infiltrative masses in the liver

18. spleen, kidney

19. Complications of transplantation include rejection, thrombosis or leak, biliary stricture or leak, infection, and neoplasia. Rejection is the most common cause of hepatic dysfunction that is confirmed by clinical diagnosis and liver biopsy. Vascular complications include thrombosis, stricture, and arterial anastomotic pseudoaneurysms. Vascular thrombosis may affect the hepatic artery, the portal vein, or less commonly, the inferior vena cava (more common in Budd-Chiari patients) and aorta. Biliary complications, stricture, and leakage affect a small percentage of transplant patients. Since the hepatic artery is the sole supply of blood to the bile ducts in transplant patients, identification of a stricture of the bile duct is an indication for assessment of hepatic artery patency. Hepatic arterial occlusion, pretransplant primary sclerosing cholangitis, choledochojejunostomy, cholangitis at liver biopsy, and young age are significantly associated with biliary strictures.

20. portal hypertension

21. thrombus, tumor

22. recanalized

23. lowered

24. smaller

25. direction of flow, velocity, and angle to flow

26. Budd-Chiari

Exercise 9

1. After evaluating Figure 6-30 in the textbook, the conclusion is fatty infiltration.

2. Based on Figure 6-34, *F,* the liver is shrunken with a coarse texture, consistent with cirrhosis. Ascites surrounds the liver. The gallbladder wall is thickened, a false positive in patients with ascites; therefore acute cholecystitis may not be ruled out by this finding alone.

3. According to Figure 6-45, the abnormality demonstrated is polycystic liver disease. The sonographer should also investigate the kidneys.

4. There is a well-defined echogenic lesion in the dome of the right lobe of the liver present in Figure 6-51 of the textbook. Color Doppler shows increased flow within the lesion. Cavernous hemangioma.

5. A large heterogeneous mass in the right lobe of the liver is visible in Figure 6-61 of the textbook. It extends from the dome of the liver, nearly filling the right lobe. With the history of cirrhosis, this most likely represents a hepatocellular carcinoma.

CHAPTER 7

Exercise 1

1. C	5. F	9. I	13. N
2. L	6. O	10. E	14. H
3. M	7. G	11. D	15. K
4. A	8. B	12. J	

Exercise 2

1. E	5. L	9. D	13. N
2. C	6. O	10. M	14. B
3. K	7. A	11. G	15. H
4. I	8. J	12. P	16. F

Exercise 3

1. See Figure 7-1 in the textbook for the answers.

2. See Figure 7-2 in the textbook for the answers.

Exercise 4

1. bile
2. common bile duct
3. ampulla of Vater
4. sphincter of Oddi
5. cystic artery
6. the transportation of bile from the liver to the intestine and the regulation of its flow

Exercise 5

1. When the gallbladder and bile ducts are functioning normally, they respond in a fairly uniform manner in various phases of digestion. Concentration of bile in the gallbladder occurs during a state of fasting. It is forced into the gallbladder by an increased pressure within the common bile duct that is produced by the action of the sphincter of Oddi at the distal end of the gallbladder. During the fasting state, very little bile flows into the duodenum. Stimulation produced by the influence of food causes the gallbladder to contract, resulting in an outpouring of bile into the duodenum. When the stomach is emptied, duodenal peristalsis diminishes, the gallbladder relaxes, the tonus of the sphincter of Oddi increases slightly, and thus very little bile passes into the duodenum. Small amounts of bile secreted by the liver are retained in the common duct and forced into the gallbladder.
2. cholesterol
3. bile salts
4. Courvoisier's sign
5. anterior, right
6. anterior, left

Exercise 6

1. 8 to 12
2. inspiration
3. decubitus
4. sonolucent
5. fossa
6. fat or fibrous
7. echogenic
8. Mickey Mouse
9. oblique
10. posterior
11. anterior
12. hepatic

Exercise 7

1. right upper abdominal quadrant
2. right
3. 3
4. cholecystitis, adenomyomatosis, cancer, acquired immunodeficiency syndrome, cholangiopathy, and sclerosing cholangitis
5. acute right upper quadrant pain (positive Murphy's sign—inspiratory arrest upon palpation of gallbladder area; may be false positive in small percentage of patients), fever, and leukocytosis
6. WES
7. emphysematous cholecystitis
8. fat, female, forty, fertile, fair
9. The patient's position should be shifted during the procedure to demonstrate the presence of movement of the stones. Patients should be scanned in the left decubitus, right lateral, or upright position. The stones should shift to the most dependent area of the gallbladder. In some cases the bile has a thick consistency, and the stones remain near the top of the gallbladder. Thus the density of the stones and the posterior shadow will be the sonographic evidence for stones.
10. The factors that produced a shadow were attributed to acoustic impedance of the gallstones; refraction through them or diffraction around them; their size, central or peripheral location, and position in relation to the focus of the beam; and the intensity of the beam.
11. choledochal cysts
12. adenomyomatosis
13. WES
14. The gallbladder wall is markedly abnormal and thickened.
15. tumor, thrombus
16. intrapancreatic obstruction, suprapancreatic obstruction, and porta hepatic obstruction
17. Mirizzi
18. cholangitis
19. calculous cholecystitis
20. air or gas
21. Caroli's

Exercise 8

1. Based on Figure 7-16 in the textbook, change the patient position to see if the sludge moves; the bile can be very viscous, and the movement of sludge may be slow.

2. According to Figure 7-19, pain in the right upper quadrant and fever are the clinical signs of acute cholecystitis. The sonographic findings include enlarged gallbladder, positive Murphy's sign, thick gallbladder wall with irregularities, presence of stones, and pericholecystic fluid. Complications would include rupture of the gallbladder, empyema, emphysematous or gangrenous cholecystitis, and perforation.

3. Based on Figure 7-20, the duodenum may lie in the area of the gallbladder, and if it is filled with fluid, may lead to confusion in the identification of the gallbladder. The sonographer can see if peristalsis is present or change the patient's position to better image the gallbladder area.

4. WES, wall echo shadow, is a finding of chronic cholelithiasis in which the gallbladder is packed with stones, based on Figure 7-23 in the textbook.

5. Multiple stones are "floating" within the gallbladder with sludge along their posterior border in Figure 7-32 in the textbook.

6. Based on your findings in Figure 7-34, there is a small echogenic structure that appears to be attached to the anterior wall of the gallbladder and most likely represents a polyp. Alterations in the patient position will show the lesion firmly attached to the gallbladder wall without movement. No shadow is apparent with the polyp.

7. How long has the patient experienced pain? Where does the pain occur? Does position change help? Has the patient noticed yellow coloration in the whites of the eyes or the skin? There is dilatation of the intrahepatic ducts. Carefully evaluate the liver and pancreas areas for possible mass.

CHAPTER 8

Exercise 1

1. E
2. A
3. G
4. J

5. O
6. N
7. K
8. L

9. H
10. D
11. C
12. M

13. I
14. B
15. F

Exercise 2

1. F
2. I
3. A

4. D
5. C
6. G

7. B
8. H
9. E

Exercise 3

1. I
2. L
3. J

4. A
5. D
6. H

7. C
8. B
9. K

10. G
11. F
12. E

Exercise 4

1. See Figure 8-2 in the textbook for the answers.
2. See Figure 8-4, *B* in the textbook for the answers.

3. See Figure 8-5 in the textbook for the answers.

Exercise 5

1. retroperitoneal
2. isoechoic, hyperechoic
3. aorta, inferior vena cava
4. anterior
5. superior mesenteric vein
6. splenic artery

7. colic flexure, transverse colon
8. duct of Wirsung
9. splenic artery, pancreaticoduodenal
10. gastroduodenal
11. common bile
12. anterior

Exercise 6

1. exocrine, endocrine
2. diabetes mellitus
3. acini cells
4. sphincter of Oddi
5. islets of Langerhans
6. insulin
7. glucagons
8. somatostatin
9. amylase, lipase
10. lipase
11. glucose

Exercise 7

1. The parenchymal texture of the pancreas depends on the amount of fat between the lobules and to a lesser extent on the interlobular fibrous tissue. The internal echoes of the pancreas consist of closely spaced elements of the same intensity with uniform distribution throughout the gland. Fat is strongly echogenic.

2. superior mesenteric artery and vein, portal and splenic veins, aorta and inferior vena cava, common bile duct, gastroduodenal artery, left renal vein, duodenal bulb, posterior wall of the stomach, and pancreatic duct

3. The patient should drink 32 to 300 ml of fluid through a straw in the erect or right lateral decubitus position. The fluid fills the duodenal cap to outline the lateral margin of the head of the pancreas. The upright position allows the air to move from the gastric antrum to the fundus of the stomach and causes the upper viscera to move downward for a better sonic window.

4. inferior vena cava

Exercise 8

1. pancreatitis
2. alcoholism, biliary tract disease
3. epigastrium, back
4. lobulations, congested vessels
5. inflammation, spasm, edema, swelling of the papilla, and pseudocyst
6. bed, pararenal, Morison's, duodenum
7. pseudocyst, phlegmon, abscess, hemorrhage, and duodenal obstruction
8. Grey Turner's
9. phlegmon
10. pancreatic ducts, chronic

11. The pancreatic enzymes that escape the ductal system cause enzymatic digestion of the surrounding tissue and pseudocyst development. The walls of the pseudocyst form in the various potential spaces in which the escaped pancreatic enzymes are found. The pseudocyst usually presents few symptoms until it becomes large enough to cause pressure of the surrounding organs.

12. lesser sac
13. pancreatic enzymes
14. adenocarcinoma
15. weight loss, painless jaundice, nausea, vomiting, and changes in stools
16. lymphoma

Exercise 9

1. The arrows in Figure 8-10, C in the textbook are pointing to the superior mesenteric vein.
2. According to Figure 8-11, the image is transverse, and the arrows are pointing to the pancreas.
3. The arrows in Figure 8-15, A are pointing to a collapsed stomach.

4. Based on Figure 8-26, the ultrasound findings are an enlarged, edematous pancreas—pancreatitis.
5. Based on Figure 8-31 in the textbook, your findings are pancreatitis with hemorrhage. The gland is enlarged and echogenic secondary to freshly clotted blood.
6. Based on Figure 8-43, your findings are adenocarcinoma of the pancreas with a dilated common bile duct. The gallbladder is dilated.

CHAPTER 9

Exercise 1

1. F	6. C	11. T	16. P
2. H	7. M	12. I	17. K
3. B	8. A	13. Q	18. L
4. J	9. N	14. O	19. R
5. D	10. E	15. S	20. G

Exercise 2

1. F   5. C
2. D   6. B
3. A   7. G
4. E

Exercise 3

1. J   4. B   7. C   10. D
2. H   5. A   8. G   11. K
3. L   6. F   9. I   12. E

Exercise 4

1. See Figure 9-1 in the textbook for the answers.
2. See Figure 9-2 in the textbook for the answers.
3. See Figure 9-4 in the textbook for the answers.
4. See Figure 9-5 in the textbook for the answers.
5. See Figure 9-6 in the textbook for the answers.

Exercise 5

1. mouth, pharynx, esophagus, stomach, small intestine (duo-denum, jejunum, and ileum), and large intestine (cecum; ascending, transverse, and descending colon; and rectum).
2. cardiac orifice
3. antrum, pyloric, pyloric
4. superior, descending, transverse, ascending
5. anterior
6. ampulla of Vater
7. thyroid, subclavian, thoracic, gastric, phrenic
8. mesentery
9. blood
10. peristalsis
11. hydrochloric acid, enzymes
12. gastrin
13. cholecystokinin, secretin
14. bacteria
15. blood
16. anemia

Exercise 6

1. The technique used to observe the upper gastrointestinal tract is for the patient to drink 10 to 40 oz of water through a straw after a baseline ultrasound study of the upper abdomen. The straw helps prevent ingestion of excess air when the water is consumed. The patient should be in an upright position for the examination; this causes air in the stomach to rise to the fundus of the stomach and not inter-fere with the ultrasound beam. The lower gastrointestinal tract requires no preparation. To image the lower colon, it may be useful to give the patient a water enema to help better delineate the colon.
2. gastroesophageal
3. antrum
4. If a patient presents with a cystic mass in the left upper quad-rant, several measurements can be taken to determine if the mass is the fluid-filled stomach or another mass arising from adjacent organs. The sonographer may give the patient a car-bonated drink to see bubbles in the stomach; ask the clini-cian to place a nasogastric tube for drainage; watch for a change in the shape or size of the "stomach" mass with the ingestion of fluids; alter the patient's position by scanning in an upright or left or right lateral decubitus position; watch for peristalsis; or ask the patient to drink water to see the swirling effect.
5. keyboard sign
6. McBurney point

Exercise 7

1. bezoars
2. polyp
3. leiomyoma
4. acute appendicitis
5. compression
6. target-shaped
7. mucocele
8. Crohn's disease

Exercise 8

1. Based on Figure 9-7, *B* and *C,* internal rugae of the stomach wall are demonstrated in this image.

2. The arrows in Figure 9-11 are pointing to a fluid-filled duodenum.

3. According to Figure 9-14, the sonographic sign demonstrated is the target or bull's-eye sign.

4. Based on Figure 9-18, appendicitis is demonstrated in the image. The technique of gradual compression should be used to further delineate the structure.

CHAPTER 10

Exercise 1

1. D	4. B	7. E	10. G
2. H	5. A	8. C	11. L
3. J	6. I	9. F	12. K

Exercise 2

1. E	5. K	9. D	13. I
2. M	6. H	10. J	14. P
3. G	7. O	11. B	15. C
4. N	8. A	12. L	16. F

Exercise 3

1. G	5. H	9. B
2. A	6. J	10. D
3. C	7. E	
4. I	8. F	

Exercise 4

1. See Figure 10-2 in the textbook for the answers.

2. See Figure 10-3 in the textbook for the answers.

3. See Figure 10-4 in the textbook for the answers.

Exercise 5

1. wastes, blood

2. lower, liver, inferiorly

3. downward

4. vascular, lymphatics

5. true capsule

6. perinephric fat

7. perinephric

8. Gerota's

9. pyramids

10. corpuscle, tubule

11. filter, urine

12. glomerulus, Bowman's capsule

13. afferent, efferent

14. where the ureter leaves the renal pelvis, where it is kinked as it crosses the pelvic brim, and where it pierces the bladder wall

15. superior mesenteric

16. lateral walls

Exercise 6

1. retroperitoneum

2. water, electrolytes

3. water, carbon dioxide

4. vascular

5. hematuria, red blood cells, pus

6. acidic, alkaline

7. specific gravity

8. low

9. hematocrit

10. elevation

Exercise 7

1. calyces, infundibula, pelvis, vessels, and lymphatics
2. pregnant
3. parenchyma
4. arcuate arteries, interlobar
5. cortex, hypoechoic
6. columns of Bertin
7. crura
8. apex, base
9. dromedary hump
10. junctional parenchymal defect
11. horseshoe kidney, lower
12. smooth, thin, well-defined border, round or oval shape, sharp interface between the cyst and renal parenchyma, anechoic, and increased posterior acoustic enhancement
13. ureterocele

Exercise 8

1. septated
2. renal hilum
3. perinatal, neonatal, infantile, and juvenile
4. Autosomal dominant polycystic kidney disease is a common genetic disease that is found in both men and women. The severity of the disease varies depending upon the genotype. The most common type is PKD1 (located on the short arm of the 16th chromosome) that affects the kidneys more severely than PKD2 (located on the long arm of the 4th chromosome). There are a number of persons who have no known genetic disposition to ADPKD; it may result by spontaneous mutations. It is a bilateral disease that is characterized by multiple cysts located in the renal cortex and medulla. The cysts vary in size and may be asymmetrical. The disease is progressive, which means it does not usually clinically manifest itself until the 4th or 5th decade. Approximately 50% of the patients by the age of 60 will have end-stage renal disease. Clinical symptoms include: pain (common complaint), hypertension, palpable mass, hematuria, headache, urinary tract infection, and renal insufficiency.
5. abnormal
6. Renal cell carcinoma is the most common of all renal tumors (85% of all kidney tumors). It is twice as common in males as in females, usually in the 6th to 7th decade of life. The classic clinical presentation is nonspecific; however, the patient may report hematuria, flank pain, and palpable mass. The tumor appears bilaterally in 0.1% to 1.5% of patients. The incidence is increased in patients with von Hippel-Lindau disease and patients on long-term dialysis.
7. adenoma
8. angiomyolipoma
9. lipomas
10. corticomedullary
11. renal atrophy
12. acute tubular necrosis
13. function
14. nephron, vascular, interstitial abnormalities
15. hydronephrosis
16. strictures, focal masses, or duplex collecting system
17. ureterovesical, urethra
18. bladder
19. There are three grades of hydronephrosis. *Grade I* entails a small separation of the calyceal pattern, also known as splaying. The sonographer must be able to rule out a peripelvic cyst (the septations may be numerous) or renal vessels in the peripelvic area. (Color flow Doppler is extremely useful.) An extrarenal pelvis would protrude outside of the renal area, and the sonographer should not confuse this pattern with hydronephrosis. *Grade II* shows the bear-claw effect, with fluid extending into the major and minor calyceal systems and thinning of the renal parenchyma. *Grade III* represents massive dilation of the renal pelvis with loss of renal parenchyma.
20. In cases of acute obstruction, the resistive index of the intrarenal vessels may be greater than 0.70 for 48 to 72 hours after obstruction. The RI returns to normal. There will be no ureteral jet on the affected side, or there will be decreased flow if the obstruction is partial.
21. color Doppler
22. pyonephrosis
23. nephrocalcinosis
24. infarction

Exercise 9

1. graft rejection
2. renal size, calyceal pattern, extrarenal fluid collections
3. hematoma, abscess, lymphocele, urinoma
4. hyperacute
5. acute
6. immunologic
7. chronic rejection
8. size and shape; appearance of the pyramids, cortex, and parenchyma; and presence of fluid collections
9. cadaveric, donor-relative
10. anuria, oliguria
11. high-velocity
12. power

Exercise 10

1. pain
2. echogenic
3. hydronephrosis, superior
4. congenital diverticulum
5. acquired
6. cystitis
7. transitional cell

Exercise 11

1. According to Figure 10-16 in the textbook, the renal veins arise from the inferior vena cava in this image.
2. The arrows in Figure 10-20 are pointing to the crura of the diaphragm.
3. The arrows in Figure 10-21 are pointing to the column of Bertin.
4. Based on Figure 10-22, a dromedary hump is demonstrated in this image.
5. The arrows in Figure 10-23 are pointing to the junctional parenchymal defect.
6. According to Figure 10-36, the finding on the right kidney is most likely a right upper pole renal cyst.
7. Based on Figure 10-46, the pathology revealed is polycystic renal disease. All of the cysts are distinct lesions and do not connect with the central renal sinus to indicate hydronephrosis.
8. Medullary sponge kidneys are demonstrated in Figure 10-50.
9. Based on the information and Figure 10-59 in the textbook, the sonographic finding is Wilms' tumor.
10. The abnormality demonstrated in Figure 10-60 is angiomyolipoma.
11. Based on Figure 10-76, this patient does not have hydronephrosis. There is an extrarenal pelvis that projects externally from the renal pelvis.
12. Figure 10-86 in the textbook shows a large complex mass with a fluid and/or debris level.
13. Figure 10-113 demonstrates a renal calculi.

CHAPTER 11

Exercise 1

1. E
2. I
3. B
4. M
5. K
6. J
7. A
8. D
9. L
10. C
11. N
12. G
13. F
14. H

Exercise 2

1. J
2. F
3. C
4. K
5. B
6. G
7. A
8. M
9. I
10. E
11. L
12. D
13. H

Exercise 3

1. K
2. O
3. G
4. N
5. I
6. A
7. C
8. D
9. H
10. B
11. M
12. J
13. F
14. L
15. E

Exercise 4

1. See Figure 11-1, *C* in the textbook for the answers.
2. See Figure 11-2 in the textbook for the answers.
3. See Figure 11-4 in the textbook for the answers.

Exercise 5

1. lymphoid
2. intraperitoneal
3. upper, inferior
4. splenic agenesis
5. accessory spleen
6. hematocrit
7. sepsis
8. leukocytosis

Exercise 6

1. low-level echo pattern

2. right

3. sickle cell anemia

4. candidiasis

5. splenic hematoma, subcapsular hematoma

Exercise 7

1. The finding in Figure 11-5 is accessory spleen.

2. Figure 11-11 demonstrates splenomegaly. In image *C*, signs of portal hypertension are present with dilatation of the splenic hilar vessels.

3. Splenic infection is found in Figure 11-18.

4. The abnormality demonstrated in Figure 11-19 is splenic infarct.

5. The finding in Figure 11-20 is subcapsular splenic hematoma.

6. The abnormality shown in Figure 11-23 is cavernous hemangioma of the spleen.

CHAPTER 12

Exercise 1

1. B

2. F

3. A

4. D

5. G

6. E

7. C

Exercise 2

1. D

2. A

3. F

4. E

5. C

6. B

Exercise 3

1. See Figure 12-9 in the textbook for the answers.

2. See Figure 12-10 in the textbook for the answers.

3. See Figure 12-11 in the textbook for the answers.

4. See Figure 12-17 in the textbook for the answers.

Exercise 4

1. parietal, posterior

2. anterior pararenal space, perirenal space, and posterior pararenal space

3. perirenal

4. anterior pararenal

5. posterior pararenal

6. superior, medial

7. anterior, posterior

8. psoas muscle

Exercise 5

1. androgens, estrogens

2. Addison's

3. mineralocorticoids, glucocorticoids, sex hormones

4. mineralocorticoids

5. aldosterone

6. glucocorticoids

7. cortisone and hydrocortisone

8. masculine

9. adrenocorticotropic

10. catecholamines

Exercise 6

1. Ultrasound patterns associated with nodes include rounded, focal, echo-poor lesions 1 to 3 cm in size and larger hypoechoic masses, which often displace the kidney laterally. The ultrasound appearance includes: a "mantle" of nodes, a "floating" or anterior displaced aorta secondary to the enlarged nodes, or the mesenteric "sandwich" sign representing the anterior and posterior node masses surrounding the mesenteric vessels.

2. Lymph nodes remain as consistent patterns, whereas bowel and the duodenum present with changing peristaltic patterns with ultrasound. As gentle pressure is applied, the lymph nodes remain constant in shape, whereas the bowel is displaced and compressed.

3. stress, asphyxia, and septicemia

4. hypertension, headaches, palpitations

5. urinoma

Exercise 7

1. Based on Figure 12-18, enlarged lymph nodes are present in the area of the peripancreatic bed and periportal area.

2. The arrows in Figure 12-24 are pointing to enlarged nodes. Color Doppler should be used to make sure the prominent nodes are not vascular structures.

3. In Figure 12-28, the abnormality shown is adrenal hemorrhage.

4. The anomaly present in Figure 12-33 is pheochromocytoma.

CHAPTER 13

Exercise 1

1. A
2. E
3. C
4. B
5. D

Exercise 2

1. H
2. D
3. B
4. K
5. F
6. C
7. I
8. A
9. G
10. E
11. J

Exercise 3

1. See Figure 13-6 in the textbook for the answers.
2. See Figure 13-7 in the textbook for the answers.
3. See Figure 13-8 in the textbook for the answers.
4. See Figure 13-10 in the textbook for the answers.
5. See Figure 13-11 in the textbook for the answers.

Exercise 4

1. coronary
2. posteromedially
3. inferior
4. ureters
5. anteriorly
6. sagittal
7. ventrally
8. inferior
9. left

Exercise 5

1. viscera, walls
2. omentum, mesenteries, ligaments
3. peritoneum
4. parietal, visceral
5. greater
6. lesser
7. epiploic
8. pelvis
9. lesser
10. greater
11. subphrenic, subhepatic
12. falciform
13. ligamentum teres
14. rectus

Exercise 6

1. location, volume, position
2. pouch of Douglas
3. floats *or* sinks
4. fine or coarse internal
5. abscess
6. through the portal system, by way of ascending cholangitis of the common bile duct, via the hepatic artery secondary to bacteremia, by direct extension from an infection, and by implantation of bacteria after trauma to the abdominal wall
7. bilomas
8. renal carbuncle
9. acute appendicitis

Exercise 7

1. infiltrative
2. multiloculated
3. urachal
4. urinoma
5. ovaries, stomach, colon
6. sandwich sign
7. symmetry

8. lymphoceles
9. hematomas
10. hernia
11. spigelian
12. (1) demonstration of an abdominal wall defect, (2) presence of bowel loops or mesenteric fat within a lesion, (3) exaggeration of the lesion with strain (Valsalva), and (4) reducibility of the lesion by gentle pressure

Exercise 8

1. Image *C* of Figure 13-16 demonstrates ascites in Morison's pouch.
2. The abnormality demonstrated in Figure 13-20 is pleural effusion.

3. Based on Figure 13-22, there is a fluid collection posterior to the renal transplant that slightly indents the posterior wall. This represents a postoperative urinoma. Other fluid collections that should be considered are a hematoma, lymphocele, abscess, or seroma.

CHAPTER 14

Exercise 1

1. I	5. G	8. J	11. F
2. D	6. K	9. A	12. H
3. M	7. C	10. L	13. E
4. B			

Exercise 2

1. C	4. E
2. A	5. B
3. D	

Exercise 3

1. acoustic emission
2. contrast enhanced sonography
3. color flow imaging
4. grayscale harmonic imaging
5. harmonic imaging

6. induced acoustic emission
7. mechanical index
8. power Doppler imaging
9. ultrasound contrast agents

Exercise 4

1. c	4. c	7. d	10. d
2. b	5. e	8. b	
3. d	6. c	9. e	

Exercise 5

1. limitations of spatial and contrast resolution on grayscale sonography and the detection of low-velocity blood flow and flow in very small vessels using Doppler flow detection modes that include color flow imaging and pulsed Doppler with spectral analysis
2. The sonographic detection of blood flow is limited by many factors, including the depth and size of a vessel, the attenuation properties of intervening tissue, or low-velocity flow. Limitations of ultrasound equipment sensitivity and the operator dependence of Doppler are also factors that may impact the results of a vascular examination.
3. scatters
4. grayscale echogenicity
5. nontoxic, have microbubbles or microparticles that are small enough to traverse the pulmonary capillary beds (i.e., less than 8 micrometers in size), and be stable enough to provide multiple recirculations

6. first generation, second generation

7. The microbubbles of these agents are removed from the blood pool and taken up by or have an affinity toward specific tissues (e.g., the reticuloendothelial system in the liver and spleen) or thrombus. Over time the presence of contrast microbubbles within or attached to the tissue changes its sonographic appearance. By changing the signal impedance (or other acoustic characteristics) of normal and abnormal tissues, these agents improve the detectability of abnormalities and permit more specific sonographic diagnoses. Tissue-specific ultrasound contrast agents are typically administered by IV injection. Some tissue-specific agents also enhance the sonographic detection of blood flow and therefore are potentially multipurpose. Because tissue-specific ultrasound contrast agents target specific types of tissues and their behavior is predictable, they can be considered in the category of molecular imaging agents.

8. microbubbles

9. reticuloendothelial

10. second

11. oscillate

12. signal-to-noise

13. perfusion imaging

14. small

15. low

CHAPTER 15

Exercise 1

1. E	4. J	7. C	9. B
2. A	5. G	8. D	10. F
3. H	6. I		

Exercise 2

1. alpha fetoprotein

2. fine-needle aspiration

3. international normalized ratio

4. prostate-specific antigen

5. prothrombin time

6. partial thromboplastin time

Exercise 3

1. The main advantage of using ultrasound for guidance is the continuous real-time visualization of the biopsy needle, which allows adjustment of the needle as needed. Also as the biopsy specimen is being obtained, the needle tip can be watched in real time to ensure that it does not slip outside the mass. This is especially important in small masses. Ultrasound also has the advantage of allowing different patient positions and approaches to be considered. The patient may be turned into a decubitus or oblique position to allow safe access to the mass. Subcostal approaches can allow the use of steep angles with the needle directed cephalad. This can help reduce the risk of a *pneumothorax* or bleeding from an injury to an intercostal artery. Using ultrasound the patient can be placed in a comfortable position and not be made to lie supine or prone. Another benefit is the ability to comfort and reassure the patient as the sonologist, sonographer, and nurse are all near the patient during the procedure. Other advantages include the ability to perform the biopsy in a single breath hold, portability, lack of radiation, decreased costs, and shorter procedure times.

2. Ultrasound guidance does have some limitations. Unfortunately, not all masses can be visualized with ultrasound because they may be isoechoic to the normal tissue. In the abdomen, bowel gas may move in and obscure the mass before or even during the procedure. The needle tip may be difficult to see or deviate from the projected path because of bending or deflection of the needle. This can bring in the sonographer's scanning skills in an attempt to maneuver the transducer to find the needle tip or correct for the deviation. Other disadvantages of using ultrasound to guide procedures include: the inexperience of ultrasound personnel, the comfort level of the radiologist and/or sonologist with other imaging modalities, overlying bowel gas that cannot be displaced, and having to use fixed angles when using needle guides on the transducers.

3. malignancy

4. Contraindications may include: an uncorrectable bleeding disorder, the lack of a safe needle path (Figure 15-6), and an uncooperative patient.

5. PTT

6. benign, malignant, infectious

7. core biopsy

8. thin

9. free hand

10. faster learning curve, allows faster placement of the needle, and keeps the needle going through the anesthetized area when multiple passes are required

11. risks

12. A member of the biopsy team should ask the patient to recite his or her full name. The patient's ID or history number is confirmed and the type and location of the procedure. This is documented usually at the bottom of the consent form. The words "timeout" may also be typed on the screen and an image documented to be part of the ultrasound examination. This is helpful because there will be a preprocedural image; the "timeout" image, which documents date and time; and then the needle tip documentation images.

13. postprocedural pain or discomfort, vasovagal reaction, hematomas

14. respiration

15. Move the needle up and down in a bobbing motion. Bob or jiggle the stylet inside the needle. Angle the transducer in a superior and inferior motion. This is helpful when the needle is bent out of the plane of the sound beam. Use harmonics or compound imaging. A last resort is to remove the needle and start again, closely watching the displacement of the tissue as the needle advances.

16. subcostal

17. upper

18. same

CHAPTER 16

Exercise 1

1. C	4. I	7. H
2. E	5. G	8. B
3. A	6. D	9. F

Exercise 2

1. See Figure 16-1 in the textbook for the answers.

2. See Figure 16-2 in the textbook for the answers.

Exercise 3

1. peritoneal lavage

2. blunt

3. intraperitoneal

4. FAST

5. hemorrhage

6. perihepatic, pararenal paracolic gutters, cul-de-sac

7. speed

8. four, pericardial

9. dependent

10. liver

11. anechoic

12. physiologic

13. acute cholecystitis

14. cholelithiasis

15. acute pancreatitis

16. hypoechoic

17. urolithiasis

18. hematuria

19. hydronephrosis

20. cephalic

21. decreased

22. dissecting aortic aneurysm

23. (1) root of the aorta with extension into the arch, (2) level of left subclavian artery with extension into descending aorta or abdominal aorta, (3) only at level of ascending aorta

24. ascending

25. systemic

26. chest

27. McBurney

28. graded

29. hernia

30. peristaltic

31. colon, omentum, fat

32. Valsalva

Exercise 4

1. The abnormality that is visible in Figure 16-9 is pleural effusion.

2. Based on Figure 16-10, the other area where the sonographer should look for fluid is in the pelvis.

3. Based on Figure 16-12, acute bleeding is suspected. The fluid is homogeneous.

4. The sonographer should look for peristalsis in Figure 16-18.

CHAPTER 17

Exercise 1

1. E	5. J	9. O	13. B
2. I	6. D	10. H	14. M
3. L	7. N	11. F	15. G
4. C	8. A	12. K	

Exercise 2

1. C	5. H	9. D	13. I
2. K	6. E	10. L	14. F
3. M	7. J	11. N	
4. B	8. G	12. A	

Exercise 3

1. G	6. F	11. A	16. R
2. O	7. Q	12. P	17. L
3. K	8. D	13. H	18. I
4. B	9. J	14. N	19. E
5. M	10. S	15. C	

Exercise 4

1. See Figure 17-2 in the textbook for the answers.
2. See Figure 17-28 (right) in the textbook for the answers.
3. See Figure 17-28 (left) in the textbook for the answers.

Exercise 5

1. sweat
2. subcutaneous layer, mammary layer, retromammary layer
3. echogenic
4. hypoechoic
5. upper outer
6. acini
7. pectoralis major
8. adipose or fatty
9. hypoechoic
10. mammary, thoracic
11. axillary

Exercise 6

1. fluid
2. ductal
3. milk
4. acini
5. menarche
6. estrogen
7. progesterone
8. prolactin
9. milk
10. oxytocin
11. cancer

Exercise 7

1. young, dense
2. differentiating
3. cyst
4. patient's age, risk factors for breast cancer, symptoms, location and clinical impression of breast lumps
5. menstrual cycle
6. round, oval
7. homogeneously solid
8. irregular
9. fibroadenomas
10. intracapsular
11. linguine
12. radial/antiradial
13. malignancies
14. devoid of internal echoes, smooth inner margins with capsule, posterior acoustic enhancement
15. Benign tumors are usually slow growing and do not invade surrounding tissue. They tend to grow horizontally within the tissue planes, parallel to the chest wall. Larger benign lesions will often cause compression of the tissue adjacent to the mass, implying that the mass is pushing against adjacent breast tissue, as opposed to infiltrating it. Malignant lesions, on the other hand, tend to grow right through the normal breast tissue. As malignant masses enlarge, they may cause retraction of the nipple or dimpling of the skin as the spiculations pull on the Cooper's ligaments.
16. benign, malignant
17. horizontally
18. parallel
19. vertical
20. height, width
21. vascularity

Exercise 8

1. fibrocystic
2. intraductal
3. cancer
4. mobile
5. fibrocystic condition
6. estrogen
7. malignant
8. acute mastitis
9. benign
10. fibrotic
11. lymphatics, blood vessels
12. encapsulated
13. terminal
14. carcinoma
15. ductal, lobular, noninvasive, invasive
16. in situ

Exercise 9

1. Figure 17-18, *B* shows a well-defined anechoic lesion with smooth borders and good through transmission.

2. According to Figure 17-19, *A* and *B,* this is a smooth, benign mass with homogeneous echogenicity. The mass is wider than tall with low-level posterior acoustic enhancement. With applied compression, the mass demonstrates decreased anteroposterior dimensions.

3. Based on Figure 17-21, *B,* the mass is heterogeneous with poorly defined and irregular borders. The lesion is higher than wide with no change in compression. This is suggestive of a malignant mass.

4. Based on Figure 17-42, the differential consideration is medullary carcinoma, fat necrosis, or fibroadenoma.

CHAPTER 18

Exercise 1

1. D
2. K
3. G
4. N
5. E
6. B
7. L
8. I
9. C
10. J
11. O
12. F
13. M
14. A
15. H

Exercise 2

1. J
2. G
3. O
4. M
5. F
6. D
7. C
8. R
9. T
10. E
11. Q
12. N
13. U
14. H
15. A
16. K
17. S
18. I
19. P
20. B
21. L

Exercise 3

1. See Figure 18-1 in the textbook for the answers.
2. See Figure 18-2 in the textbook for the answers.

Exercise 4

1. carotid, jugular
2. strap
3. posterior medial
4. calcium-sensing
5. parathyroid hormone (PTH)
6. decreases
7. bone, kidney
8. hypercalcemia
9. adenoma
10. secondary

Exercise 5

1. metabolism, growth, development
2. T_3, T_4, calcitonin
3. iodine
4. TSH
5. hypothalamus
6. calcitonin
7. hypothyroidism
8. hyperthyroidism
9. nuclear medicine
10. goiter
11. multinodular goiter
12. Graves' disease
13. adenoma
14. papillary cancer

Exercise 6

1. homogeneous
2. cystic hygroma
3. homogeneous
4. longus colli

Exercise 7

1. The arrows in Figure 18-6 are pointing to the isthmus.
2. The arrows in Figure 18-7 are pointing to thyroid adenoma with the hypoechoic halo.
3. Based on Figure 18-9, *A*, multinodular goiter with a complex sonographic pattern is present.
4. In Figure 18-22, a solid mass of the thyroid is present.

CHAPTER 19

Exercise 1

1. F
2. N
3. A
4. J
5. L
6. C
7. H
8. O
9. B
10. Q
11. E
12. K
13. P
14. G
15. M
16. I
17. D

Exercise 2

1. D
2. A
3. C
4. E
5. B

Exercise 3

1. G
2. C
3. F
4. J
5. D
6. H
7. I
8. A
9. E
10. B

Exercise 4

1. scrotum
2. rete testis
3. head
4. vas deferens
5. tunica albuginea
6. mediastinum
7. hydroceles
8. vas deferens, epididymis
9. seminal vesicles
10. abdominal aorta
11. pampiniform
12. slow

Exercise 5

1. rupture
2. echogenic
3. epididymo-orchitis
4. little
5. increased
6. anterolateral
7. torsion
8. bell clapper
9. adolescents
10. absence
11. albuginea
12. varicoceles
13. echogenic
14. hydrocele
15. 20 to 34
16. undescended
17. extratesticular, intratesticular
18. undescended testis or cryptorchidism

Exercise 6

1. The arrows in Figure 19-1 are pointing to the testis mediastinum.

2. In Figure 19-2, the closed arrow is pointing to the upper pole, and the open arrow is pointing to the body.

3. In Figure 19-3, the arrow is pointing to the appendix testis.

4. Based on Figure 19-14, the image demonstrates a large heterogeneous mass adjacent to the left testis representing a complex hematoma.

5. The abnormality demonstrated in Figure 19-15 is severe epididymitis with an enlarged epididymis with a heterogeneous echo pattern. The focal hyperechoic areas within the epididymis may represent hemorrhage. A complex hydrocele with numerous septations is seen near the epididymal head. Doppler shows increased diastolic flow associated with inflammation.

6. Figure 19-16 shows an enlarged left testis and normal right testis. A complex hydrocele surrounds the left testis. Marked skin thickening is present on the left side. Color Doppler shows hyperemic flow.

7. Figure 19-19 shows a left spermatic cord torsion. The left testis is enlarged and heterogeneous. The infarcted testis has a mixed echo pattern caused by the hemorrhage, necrosis, and vascular congestion associated with spermatic cord torsion exceeding 24 hours. No flow was shown in the left testis.

8. Figure 19-34 shows a germ cell testicular tumor. In *A* the normal testis is heterogeneous whereas the mass is hypoechoic. *B* shows distortion of the normal vessel architecture within the testis. In *C* power Doppler shows the distorted vasculature of the testis within the mass. *D* shows a low resistance Doppler flow pattern with prominent end-diastolic velocities characteristic of tumor flow.

CHAPTER 20

Exercise 1

1. E
2. H
3. B
4. K
5. F
6. A
7. I
8. D
9. L
10. C
11. G
12. J

Exercise 2

1. D
2. F
3. A
4. K
5. I
6. B
7. E
8. G
9. C
10. J
11. H

Exercise 3

1. See Figure 20-1 in the textbook for the answers.
2. See Figure 20-24 in the textbook for the answers.

Exercise 4

1. fibers
2. muscle
3. multipennate, circumpennate
4. tendon
5. synovial
6. shoulder, hand, wrist, ankle
7. ligaments
8. bursa
9. nine
10. paratenon
11. epitendineum
12. parallel
13. longitudinal
14. origin, insertion

15. hyperechoic, hypoechoic

16. friction

17. communicating

18. anisotropic

19. edge

20. refractile

21. time of flight

Exercise 5

1. C	4. B	7. A	10. D
2. I	5. E	8. J	
3. G	6. H	9. F	

Exercise 6

1. internal
2. left, right
3. biceps
4. anteromedially
5. supraspinatus
6. glenoid labrum
7. superficial, posterior
8. carpal, flexor
9. radial
10. Achilles
11. transverse humeral ligament, abnormal development of the bicipital groove, supraspinatus and/or subscapularis tears
12. partial
13. full-thickness
14. flattens
15. double-effusion
16. synovial
17. halo
18. distraction
19. compression

Exercise 7

1. The arrow in Figure 20-30 is pointing to the supraspinatus tendon.

2. The abnormality shown in Figure 20-49 is tendon inflammation and focal areas of tendonitis.

3. Based on Figure 20-50, the sonographic imaging of the large abductor pollicis longus and small extensor pollicis brevis tendon reveal hypoechoic tendons and synovium.

4. In Figure 20-51, intramuscular hematoma is found.

5. The abnormality shown in Figure 20-53 is that the right median nerve is flattened; the left median nerve is also mildly flattened.

CHAPTER 21

Exercise 1

1. I	6. M	11. C	16. L
2. O	7. G	12. Q	17. F
3. D	8. A	13. J	18. N
4. K	9. R	14. B	
5. E	10. H	15. P	

Exercise 2

1. G	4. L	7. H	10. K
2. D	5. J	8. F	11. E
3. A	6. C	9. B	12. I

Exercise 3

1. See Figure 21-2, *B* in the textbook for the answers.

2. See Figure 21-3, *D* in the textbook for the answers.

3. See Figure 21-4 in the textbook for the answers.

4. See Figure 21-5 in the textbook for the answers.

5. See Figure 21-6 in the textbook for the answers.

6. See Figure 21-7 in the textbook for the answers.

7. See Figure 21-8 in the textbook for the answers.

8. See Figure 21-9 in the textbook for the answers.

9. See Figure 21-10 in the textbook for the answers.

10. See Figure 21-11 in the textbook for the answers.

11. See Figure 21-13 in the textbook for the answers.

Exercise 4

1. neural
2. neural tube
3. massa intermedia
4. choroid plexus
5. falx cerebri
6. fourth ventricle
7. fontanelles
8. anterior
9. dura mater
10. tentorium cerebelli
11. lateral

12. corpus callosum
13. thalamus, nucleus
14. aqueduct of Sylvius
15. Luschka
16. cerebrospinal fluid
17. choroid plexus
18. sylvian fissure
19. thalamus
20. medulla oblongata
21. cerebellar peduncles

Exercise 5

1. supratentorial
2. infratentorial
3. coronal
4. anteriorly

5. posteriorly
6. echogenic
7. higher
8. fourth

Exercise 6

1. Chiari
2. hydrocephalus
3. holoprosencephaly
4. fourth
5. cisterna magna
6. corpus callosum
7. hydrocephalus
8. communicating
9. aqueductal stenosis

10. subependymal-intraventricular
11. germinal matrix
12. posterior
13. echogenic
14. hypoxia
15. periventricular
16. echolucencies
17. ventriculitis
18. ependymitis

Exercise 7

1. In Figure 21-27, Chiari malformation with hydrocephaly is present.
2. Figure 21-30, A shows alobar holoprosencephaly with a single ventricular cavity. B shows semilobar holoprosencephaly with partial separation of the thalami.
3. Based on Figure 21-33, posterior fossa cyst and splaying of the cerebellar hemispheres without hydrocephalus are visible in A and B. In images C and D, hydrocephalus is noted with a large posterior cyst (Dandy-Walker malformation).
4. The abnormality present in Figure 21-35 is agenesis of the corpus callosum with semilobar holoprosencephaly.
5. The arrow in Figure 21-38 is pointing to a small subependymal bleed.
6. Based on Figure 21-39, this premature infant would be considered Grade II; bleed is still within the ventricular cavity.
7. The abnormality present in Figure 21-42 is periventricular leukomalacia.

CHAPTER 22

Exercise 1

1. G
2. K
3. D
4. B
5. J
6. A
7. F
8. M
9. H
10. N
11. I
12. E
13. C
14. L

Exercise 2

1. See Figure 22-14 in the textbook for the answers.

Exercise 3

1. 1
2. 1, 2, 4, 7
3. kidney
4. hepatitis, biliary atresia, choledochal cyst
5. persistent jaundice, acholic stools, dark urine, distended abdomen from hepatomegaly
6. choledochal cyst
7. fusiform dilation, intrahepatic
8. hemangioendothelioma
9. hypoechoic, hepatomegaly
10. hepatoblastoma
11. pyloric canal
12. hypertrophic pyloric stenosis
13. projectile
14. 3.5, 17, 20 mm
15. perforation
16. noncompressible
17. localized pain
18. intussusception
19. target *or* donut
20. hydrostatic

Exercise 4

1. Based on Figure 22-7, images *A* through *D* show the gallbladder contracted after eating. Two hours later the gallbladder does not enlarge or change in appearance. Biliary atresia is present.
2. In Figure 22-8, the cystic structure superior to the gallbladder is a choledochal cyst.
3. Based on Figure 22-9, the image shows infantile hemangioma with focal areas of calcification.
4. Based on Figures 22-18, 22-19, and 22-20, hypertrophic pyloric stenosis is present.
5. According to Figure 22-21, appendicitis is present.
6. Based on Figure 22-24, intussusception is present.

CHAPTER 23

Exercise 1

1. R
2. J
3. K
4. W
5. E
6. V
7. N
8. P
9. B
10. C
11. T
12. A
13. H
14. D
15. Q
16. G
17. U
18. F
19. O
20. I
21. L
22. S
23. M

Exercise 2

1. renunculi
2. column of Bertin
3. lobes
4. cortex, pyramids
5. fat
6. medullary pyramids
7. liver
8. arcuate
9. junctional parenchymal
10. superior
11. 3

Exercise 3

1. hydronephrosis
2. ureteropelvic junction obstruction
3. proximal
4. posterior urethral
5. ascites, urinoma
6. ureterocele
7. prune-belly
8. multicystic dysplastic kidney
9. noncommunicating
10. autosomal recessive polycystic kidney disease
11. Wilms' tumor
12. neuroblastoma
13. adrenal
14. hemorrhage

Exercise 4

1. Based on Figure 23-1, that patient has nonobstructive dilation of the distal ureter.

2. The arrow in Figure 23-4 is pointing to the adrenal gland.

3. In Figure 23-6, there is major obstruction present with loss of the renal parenchyma.

4. The abnormality demonstrated in Figure 23-7, *A* is posterior urethral valves with a thick bladder wall.

5. In Figure 23-10, the sonograph shows evidence of multicystic dysplastic kidney disease. There is no apparent renal pelvis.

6. In Figure 23-12, infantile autosomal recessive polycystic kidney disease is present.

7. Based on Figure 23-16, the finding is Wilms' tumor with extension into the IVC.

8. Based on Figure 23-17, the finding is an adrenal hemorrhage.

CHAPTER 24

Exercise 1

1. C	4. A	7. F	10. G
2. H	5. I	8. B	
3. D	6. J	9. E	

Exercise 2

1. gonads	15. heterogeneous
2. oogonium	16. ovarian
3. oocytes	17. kidneys
4. genital	18. atresia
5. 9th	19. cigar
6. 12th	20. uterus didelphys
7. urinary bladder	21. bicornuate uterus
8. echogenic	22. diethylstilbestrol
9. smaller	23. ambiguous genitalia
10. decrease	24. hermaphrodites
11. larger	25. isosexual
12. puberty	26. gonad
13. uterine	27. steroids
14. myometrial	

Exercise 3

1. follicles	5. vascular pedicle
2. follicle-stimulating hormone	6. hemorrhagic infarction
3. hemorrhage, salpingotorsion	7. teratoma
4. two	8. ovarian teratomas

Exercise 4

1. See Figure 24-5 in the textbook for the answers.

CHAPTER 25

Exercise 1

1. C	3. B	5. A	7. H
2. F	4. G	6. E	8. D

Exercise 2

1. D	3. A	5. B
2. F	4. C	6. E

Exercise 3

1. See Figure 25-3, *A* in the textbook for the answers.
2. See Figure 25-3, *B* in the textbook for the answers.

Exercise 4

1. sacroiliac
2. ilium, ischium, pubis
3. femur
4. profunda femoris
5. sciatic
6. fascia lata
7. femoral triangle
8. canal, vein, artery, nerve
9. sheath
10. pectineus, iliacus
11. hip joint
12. minimus
13. piriformis
14. acetabulum
15. iliofemoral ligament

Exercise 5

1. C
2. E
3. A
4. F
5. B
6. D

Exercise 6

1. psoas, iliacus, rectus
2. medially, laterally
3. medius, minimus
4. piriformis, obturator internus, quadratus femoris, gluteus maximus

Exercise 7

1. 2, 8
2. linear-array
3. hypoechoic
4. echogenic
5. labrum
6. (1) coronal/neutral, (2) coronal/flexion, (3) transverse/flexion, and (4) transverse/neutral
7. alpha
8. beta
9. beta, alpha
10. coronal/neutral
11. coronal/flexion
12. femoral head, acetabulum
13. transverse/flexion
14. transverse/neutral

Exercise 8

1. acquired
2. teratogenic
3. developmental displacement of the hip
4. It usually affects the firstborn child with females affected more frequently than males. The left hip is most commonly affected with only a small number of cases affecting both hips. The condition affects Caucasians more than the African-American population. A breech birth is also a risk factor in DDH as is low birth weight. Other risk factors include maternal hypertension, fetal growth restriction, oligohydramnios, premature rupture of membranes, prolonged gestation, increased birth weight, Potter's syndrome, and neonatal intensive care.
5. The Barlow maneuver determines if the hip can be dislocated. The Ortolani maneuver determines if the dislocated femoral head can be reduced back into the acetabulum.
6. A shallow dysplastic acetabulum, delayed ossification of the femoral head (in either a lateral or posterior direction), increased thickness of the acetabular cartilage, an alpha angle greater than 60 degrees, and a beta angle of less than 55 degrees. A "normal" sonogram does not absolutely exclude DDH, although the sensitivity and specificity of sonography approaches 100%.
7. subluxatable
8. dislocatable
9. dislocated

Exercise 9

1. In Figure 25-10, the image is the coronal/neutral view.
2. The arrow in Figure 25-11, *A* is pointing to the fibrocartilaginous tip of the labrum.
3. The abnormality demonstrated in Figure 25-12 is a dislocation of the hip.

4. Based on Figure 25-14, *A* shows a normal coronal/flexion view, and *B* shows dislocation of the hip.

5. Based on Figure 25-18, *A* shows the normal U-shaped configuration that is not present in *B* with the dislocated hip.

6. The transverse/neutral view is demonstrated in Figure 25-20, *A*.

CHAPTER 26

Exercise 1
1. B
2. D
3. F
4. C
5. A
6. E

Exercise 2
1. F
2. C
3. A
4. E
5. B
6. D
7. G

Exercise 3
1. See Figure 26-2 in the textbook for the answers.
2. See Figure 26-3, *C* in the textbook for the answers.
3. See Figure 26-4, *B* in the textbook for the answers.
4. See Figure 26-5, *B* in the textbook for the answers.

Exercise 4
1. dimple
2. hemangioma, hairy
3. one inch
4. dysraphism
5. 8.5
6. mesoderm
7. diastematomyelia
8. myelomeningocele
9. meninges

Exercise 5
1. anteriorly, posteriorly
2. foramen
3. laminae
4. sacroiliac
5. hiatus
6. intervertebral
7. fibrosus, pulposus
8. third
9. medullaris, terminale
10. median
11. cauda equina
12. dura, arachnoid, pia
13. dura
14. arachnoid
15. pia

Exercise 6
1. hypoechoic
2. canal
3. oscillate
4. tethered
5. eccentrically
6. echogenic
7. myelomeningocele
8. meningocele
9. hemangiomas

Exercise 7
1. In Figure 26-6, the structures are: (1) posterior elements or spinous processes, (2) posterior arachnoid-dural layer, (3) subarachnoid space, (4) posterior margin of spinal cord, (5) spinal cord with central echo complex, and (6) anterior margin of spinal cord

2. In Figure 26-9, the structures are: (1) posterior elements or spinous processes, (2) cauda medullaris, (3) filum terminale, and (4) cauda equina and nerve roots.

3. Based on Figure 26-10, a tethered spinal cord is demonstrated.

4. Based on Figure 26-11, the mass would more likely be a leptomyelolipoma.

5. The abnormality present in Figure 26-12 is diastematomyelia.

CHAPTER 27

Exercise 1

1. D	3. A	5. C
2. B	4. E	6. F

Exercise 2

1. H	4. B	6. I	8. G
2. D	5. A	7. E	9. C
3. F			

Exercise 3

1. See Figure 27-4 in the textbook for the answers.
2. See Figure 27-5 in the textbook for the answers.
3. See Figure 27-6 in the textbook for the answers.
4. See Figure 27-7 in the textbook for the answers.
5. See Figure 27-9 in the textbook for the answers.
6. See Figure 27-10 in the textbook for the answers.
7. See Figure 27-11 in the textbook for the answers.
8. See Figure 27-12 in the textbook for the answers.
9. See Figure 27-13 in the textbook for the answers.

Exercise 4

1. E	3. G	5. D	7. F
2. C	4. A	6. B	

Exercise 5

1. oxygenated, waste
2. diaphragm
3. angle of Louis
4. pleural sac
5. costophrenic sinus
6. left
7. anterior
8. anterior, right
9. posterior
10. parietal
11. pericardial cavity
12. endocardium
13. myocardium
14. filling
15. all of the body, lungs
16. superior vena cava, inferior vena cava
17. interatrial
18. atrioventricular
19. eustachian, thebesian
20. coronary sinus
21. tricuspid
22. supraventricularis
23. infundibulum
24. mitral
25. chordae tendineae
26. apex, base
27. membranous, inflow, trabecular, infundibular
28. membranous
29. main coronary arteries

Exercise 6

1. 70
2. systole, diastole
3. right atrium
4. pulmonary veins
5. rising
6. Valsalva
7. sinoatrial, atrioventricular, atrioventicular bundle, Purkinje
8. sinoatrial
9. atrioventricular
10. P
11. QRS
12. P-R
13. T
14. Frank Starling
15. preload
16. afterload

Exercise 7

1. laminar
2. disturbed
3. viscosity, momentum
4. parabolic flow velocity
5. flat flow velocity
6. systole
7. diastole
8. high fluid
9. high
10. 67
11. lowered

CHAPTER 28

Exercise 1

1. E
2. C
3. B
4. A
5. G
6. D
7. F

Exercise 2

1. G
2. D
3. B
4. A
5. F
6. E
7. C

Exercise 3

1. third, fifth
2. hemodynamic
3. parallel
4. above, positive
5. Nyquist
6. spectral analysis
7. directly

Exercise 4

1. In Figure 28-11, *B,* the parasternal long axis is demonstrated.
2. In Figure 28-15, *B,* the parasternal high short axis at the level of pulmonary bifurcation is demonstrated.
3. In Figure 28-16, *B,* the parasternal high short axis at the level of aortic valve is demonstrated.
4. In Figure 28-17, *B,* the parasternal short axis at the level of mitral valve is demonstrated.
5. In Figure 28-18, *B,* the parasternal short axis at the level of papillary muscles is demonstrated.
6. In Figure 28-24, *B,* the apical four-chamber view is demonstrated.
7. In Figure 28-25, *C,* the apical two-chamber view is demonstrated.
8. In Figure 28-31, *B,* the subcostal four-chamber view is demonstrated.
9. In Figure 28-37, the M-mode sweep from the tip of the mitral valve to the base of the annulus is demonstrated.

CHAPTER 29

Exercise 1

1. E
2. C
3. G
4. A
5. D
6. B
7. H
8. F

Exercise 2

1. F
2. J
3. D
4. H
5. K
6. E
7. I
8. B
9. C
10. A
11. G

Exercise 3

1. See Figure 29-3, *B* and *D* in the textbook for the answers.
2. See Figure 29-4, *C, D,* and *E* in the textbook for the answers.
3. See Figure 29-5 in the textbook for the answers.

Exercise 4

1. 3rd, 5th
2. yolk sac
3. cardinal, vitelline
4. umbilical
5. endocardial cushions
6. septum primum
7. septum secundum
8. foramen ovale
9. bulbus cordis
10. fossa ovale, ductus arteriosus
11. crista dividens
12. septum secundum
13. tricuspid valve, right ventricle, main pulmonary artery
14. ductus arteriosus
15. posterior
16. left ventricle, mitral valve, ascending aorta
17. floor
18. ductus arteriosus
19. 120 and 160
20. bradycardia, tachycardia

Exercise 5

1. horizontal
2. larger
3. toward
4. moderator band
5. inferior
6. atrioventricular
7. anterior, left
8. inflow, outflow
9. septum, anterior
10. systole, diastole
11. anterior
12. descending aorta and arch
13. innominate, carotid, left subclavian
14. patent ductus arteriosus

Exercise 6

1. In Figure 29-10, *F,* the right lower pulmonary vein is not shown.
2. Based on Figure 29-10, *G,* the mitral annulus is the structure.
3. In Figure 29-15, *C,* the end-diastole stage of the cardiac cycle is shown.
4. In Figure 29-16, *B,* the main pulmonary artery with the bifurcation is anterior and to the left of the circular aorta, making this a normal relationship and ruling out transposition of the great vessels.
5. In Figure 29-17, *A,* the aortic arch with the head and neck vessels is shown.
6. In Figure 29-18, *A,* the structure of the patent ductus arteriosus is shown.

CHAPTER 30

Exercise 1

1. K	5. G	9. J	13. M
2. N	6. B	10. C	14. L
3. F	7. I	11. H	
4. A	8. E	12. D	

Exercise 2

1. H	4. G	7. J	10. D
2. E	5. A	8. B	11. F
3. I	6. C	9. K	

Exercise 3

1. E	4. G	7. J	10. C
2. B	5. A	8. F	
3. H	6. D	9. I	

Exercise 4

1. ventricular septal defect
2. dextroposition
3. 2 mm
4. ostium secundum
5. ostium primum
6. arrhythmias
7. membranous, aneurysmal, supracristal
8. aneurysm
9. incomplete
10. complete
11. left, right
12. atrialized
13. pulmonary stenosis
14. acyanotic, cyanotic
15. double-outlet right
16. domed
17. bicuspid aortic valve
18. subvalvular aortic stenosis
19. hypoplastic left heart syndrome
20. transposition of the great arteries
21. truncus arteriosus
22. pulmonary artery
23. rhabdomyoma
24. cor triatriatum
25. azygous
26. TAPVR—total anomalous pulmonary venous return

Exercise 5

1. premature atrial and ventricular contractions
2. simultaneously
3. systolic, atrial
4. supraventricular tachyarrhythmias
5. atrial
6. atrial fibrillation
7. suboptimal
8. atrioventricular block
9. complete

Exercise 6

1. Based on Figure 30-3:
   a. 4 o'clock
   b. dilated with a "rounded" shape
   c. The ratio of the cardiac circumference is greater than 50% of the thoracic circumference.
   d. Contractility would be expected to be very low.
2. In Figure 30-12, A, a ventricular septal defect is demonstrated.
3. Based on Figure 30-14, C, D, and E, large defect in the center of the heart; the membranous and primum septum defects are seen with the cleft mitral valve. There is a common leaflet from the anterior mitral leaflet to the septal tricuspid leaflet. D, The chordal attachments from the medial portion of the cleft mitral leaflet are related to the papillary muscle on the right side of the septal defect. E, There is a large defect in the center of the heart with a free-floating common atrioventricular leaflet.
4. Atrioventricular septal defect (primum ASD and membranous VSD) is demonstrated in Figure 30-15, A.
5. The anomaly present in Figure 30-19, B is Ebstein's anomaly.
6. The anomaly present in Figure 30-20, A is hypoplastic right heart.
7. The anomaly present in Figure 30-30 is critical aortic stenosis.
8. Based on Figure 30-36, A, the illustration shows transposition of the great arteries. The aorta is anterior and emptying the right ventricle, and the pulmonary artery is posterior, arising from the left ventricle.
9. Based on Figure 30-39, the illustration shows truncus arteriosus.
10. According to Figure 30-41, B shows a long segment narrowing of the isthmus of the aorta.

CHAPTER 31

Exercise 1

1. I
2. M
3. E
4. C
5. L
6. B
7. N
8. Q
9. A
10. D
11. O
12. K
13. G
14. J
15. P
16. H
17. F

Exercise 2

1. See Figure 31-1 in the textbook for the answers.

Exercise 3

1. left
2. brachiocephalic, left, left
3. innominate
4. medial
5. longer
6. bifurcation
7. smaller
8. ICA
9. cervical, petrous, cavernous, cerebral
10. posterolateral
11. subclavian
12. extravertebral

Exercise 4

1. interruption
2. ischemic
3. age, sex, race
4. hypertension, atrial fibrillation, cardiac disease, diabetes mellitus, elevated cholesterol, smoking, sedentary lifestyle
5. contralateral
6. ipsilateral
7. amaurosis fugax, hemiparesis, dysarthria, aphasia, dysphagia, ataxia, diplopia, vertigo

Exercise 5

1. ≥20 mm Hg
2. low
3. positive
4. continuous, above
5. continuous
6. pulsatile
7. faster
8. laterally

Exercise 6

1. highest
2. subclavian steal
3. multiphasic
4. (1) the location of the stenosis, (2) the extent of the plaque and patency of the distal ICA, (3) the presence of tortuosity or kinking of the vessels, and (4) plaque characteristics (smooth versus irregular surface, calcification)
5. residual, recurrent

Exercise 7

1. homogeneous, heterogeneous
2. calcified
3. decreased, increased
4. multiple
5. fibromuscular dysplasia

Exercise 8

1. Based on Figure 31-3, the external carotid artery demonstrates a higher resistance flow pattern.
2. Figure 31-7 demonstrates irregular plaque along the posterior surface.
3. Figure 31-12 shows bright echoes from the lumen of the stent.
4. Doppler aliasing from the narrowed lumen—carotid stenosis is demonstrated in Figure 31-13.

CHAPTER 32

Exercise 1

1. E
2. B
3. G
4. A
5. H
6. I
7. F
8. C
9. D

Exercise 2

1. E   3. C   5. F   7. G
2. H   4. A   6. B   8. D

Exercise 3

1. See Figure 32-1 in the textbook for the answers.
2. See Figure 32-16 in the textbook for the answers.

Exercise 4

1. carotid, vertebral
2. ophthalmic
3. posterior communicating
4. middle cerebral
5. anterior, posterior
6. anterior cerebral
7. anterior communicating
8. vertebral
9. basilar
10. posterior cerebral
11. circle of Willis

Exercise 5

1. hematocrit
2. flow
3. hyperventilation
4. hypoventilation

Exercise 6

1. transtemporal
2. suboccipital
3. foramen magnum, occipital
4. transorbital
5. submandibular

Exercise 7

1. subarachnoid
2. increase
3. ischemia, infarction
4. stenoses
5. increased
6. subclavian steal
7. basilar
8. away, toward

Exercise 8

1. In Figure 32-18, there is intracranial arterial narrowing with increased velocities in the middle cerebral artery.

CHAPTER 33

Exercise 1

1. N   6. A   11. D   16. O
2. G   7. L   12. B   17. E
3. R   8. S   13. M   18. F
4. C   9. P   14. Q   19. J
5. K   10. H   15. I

Exercise 2

1. See Figure 33-1 in the textbook for the answers.
2. See Figure 33-2 in the textbook for the answers.

Exercise 3

1. thoracic, abdominal
2. bifurcation
3. hypogastric
4. common femoral
5. profunda femoris
6. popliteal
7. anterior, peroneal
8. dorsalis pedis
9. peroneal
10. subclavian
11. axillary
12. brachial

Exercise 4

1. increasing age, hypertension, diabetes mellitus, elevated cholesterol, tobacco smoking, documented atherosclerosis in the coronary or carotid system, and a family history of atherosclerosis
2. claudication, rest
3. distal

Exercise 5

1. 15
2. supine, heart
3. 20%
4. elevated, lower
5. segmental

Exercise 6

1. increase, decrease
2. symptomatic cardiac disease, severe pulmonary disease, severe hypertension, inability to walk on the treadmill, and in cases of calcified vessels (unreliable pressure measure-ments), the use of pulse volume recordings may be helpful in some patients.
3. healing

Exercise 7

1. hemodynamics
2. occlusion, patency, pseudoaneurysms
3. 60
4. triphasic
5. forward, reversal
6. decreases
7. (1) an increase in peak systolic velocities (greater than 100%), (2) marked spectral broadening because of turbulence, and (3) the loss of the reversal of blood flow during diastole
8. thrombus
9. neck
10. systole, diastole

Exercise 8

1. Based on Figure 33-5, the triphasic Doppler flow signal demonstrates a fast upstroke to peak systole, reversal of blood flow during early diastole, and a forward flow component during late diastole.
2. Based on Figure 33-6, the peak-systolic velocity is 55 cm per second, and the waveform shape is abnormal.
3. At the site of the narrowing in Figure 33-7, the peak-systolic velocity increases to over 450 cm per second.
4. The abnormality demonstrated in Figure 33-10 is popliteal artery aneurysm.

CHAPTER 34

Exercise 1

1. J
2. D
3. F
4. L
5. A
6. H
7. C
8. K
9. E
10. B
11. I
12. G

Exercise 2

1. F	4. D	7. L	10. I
2. K	5. J	8. C	11. B
3. A	6. H	9. E	12. G

Exercise 3

1. See Figure 34-1 in the textbook for the answers.
2. See Figure 34-2 in the textbook for the answers.
3. See Figure 34-3 in the textbook for the answers.
4. See Figure 34-4 in the textbook for the answers.
5. See Figure 34-5 in the textbook for the answers.

Exercise 4

1. pulmonary embolism
2. postthrombotic
3. (1) a hypercoagulable state, (2) venous stasis (blood pools in the veins), and (3) vein wall injury (endothelium of the vein is damaged exposing the subendothelium to blood, triggering platelet adhesion and aggregation, which promotes blood coagulation).
4. superficial
5. superficial, deep, communicating
6. superficial, deep
7. superficial, deep
8. unidirectional

Exercise 5

1. area, calf
2. distention
3. externally, flexed
4. collapse, change
5. greater saphenous
6. reduce
7. posterior, decubitus, prone
8. superficial

Exercise 6

1. The patent vein is free of echogenic material, compresses fully with transducer pressure on the skin, and exhibits a normal, venous Doppler signal.
2. pressure
3. compress
4. echogenic, anechoic
5. bypass conduit
6. incompetent
7. superficial

Exercise 7

1. Based on Figures 34-7 and 34-8, *B* is with transducer pressure.
2. Based on Figure 34-10, the vein walls do not coapt, and echogenic material fills the lumen of the vein suggestive of thrombus.
3. In Figure 34-12, a floating clot within the lumen of the femoral vein was found.

CHAPTER 35

Exercise 1

1. E	4. H	7. F	10. G
2. J	5. D	8. A	11. C
3. B	6. K	9. I	

Exercise 2

1. S	7. C	13. F	19. B
2. I	8. N	14. P	20. V
3. M	9. H	15. D	21. R
4. G	10. T	16. W	22. J
5. Q	11. A	17. K	23. E
6. L	12. X	18. U	24. O

Exercise 3

1. D	4. I	7. H	10. C
2. G	5. A	8. E	11. F
3. B	6. L	9. J	12. K

Exercise 4

1. See Figure 35-7 in the textbook for the answers.
2. See Figure 35-8 in the textbook for the answers.
3. See Figure 35-9 in the textbook for the answers.
4. See Figure 35-10 in the textbook for the answers.
5. See Figure 35-11 in the textbook for the answers.
6. See Figure 35-14 in the textbook for the answers.
7. See Figure 35-15 in the textbook for the answers.
8. See Figure 35-17 in the textbook for the answers.

Exercise 5

1. vesicouterine
2. rectouterine
3. Douglas
4. Retzius
5. anterior
6. posteriorly
7. ovulation

Exercise 6

1. 28
2. hypothalamus
3. ovum
4. 14
5. follicle-stimulating hormone
6. follicular
7. luteinizing
8. luteal
9. proliferative
10. secretory

Exercise 7

1. transabdominal
2. endovaginal
3. wider
4. distended
5. labia, majora, minora
6. innominate, sacrum, coccyx
7. piriformis, coccygeus
8. obturator internus
9. levator ani, coccygeus
10. perineum
11. psoas, iliacus
12. puborectalis
13. vagina
14. posterior, anterior
15. uterus
16. cornua
17. internal, external
18. isthmus
19. perimetrium, myometrium, endometrium
20. functionalis, basalis
21. broad, round, uterosacral, cardinal
22. anteverted, anteflexed
23. fallopian tubes
24. infundibulum, ampulla, isthmus, interstitial portion
25. infundibulum
26. medial, anterior
27. tunica albuginea
28. medulla
29. estrogen, progesterone
30. iliac
31. internal
32. radial
33. spiral

CHAPTER 36

Exercise 1

1. B	5. L	9. C	12. K
2. H	6. A	10. M	13. E
3. F	7. N	11. G	14. I
4. D	8. J		

Exercise 2

1. G	4. H	7. I
2. E	5. C	8. D
3. A	6. F	9. B

Exercise 3

1. See Figure 36-10 in the textbook for the answers.

Exercise 4

1. displaces, flattens
2. triangular
3. iliac
4. right upper quadrant, renal
5. anterior, posterior
6. length, width, axial
7. sagittal
8. symmetric
9. obturator internus
10. levator ani
11. piriformis
12. lateral
13. low-velocity
14. decreases
15. myometrium
16. endometrium
17. arcuate
18. internal os
19. flexion, version
20. transabdominal
21. endometrial
22. hyperechoic
23. single thin
24. functionalis
25. basalis
26. secretory
27. echogenic
28. fluid
29. lateral, anteromedial
30. follicular cyst
31. rectouterine recess
32. sonohysterography

Exercise 5

1. In Figure 36-13, *A* in the textbook, the fundus is to the left of the image, and the cervix is to the right of the image.
2. The structure in the center of Figure 36-14, *B* is the endometrial cavity.
3. Based on Figure 36-15, *B,* the visible structures are the multiple anechoic follicles.
4. The secretory phase is demonstrated in Figure 36-36.

CHAPTER 37

Exercise 1

1. C	4. D	7. H
2. F	5. I	8. E
3. A	6. B	9. G

Exercise 2

1. B	4. C
2. D	5. A
3. E	6. F

Exercise 3

1. D
2. I
3. B
4. F
5. H
6. C
7. E
8. G
9. A

Exercise 4

1. nabothian cysts
2. cervical polyps
3. cervical stenosis
4. cuff
5. Gartner's duct
6. imperforate hymen
7. leiomyoma
8. estrogen
9. submucosal, intramural, subserosal
10. submucosal
11. myomas
12. myomas, arcuate
13. adenomyosis
14. arteriovenous
15. endometrial hyperplasia
16. sequential
17. polyps
18. endometritis
19. synechiae
20. endometrial carcinoma
21. cancer
22. intrauterine contraceptive

Exercise 5

1. In Figure 37-1 in the textbook, multiple nabothian cysts are demonstrated.
2. Based on Figure 37-4, cervical stenosis with a large endometrial fluid collection is demonstrated.
3. According to Figure 37-10, A and B show a small submucosal myoma. In B an anechoic follicular cyst is seen along the posterior border compressing the uterine wall.
4. A large myoma is shown posterior to the endometrium in Figure 37-12.
5. Multiple subendometrial cysts and an echogenic nodule are shown in Figure 37-17, E, typical of adenomyosis.
6. The endometrium is very large—patient had endometrial hyperplasia in Figure 37-23.

CHAPTER 38

Exercise 1

1. C
2. F
3. A
4. E
5. D
6. G
7. B

Exercise 2

1. L
2. G
3. P
4. B
5. I
6. E
7. N
8. K
9. C
10. M
11. H
12. O
13. A
14. F
15. J
16. D

Exercise 3

1. See Figure 38-1 in the textbook for the answers.

Exercise 4

1. laterally, posterolaterally
2. medially
3. homogeneous
4. peripherally
5. proliferative
6. cumulus oophorus
7. follicular
8. luteal
9. corpus luteum
10. cyst
11. malignant
12. 10
13. benign
14. diastolic
15. ruptured
16. theca-lutein cysts

17. ovarian hyperstimulation syndrome

18. polycystic ovarian syndrome

19. broad

20. endometrial

21. chocolate cyst

22. blood

23. complete

24. edematous

25. benign

26. malignant

27. cystic

28. increased

29. angiogenesis

30. dermoid plug, fat-fluid level, shadowing, internal

31. ovaries

Exercise 5

1. In Figure 38-9, *D, E,* and *F,* a hemorrhagic cyst is represented.

2. Molar pregnancy with theca-lutein cysts is shown in Figure 38-10.

3. Figure 38-11 shows ovarian hyperstimulation with an enlarged ovary with multiple complicated cysts.

4. Endometriosis is shown in Figure 38-16.

5. Based on Figure 38-19, *A, C, F,* and *G,* ovarian carcinoma with bilateral metastases is shown.

6. The abnormality represented in Figure 38-27 is a dermoid tumor.

CHAPTER 39

Exercise 1

1. N
2. L
3. C
4. G
5. E
6. A
7. M
8. H
9. J
10. D
11. K
12. O
13. F
14. B
15. I

Exercise 2

1. Fitz-Hugh-Curtis
2. mucosa
3. endometritis, salpingitis
4. pyosalpinx
5. pain, vaginal
6. hydrosalpinx
7. thick, echogenic
8. tuboovarian
9. peritonitis
10. adenomyosis, endometriosis
11. anechoic, solid
12. bleeding, hematomas, abscess

Exercise 3

1. In Figure 39-3, a dilated fallopian tube is found (hydrosalpinx).

2. Based on Figure 39-7, the mass does appear to be separate from the uterus (extrauterine). Careful angulation of the transducer to separate the mass from the uterus and cervical area, along with bladder filling, will help to determine the location of the mass.

3. The mass in Figure 39-8, *A* and *B* is extrauterine.

4. There is a large complex tuboovarian abscess that is seen posterior to the distended urinary bladder in Figure 39-13. The uterus is not shown.

CHAPTER 40

Exercise 1

1. D
2. G
3. B
4. L
5. H
6. K
7. I
8. A
9. C
10. J
11. E
12. F

Exercise 2

1. 12
2. nonhostile
3. postcoital
4. thickness, echogenicity, intracavitary
5. bicornuate, didelphys
6. bicornuate

7. patency

8. dominant

9. 22

10. basal body temperature

11. elevated

12. 12 to14

13. hyperstimulation, gestations, ectopic

14. ovarian hyperstimulation syndrome

15. heterotopic

Exercise 3

1. A submucosal fibroid is demonstrated in Figure 40-5.

2. Uterine synechia is demonstrated in Figure 40-8.

3. The ovarian follicular phase is shown in Figure 40-10.

4. Polycystic ovarian syndrome is shown in Figure 40-12.

5. The complication in Figure 40-15 is associated with ovarian hyperstimulation syndrome.

CHAPTER 41

Exercise 1

1. F
2. J
3. D
4. H

5. C
6. A
7. B
8. L

9. G
10. I
11. K
12. E

13. P
14. N
15. M
16. O

Exercise 2

1. H
2. E
3. A

4. D
5. C
6. G

7. L
8. I
9. K

10. F
11. J
12. B

Exercise 3

1. estimation of gestational age

2. evaluation of fetal growth

3. vaginal bleeding of undetermined cause in pregnancy

4. determination of fetal presentation when the presenting part cannot be adequately determined in labor or the fetal presentation is variable in late pregnancy

5. suspected multiple gestation based on detection of more than one fetal heartbeat pattern, fundal height larger than expected for dates, or prior use of fertility drugs

6. adjunct to amniocentesis

7. significant discrepancy between uterine size and clinical dates

8. pelvic mass detected clinically, sonography

9. suspected hydatidiform mole on the basis of clinical signs of hypertension, proteinuria, or the presence of ovarian cysts felt on pelvic examination or failure to detect fetal heart tones with a Doppler ultrasound device after 12 weeks

10. adjunct to cervical cerclage placement

11. suspected ectopic pregnancy or when pregnancy occurs after tuboplasty or prior ectopic gestation

12. adjunct to special procedures, such as cordocentesis, intrauterine transfusion, shunt placement, in vitro fertilization, embryo transfer, or chorionic villus sampling

13. suspected fetal death

14. suspected uterine abnormality (e.g., clinically significant leiomyomata, congenital structural abnormalities, such as bicornuate uterus or uterus didelphys)

15. intrauterine contraceptive device (IUD) localization

16. ovarian follicle development surveillance

17. biophysical evaluation for fetal well-being after 28 weeks of gestation

18. observation of intrapartum events (e.g., version or extraction of second twin, manual removal of placenta)

19. suspected polyhydramnios or oligohydramnios

20. suspected abruptio placentae

21. adjunct to external version from breech to vertex presentation

22. estimation of fetal weight and presentation in premature rupture of the membranes or premature labor

23. abnormal maternal serum alpha fetoprotein (MSAFP) value for clinical gestational age when drawn

24. follow-up observation of identified fetal anomaly

25. follow-up evaluation of placenta location for identified placenta previa

26. serial evaluation of fetal growth in multiple gestation

Exercise 4

1. increased maternal age, abnormal triple screen biochemistry values, maternal disease (e.g., diabetes mellitus, systemic lupus erythematosus), a pregnant uterus that is either too small or too large for dates

2. chromosomal, teratogenic

3.
   a. The sonographer first tries to determine the clinical dates of the pregnancy.
   b. Does the patient have any latex allergies?
   c. When was the first date of the last menstrual period (LMP or LNMP)?
   d. The sonographer also needs to know if the patient is currently taking any medication.
   e. Has the patient experienced clinical problems with the pregnancy, such as bleeding, decreased fetal movement, or pelvic pain?
   f. If the patient has had problems with previous pregnancies, such as incompetent cervix, fibroids, fetal macrosomia or growth restriction, congenital or chromosomal fetal anomalies, this should be documented on the record as well.

Exercise 5

1.
   a. qualifications of personnel performing the examination
   b. documentation
   c. equipment specifications
   d. fetal safety
   e. quality control
   f. safety, infection control
   g. patient education concerns

2. certification

3. permanent

4. patient's name, date, image orientation

5.
   a. The uterus and adnexa should be evaluated for the presence of a gestational sac, yolk sac, and embryo.
   b. Presence or absence of cardiac activity should be reported.
   c. Fetal number should be documented.
   d. Evaluation of the uterus, adnexal structures, and cul-de-sac should be performed.

6.
   a. Fetal life, number, presentation, and activity should be documented.
   b. Estimation of the quantity of amniotic fluid should be done.
   c. Placental localization, appearance, and relationship to the internal cervical os should be recorded.
   d. Multiple sonographic parameters can be used to estimate gestational age in the second and third trimesters (IC, BPD, HC, AC, FL).
   e. Uterine, adnexal, and cervical evaluation should be performed to document the presence, location, and size of uterine or adnexal masses that may complicate obstetric management. The normal maternal ovaries may not be imaged during the second and third trimester.
   f. Fetal anatomy may be adequately assessed after 18 weeks of gestation. Anatomy may be difficult to image because of fetal movement, size, or position and/or maternal scars, or increased wall thickness. When anatomy is not seen because of technical limitation, the sonographer should note the reason. A follow-up examination may be ordered.

7. Anatomic areas recommended include the following:
   a. head and neck
      cerebellum, choroid plexus, cisterna magna, lateral cerebral ventricles, midline falx, and cavum septi pellucidi
   b. chest
      four-chamber view of the fetal heart and, if technically feasible, an extended basic cardiac examination that includes both outflow tracts may be attempted
   c. abdomen
      stomach (presence, size, and situs), kidneys, bladder, umbilical cord insertion into the fetal abdomen, and umbilical cord number
   d. spine
      cervical, thoracic, lumbar, and sacral spine
   e. extremities
      presence and absence of arms and legs
   f. gender
      medically indicated in low-risk pregnancies only for assessment of multiple pregnancies

CHAPTER 42

Exercise 1

1. F	4. A	7. J	10. E
2. B	5. K	8. H	11. C
3. I	6. G	9. D	

Exercise 2

1. morality
2. right and wrong, good and bad
3. values
4. freedom, autonomy
5. ethics
6. first do no harm
7. nonmaleficence
8. education
9. beneficence
10. minimum
11. privacy
12. competency, knowledge, sonographic
13. autonomy
14. consent
15. veracity
16. justice
17. timing
18. beneficence

CHAPTER 43

Exercise 1

1. E
2. A
3. D
4. I
5. G
6. B
7. F
8. C
9. H
10. J

Exercise 2

1. K
2. C
3. G
4. M
5. B
6. J
7. E
8. A
9. H
10. D
11. L
12. I
13. F

Exercise 3

1. See Figure 43-1 in the textbook for the answers.
2. See Figure 43-6 in the textbook for the answers.
3. See Figure 43-12, *A* in the textbook for the answers.

Exercise 4

1. gestation
2. embryo
3. fetus
4. 2
5. zygote
6. 7 to 9
7. cardiovascular
8. proportionately
9. plateau
10. 1000 to 2000
11. ectopic
12. double decidual sac
13. 1
14. yolk
15. 6th
16. 5th through 7th
17. 12th
18. 11th
19. 8th to 11th
20. lateral

Exercise 5

1. length, width, height
2. 8
3. 10 to 15
4. 0.1

Exercise 6

1. 5.5 and 6.5
2. two
3. one, two, two, two
4. one, one

Exercise 7

1. Based on Figure 43-4, the age and appearance in *A* is a 4-week gestational sac within the fundus of the uterus. *B*, 5-week gestational sac with the characteristic trophoblastic ring surrounding the sac. *C*, 6-week gestational sac within the fundus of the uterus.

2. The arrows in Figure 43-10 are pointing to the amniotic membrane.

3. In Figure 43-11, the structure in *A* is the embryo, and the structure labeled *C* in image *B* is the embryonic cranium.

4. The curved arrow in Figure 43-12, *B* is pointing to the amniotic membrane, and the straight arrows are pointing to the umbilical cord.

5. Figure 43-25 represents the crown-rump length.

6. The type of multiple gestation predicted from Figure 43-26 is diamniotic-dichorionic pregnancy.

7. The type of multiple gestation predicted from Figure 43-28 is monoamniotic-monochorionic pregnancy.

CHAPTER 44

Exercise 1

1. I	4. B	7. K	10. D
2. C	5. J	8. G	11. H
3. F	6. E	9. A	

Exercise 2

1. D	4. E	7. F
2. H	5. I	8. A
3. B	6. C	9. G

Exercise 3

1. choroid plexus
2. ossification
3. anencephaly
4. ventriculomegaly
5. Dandy-Walker malformation
6. 10 to 12
7. cystic hygroma
8. pseudomembrane
9. subchorionic
10. corpus luteum
11. previous pelvic infections, IUCD, fallopian tube surgery, infertility treatments, and previous ectopic pregnancies
12. empty, mass
13. pseudogestational sac
14. interstitial pregnancy
15. 90
16. subchorionic
17. complete
18. incomplete
19. gestational trophoblastic
20. elevated
21. snowstorm
22. theca lutein

Exercise 4

1. Based on Figure 44-3, acrania is found. The fetal head is not completely formed with the fetal brain uncovered by the incomplete fetal skull development.

2. Ventriculomegaly is found in Figure 44-4.

3. There is a mass projecting from the fetal abdomen in Figure 44-6. At this stage, this could be normal bowel migration; however, a membrane is seen, and on subsequent scans in the second trimester an omphalocele is demonstrated.

4. The arrows in Figure 44-8 are pointing to the amniotic membrane.

5. Intrauterine 8-week gestation with a leiomyoma tumor in the lower uterine segment is evident in Figure 44-14.

6. Empty uterus, fluid in the cul-de-sac, and an ectopic gestational sac in the right adnexal area are present in Figure 44-19.

7. Subchorionic hemorrhage of the placenta is demonstrated in Figure 44-24.

CHAPTER 45

Exercise 1

1. E	4. D
2. C	5. B
3. A	

Exercise 2

1. F	4. B	7. A	10. C
2. J	5. H	8. K	11. I
3. D	6. G	9. E	

Exercise 3

1.

a. observation of fetal viability by visualization of cardiovascular pulsations

b. demonstration of presentation (fetal lie)

c. Demonstration of the number of fetuses. In multiple gestations, anatomy images are obtained on each fetus, growth parameters of each fetus are obtained and compared, placenta and membrane structures are assessed, and amniotic fluid levels in each sac are documented.

d. characterization of the quantity of amniotic fluid as normal or abnormal by subjective visualization or by quantitative estimation techniques

e. Characterization of the placenta including localization and relationship to the internal cervical os. Placenta previa should be excluded by examination of the cervical area.

f. visualization of the cervix and extension of the examination to include transperineal or transvaginal imaging if the cervix appears shortened or the patient complains of regular uterine contractions

g. Assessment of fetal age. Multiple growth parameters are evaluated. Fetal growth studies may include a serial growth analysis when serial examinations are performed at intervals that are 3 weeks apart.

h. biometric parameters, such as the following:
- biparietal diameter
- head circumference
- femur length, humerus length
- abdominal circumference
- fetal weight
- head circumference to abdominal circumference ratio (used in cases in which disproportionate growth is suspected or unusual head or body contours are observed)
- measurement ratios related to head shape or growth

i. Evaluation of uterus, adnexa, and cervix to exclude masses that may complicate obstetric management. Maternal ovaries may not be visualized during the second and third trimesters of pregnancy.

j. Survey of fetal anatomy to exclude major congenital malformations. Targeted studies may be necessary when a fetal anomaly is suspected.

k. Standard obstetric antepartum sonography examinations should strive to evaluate the anatomic areas listed below. Targeted or repeat studies may be appropriate if anatomy is not well visualized. Technical difficulty should be reported, and images should be preserved that document visualization of the following:
- cerebral ventricles (to reduce risk of ventriculomegaly)
- posterior fossa of the fetal head including the cerebellum, cisterna magna, and nuchal skin fold
- choroid plexus
- midline falx and cavum septi pellucidi
- spine views including the cervical, thoracic, lumbar, and sacral spine (to reduce risk of spinal defects)
- stomach (to reduce risk of gastrointestinal obstruction)

Exercise 4

1. human chorionic gonadotropin
2. gravidity
3. parity
4. two, one, no, three

Exercise 5

1. mother
2. cardiac
3. left and right
4. 34
5. transverse
6. vertex, breech
7. footling
8. down, up

Exercise 6

1. hypoechoic
2. large, small
3. ossify
4. dura, pia arachnoid
5. round or oval, smooth
6. falx cerebri
7. central nervous
8. glomus of the choroid plexus
9. 10
10. midline echo complex
11. third
12. Willis
13. cerebellum
14. cisterna magna
15. 3 to 11
16. cerebellum

Exercise 7

1. positioning, amniotic fluid, acoustic
2. one third
3. swallowing
4. periphery
5. cervical, thoracic, lumbar, sacral
6. three
7. railway
8. equidistant
9. center
10. transverse
11. homogeneous
12. In four-chamber views of the heart, it is important to assess the following:

    - Cardiac position, situs, and axis. The apex of the heart should point to the fetal left side.

- Presence of the right ventricle (the ventricle found when a line is drawn from the spine to the anterior chest wall) and left ventricle
- Equal-size ventricles. By the end of pregnancy, the right ventricle may be larger than the left ventricle because it is the chamber that pumps blood through the ductus arteriosus to the descending aorta and to the placenta.
- Presence of equal-size right and left atria, with the foramen ovale opening toward the left atrium as blood is shunted from the right atrium, bypassing the lungs
- An interventricular septum that appears uninterrupted. The septum appears wider toward the ventricles and thins as it courses cephalad within the heart.
- Normal placement of the tricuspid and mitral valves. The tricuspid valve inserts lower, or closer to the apex, than the mitral valve. Both valves should open during diastole and close during systole.
- Normal rhythm and rate (120 to 160 beats per minute)
- Guidelines recommend that the standard antepartum obstetric examination include views of the ventricular outflow tracts when it is technically feasible.

Exercise 8

1. longitudinal
2. swallowed
3. pulsations
4. right
5. oxygenation
6. higher
7. bypasses
8. away
9. directly
10. ductus venosus
11. umbilical
12. falciform
13. hepatic
14. foramen
15. foramen ovale, ductus venosus, ductus arteriosus
16. left
17. gallbladder
18. stomach
19. 11th, 16th
20. meconium
21. 15th
22. pelvocaliceal
23. 10
24. echogenic
25. once
26. normal
27. abducted
28. 12 to 16, 20th to 22nd
29. 12th
30. soft tissue

Exercise 9

1. bowing, fractures
2. humerus
3. 39th
4. ulna
5. opened
6. 33 to 35

Exercise 10

1. The breech position is demonstrated in Figure 45-6 in the textbook.
2. In Figure 45-12, A, the choroid plexus is the structure within the ventricle. The structure in the center of the fetal head is the thalamus in Figure 45-12, B, and the cerebellum is measured in Figure 45-12, C. The biparietal diameter should be measured at the level of the thalamus, image B.
3. In Figure 45-19, the f denotes the frontal bone, the t denotes the tongue, and the c denotes the chin.
4. The right side is closest to the transducer in Figure 45-42, A.
5. The L in Figure 45-48, A is pointing to the labia majora.
6. The scrotum and penis are demonstrated in Figure 45-50.
7. Based on Figure 45-53, the radius is anterior, and the ulna is posterior.

CHAPTER 46

Exercise 1

1. K
2. D
3. H
4. F
5. C
6. J
7. A
8. L
9. I
10. M
11. E
12. B
13. G

Exercise 2

1. J
2. G
3. A
4. D
5. H
6. B
7. K
8. F
9. I
10. C
11. E

Exercise 3

1. decidua
2. anteroposterior, transverse, longitudinal
3. 10
4. 8
5. 6, 8
6. 16
7. 1 to 2
8. crown-rump length
9. 8
10. anembryonic
11. CRL in cm + 6

Exercise 4

1. biparietal, head, abdominal, femur
2. 1
3. 3, 1.8
4. axial
5. thalamus, cavum septi pellucidi
6. falx, cavum septi pellucidi, choroid plexus
7. ovoid
8. leading, leading
9. transverse
10. perpendicular
11. underestimate, overestimate
12. growth parameter
13. liver, umbilical
14. circular
15. femur
16. distal femoral point
17. femur
18. abdomen
19. elbow

Exercise 5

1. The structure in Figure 46-2 is the yolk sac in a 4-week gestational sac.
2. In Figure 46-10, the *f* is falx, the *t* is thalamic nuclei and the *3v* is the third ventricle.
3. Image *C* of Figure 46-12 shows the cerebellum.
4. In Figure 46-21, the *sp* is the spine and the *st* is the stomach. The fetal abdominal circumference is made at this level.
5. The arrow in Figure 46-22 is pointing to the distal femoral point; femur.

CHAPTER 47

Exercise 1

1. L
2. F
3. A
4. I
5. D
6. M
7. G
8. K
9. C
10. H
11. E
12. B
13. J

Exercise 2

1. 10
2. previous fetus with IUGR, maternal hypertension or smoking, presence of a uterine anomaly, and significant placental hemorrhage
3. BPD, HC, AC, and FL
4. symmetric
5. asymmetric
6. small
7. AC

Exercise 3

1. head-sparing
2. head
3. liver
4. oligohydramnios

Exercise 4

1. cardiac non-stress test (NST), observation of fetal breathing movements (FBM), gross fetal body movements (FM), fetal tone (FT), and amniotic fluid volume (AFV)
2. increase, decreases
3. resistance
4. 4000
5. diabetes mellitus

Exercise 5

1. Serial ultrasound evaluations should be made to determine fetal growth assessment according to Figure 47-1.
2. Figure 47-2 is demonstrating the four quadrant assessment of amniotic fluid.
3. Figure 47-7 represents normal umbilical artery flow.
4. Figure 47-9 represents high resistance, and it is associated with adverse perinatal outcome.

CHAPTER 48

Exercise 1

1. T
2. L
3. D
4. J
5. B
6. P
7. H
8. O
9. R
10. E
11. N
12. I
13. A
14. K
15. Q
16. F
17. S
18. C
19. M
20. G

Exercise 2

1. advanced maternal age
2. nuchal
3. quad
4. targeted
5. hydrops fetalis
6. anasarca, ascites, pericardial effusion, pleural effusion, placental edema, polyhydramnios
7. antigen
8. scalp, pleural, pericardial, ascites, polyhydramnios, thickened
9. cordocentesis
10. thrombocytopenia
11. nonimmune hydrops
12. functional, structural
13. macrosomic
14. shoulder dystocia
15. transposition of the great arteries, tetralogy of Fallot
16. diabetic
17. small
18. eclampsia
19. systemic lupus erythematosus
20. hyperemesis gravidarum
21. Progesterone has a dilatory effect on the smooth muscle of the ureter, and enlarging uterus compresses the ureters at the pelvic brim—hydronephrosis.

Exercise 3

1. one half
2. 10 to 12
3. 20
4. 16 and 20
5. (1) absent heartbeat, (2) absent fetal movement, (3) overlap of skull bones (Spalding's sign), (4) an exaggerated curvature of the fetal spine, and (5) gas in the fetal abdomen

Exercise 4

1. preeclampsia, third-trimester bleeding, prolapsed cord
2. five
3. gestational
4. dizygotic, diamniotic, dichorionic
5. monozygotic
6. early, late
7. early
8. 4 to 8
9. monochorionic, monoamniotic
10. conjoined
11. poly-oli
12. arteriovenous
13. acardiac
14. amniotic
15. smaller
16. reverse

Exercise 5

1. Scalp edema is shown in Figure 48-2. Pleural effusion is shown in Figure 48-3, and abdominal ascites is shown in Figure 48-4.
2. Polyhydramnios is demonstrated in Figure 48-5.
3. In Figure 48-10, *A,* abdominal ascites is demonstrated. In Figure 48-10, *B,* the umbilical vein is denoted with the *v.*
4. In Figure 48-21, this is fetal demise with the fetus curled up; no cardiac activity or fetal motion is noted. Scalp edema is present.
5. Dichorionic, diamniotic twin gestation is represented in Figure 48-27.
6. Monochorionic, monoamniotic twinning is depicted in Figure 48-31.
7. Conjoined twins at the thorax are present in Figure 48-33.

CHAPTER 49

Exercise 1

1. K
2. B
3. E
4. G
5. C
6. H
7. J
8. A
9. F
10. I
11. D

Exercise 2

1. 3
2. chorionic villus sampling
3. embryoscopy
4. amniocentesis
5. each
6. cordocentesis
7. alpha fetoprotein
8. amniotic fluid
9. neural tube defects
10. omphalocele, gastroschisis
11. twin
12. AFP, human chorionic gonadotropin, unconjugated estriol

Exercise 3

1. 46, 22
2. aneuploidy
3. Down
4. 50
5. 25
6. boys
7. sons, daughters
8. multifactorial
9. mosaicism

Exercise 4

1. aneuploidy
2. 3
3. neck, nuchal
4. 3, 4
5. nuchal fold of 6 mm or greater, extremity anomalies (hypoplasia of the middle phalanx or clinodactyly of the fifth finger, space between first and second toes), shortened femur or short humerus, duodenal atresia, heart defects (present in approximately 30% to 40%), intrauterine growth restriction (IUGR), mild pyelectasis (4 mm in anteroposterior diameter), echogenic bowel, mild ventriculomegaly, echogenic intracardiac focus, and absence of the nasal bone between 11 to 14 weeks
6. Physical features that have been identified in fetuses with trisomy 18 include cardiac anomalies, which are present in the majority of fetuses with this chromosomal anomaly. Cranial anomalies that have been identified are dolichocephaly, microcephaly, hydrocephalus, agenesis of the corpus callosum, cerebellar hypoplasia, a strawberry-shaped head, and

choroid plexus cysts. Facial abnormalities include low-set ears, micrognathia, and cleft lip and palate. Abnormal extremities identified with trisomy 18 include persistently clenched hands, talipes, rocker-bottom feet, and radial aplasia. Other anomalies associated with Edward's syndrome include omphalocele, congenital diaphragmatic hernia, neural tube defects, cystic hygroma, and renal anomalies. Sonographic features also include polyhydramnios, IUGR, single umbilical artery, and nonimmune hydrops.

7. The physical features characteristic of trisomy 13 include holoprosencephaly, which is a common finding in fetuses with trisomy 13. Other cranial anomalies include agenesis of the corpus callosum and microcephaly. Facial anomalies may be associated with the presence of holoprosencephaly and include hypotelorism, proboscis, cyclopia, and nose with a single nostril. Cleft lip and palate, microphthalmia, and micrognathia may also be present. Heart defects are present in 90% of fetuses and may include ventricular septal defect, atrial septal defect, and hypoplastic left heart. Other anomalies associated with trisomy 13 include omphalocele, renal anomalies, and meningomyelocele. Associated limb anomalies include polydactyly, talipes, rocker-bottom feet, and overlapping fingers. Cystic hygroma and echogenic chordae tendineae may also be identified.

8. Physical features of triploidy include heart defects, renal anomalies, omphalocele, and meningomyelocele. Cranial defects associated with triploidy include holoprosencephaly, agenesis of the corpus callosum, hydrocephalus, and Dandy-Walker malformation. Facial anomalies may be present and include low-set ears, hypertelorism, cleft lip and palate, and micrognathia. Cryptorchidism, ambiguous genitalia, syndactyly, and talipes may also be observed. Sonographic features of triploidy include severe IUGR and placental changes (hydatidiform degeneration). Oligohydramnios is often present and may hamper adequate visualization of the fetus.

9. Turner's

10. cystic hygroma, coarctation of the aorta

Exercise 5

1. Based on Figure 49-13, the finding in *A* is a thickened nuchal fold. In *B* or Figure 49-14, double bubble sign is present—duodenal atresia is demonstrated. In Figure 49-15 or *C*, endocardial cushion defect with common atrioventricular valve is shown and in Figure 49-16 or *D*, echogenic bowel is shown.

2. In Figure 49-21, image *A* shows a clubbed hand, and image *C* shows ascites within the defect.

3. In Figure 49-24, image *A* shows a proboscis; image *B* shows a fused thalamus and thickened nuchal fold; image *C* shows polydactyly; and image *D* shows a ventricular septal defect.

4. Facial anomalies of cyclopia and absent nose are demonstrated in Figure 49-25.

5. In Figure 49-30, image *A* shows a cystic hygroma in the nuchal area; image *B* shows hydrops; image *C* shows edema around fetal head and pleural effusions.

CHAPTER 50

Exercise 1

1. D
2. I
3. B
4. G
5. C
6. E
7. A
8. F
9. H

Exercise 2

1. echo data must process along an ultrasound beam, ultrasound beam must move over the area of interest, translation and rotation of the axis from the ultrasound beam and the time of the reflected sound waves creates the 3-D data set, which is converted into distance information by the assumption of the speed of sound within the volume of interest, storage of the data and the gap-filling procedure, and visualization of the data obtained

2. automated

3. free-hand

4. manually

5. planar reconstruction, volume-rendering

6. surface-light

7. transparent

CHAPTER 51

Exercise 1

1. D
2. G
3. A
4. H
5. C
6. F
7. E
8. B

Exercise 2

1. M	5. L	9. C	13. K
2. D	6. B	10. I	14. E
3. O	7. G	11. N	15. H
4. J	8. A	12. F	

Exercise 3

1. See Figure 51-1, *A* in the textbook for the answers.

2. See Figure 51-1, *B* in the textbook for the answers.

3. See Figure 51-2 in the textbook for the answers.

Exercise 4

1. oxygenated, deoxygenated

2. posterior, umbilical cord

3. chorionic plate

4. basal plate

5. chorionic villus

6. protection, nutrition, respiration, excretion

7. spiral

8. hypotension, renal, placental

9. metabolism, endocrine, transfer

10. center

11. blood

12. excrete, swallows

Exercise 5

1. subplacental

2. 45-50 mm

3. position

4. full bladder

5. succenturiate

6. high, low

7. placentomegaly

8. previa

9. complete

10. transperineal, translabial

11. vasa

12. placenta

13. cesarean section

14. increta

15. circumvallate

16. abruption

17. retroplacental

18. marginal

19. infarction

20. gestational trophoblastic

21. chorioangioma

Exercise 6

1. In Figure 51-6, *A,* echolucent areas are shown along the inner margin of the chorionic plate. In Figure 51-6, *B,* intervillous lakes are shown.

2. An edematous placenta may be seen in the Rh-sensitized pregnancy or in diabetic pregnancies in Figure 51-7.

3. Placenta previa is found in Figure 51-11.

4. Retroplacental abruption of the placenta is found in Figure 51-22.

5. Chorioangioma of the placenta is found in Figure 51-25. There is right heart enlargement with pleural effusion.

CHAPTER 52

Exercise 1

1. H	6. M	10. K	14. F
2. D	7. A	11. I	15. O
3. C	8. L	12. Q	16. G
4. J	9. B	13. N	17. E
5. P			

Exercise 2

1. oxygen
2. herniate
3. two, one, Wharton's
4. bladder, liver
5. ductus venosus
6. portal, systemic
7. venosum
8. lateral
9. 2.6 to 6.0 cm

Exercise 3

1. true
2. false
3. nuchal
4. battledore
5. velamentous
6. prolapse
7. compression
8. single

Exercise 4

1. The arrows in Figure 52-2 are pointing to the umbilical arteries.
2. Gastroschisis is the abnormality in Figure 52-11.
3. Umbilical hernia is present in Figure 52-12.
4. The arrows in Figure 52-13, *B* are pointing to a clot in the umbilical arteries.
5. Multiple knots in the cord are demonstrated in Figure 52-14.
6. The nuchal cord around the fetal neck is found in Figure 52-16.

CHAPTER 53

Exercise 1

1. D
2. I
3. L
4. M
5. F
6. B
7. G
8. A
9. H
10. E
11. C
12. K
13. J

Exercise 2

1. amniotic fluid
2. amniotic, yolk
3. membranes, lungs, kidneys
4. chorion frondosum
5. keratinization
6. 8 and 11
7. swallows, produces
8. kidney
9. exchange
10. oligohydramnios
11. 25, 50
12. generous
13. isolated
14. decreased, increased
15. echo-free

Exercise 3

1. subjective assessment
2. four quadrant
3. single pocket assessment
4. 5 to 10, 20 to 24
5. perpendicular
6. maximum vertical pocket
7. oligohydramnios

Exercise 4

1. polyhydramnios
2. central nervous system, gastrointestinal
3. depressed
4. blockage
5. oligohydramnios
6. 2, 5
7. congenital anomalies, IUGR, postterm pregnancy, ruptured membranes, iatrogenic
8. IUGR
9. blood flow
10. compression

Exercise 5

1. amniotic band syndrome

2. birth

3. synechiae

Exercise 6

1. The arrows in Figure 53-2, *A* are pointing to implantation bleed and in *B*, the arrow is pointing to the amnion.

2. Premature rupture of membranes with marked oligohydramnios is evident in Figure 53-12.

3. In Figure 53-13, *A*, renal agenesis is present and in *B*, infantile polycystic kidney disease is present.

CHAPTER 54

Exercise 1

1. F	5. E	9. H	13. J
2. I	6. K	10. O	14. N
3. L	7. A	11. D	15. C
4. B	8. M	12. G	

Exercise 2

1. J	5. F	9. C	13. E
2. D	6. N	10. K	14. H
3. M	7. G	11. B	
4. I	8. A	12. L	

Exercise 3

1. See Figure 54-1, *A* in the textbook for the answers.

2. See Figure 54-1, *B* in the textbook for the answers.

3. See Figure 54-2 in the textbook for the answers.

Exercise 4

1. branchial apparatus

2. six

3. mandibular

4. neural, mesoderm

5. ectoderm

6. medially, upper

Exercise 5

1. family, congenital

2. chromosomal

3. curvilinear

4. hypertelorism

5. craniosynostosis

6. kleeblattschädel

7. thanatophoric dysplasia, ventriculomegaly

8. trigonocephaly

9. frontal bossing

10. midface, maxillary

11. 21

12. frontonasal dysplasia

13. 11, 13, 6

14. 45, 84

15. Beckwith-Wiedemann

16. rami, rami

17. mentum, bisection

18. chromosome, skeletal, mandibular

19. microphthalmia, anophthalmia

20. hypotelorism

21. hypertelorism

22. profile

23. (1) nostril symmetry, (2) nasal septum integrity, (3) continuity of the upper lip to exclude cleft lip and palate

24. cleft

25. hard and soft

26. left

27. swallowing

Exercise 6

1. cystic hygroma
2. dystocia
3. goiter
4. Turner's

5. fetal cystic hygroma
6. hydrops
7. goiter

Exercise 7

1. The arrows in Figure 54-7 are pointing to the lens in *A* and the eyelids in *B*.

2. In Figure 54-8, the *t* denotes the tongue in *A*. In *B,* coronal view is demonstrated.

3. Thanatophoric dysplastic fetus with a cloverleaf skull (klee-blattschädel) is demonstrated in Figure 54-10.

4. The arrow in Figure 54-13 is pointing to the absent nasal bone in a fetus with trisomy 21.

5. Holoprosencephaly with a proboscis is demonstrated in Figure 54-26.

6. Unilateral cleft lip with extension into the nasal cavity is demonstrated in Figure 54-31.

7. In Figure 54-40, cystic hygroma is present.

CHAPTER 55

Exercise 1

1. M
2. B
3. L
4. F

5. J
6. N
7. C
8. P

9. G
10. I
11. A
12. O

13. H
14. D
15. K
16. E

Exercise 2

1. forebrain, spinal

2. prosencephalon, mesencephalon, rhombencephalon

3. anencephaly

4. absence of the brain and cranial vault, rudimentary brain tissue characterized as the cerebrovasculosa, and bulging fetal orbits, giving the fetus a froglike appearance

5. the presence of brain tissue without the presence of a calvarium, disorganization of brain tissue, and prominent sulcal markings

6. cephalocele

7. encephalocele

8. meningocele

9. Chiari Type II

10. splaying of the posterior ossification centers with a V or U configuration, protrusion of a saclike structure that may be anechoic (meningocele) or contain neural elements (myelomeningocele), a cleft in the skin, and ventriculomegaly

11. a posterior fossa cyst that can vary considerably in size, splaying of the cerebellar hemispheres as a result of the complete or partial agenesis of the cerebellar vermis, an enlarged cisterna magna caused by the cerebellar vermis anomaly and posterior fossa cyst, and ventriculomegaly

12. alobar

13. semilobar

14. lobar

15. corpus callosum

16. absence of the corpus callosum, elevation and dilation of the third ventricle, widely separated lateral ventricular frontal horns with medial indentation of the medial walls, dilated occipital horns (colpocephaly), giving the lateral ventricles a teardrop shape, and absence of the cavum septi pellucidi

17. aqueductal stenosis

18. porencephalic

19. schizencephaly

20. obstruction

21. occipital, frontal

22. 10

Exercise 3

1. In Figure 55-1, an anencephalic fetus is found.

2. The abnormality demonstrated in Figure 55-13 is a large spinal defect at the thoracic level.

3. The abnormality in the fetus in Figure 55-15 is a meningomyelocele with splaying of the spinal canal.

4. In Figure 55-17, spina bifida with a U-shaped configuration and an open cleft in the skin is visible.

5. An abnormally shaped cerebellum "banana sign" is visible in Figure 55-18.

6. The abnormality demonstrated in Figure 55-32 is agenesis of the corpus callosum in this fetus with an absent cavum septi pellucidi.

7. In Figure 55-39, hydranencephaly with massive collection of cerebrospinal fluid is visible.

CHAPTER 56

Exercise 1

1. I
2. D
3. G
4. B
5. J
6. E
7. K
8. A
9. F
10. C
11. H

Exercise 2

1. fluid
2. bell, ribs, clavicles, diaphragm
3. smaller
4. hypoplasia
5. mass, effusion, malformation
6. echogenicity
7. liver
8. second, third
9. 20

Exercise 3

1. heart position, orientation of the cardiac axis, and measure the thoracic circumference
2. hypoplasia
3. reduction
4. four-chamber
5. bronchogenic
6. hydrothorax
7. sequestration, intralobar, extralobar
8. thoracic aorta
9. echo-dense
10. congenital cystic adenomatoid
11. abdominal
12. Bochdalek
13. Morgagni
14. malformations
15. left
16. right
17. hypoplasia
18. ECMO

Exercise 4

1. As seen in Figure 56-1, the fetal lungs are more echogenic than the homogeneous fetal liver.
2. The apex of the heart points toward the left side of the abdomen in Figure 56-3. The heart axis is normal.
3. In Figure 56-12, the fetal lungs are very echogenic compared with the liver. There is pleural effusion and ascites. The fetus has tracheal atresia.
4. The type of cystic adenomatoid shown in Figure 56-13 is Type I CAM.
5. A diaphragmatic hernia is also seen in Figure 56-18. Displacement of the heart to the right chest is shown in image *A*. Herniated bowel is seen (arrows).
6. In Figure 56-19, there is a large left-sided hernia. The stomach and bowel are seen within the thoracic cavity.

CHAPTER 57

Exercise 1

1. B
2. G
3. D
4. J
5. H
6. A
7. E
8. C
9. I
10. F

Exercise 2

1. ectoderm, mesoderm, endoderm
2. bowel
3. 12th
4. gastroschisis, omphalocele, umbilical hernia
5. distortion
6. omphalocele
7. membrane
8. chromosomal
9. liver
10. right
11. small
12. alpha fetoprotein

13. without

14. amniotic band syndrome

15. Beckwith-Wiedemann

16. exstrophy

17. pentalogy of Cantrell

18. ectopia cordis

19. limb body wall complex

Exercise 3

1. The arrows in Figure 57-3 are pointing to a small omphalocele.

2. In Figure 57-5, a bowel omphalocele is shown in *A,* and an umbilical cord cyst is shown in *B.*

3. A liver-filled omphalocele and ascites are visible in Figure 57-14. Bowel is displaced into the chest.

4. In Figure 57-20, gastroschisis with a herniated large intestine with meconium is visible.

CHAPTER 58

Exercise 1

1. G
2. C
3. D
4. A
5. F
6. H
7. E
8. B
9. I

Exercise 2

1. M
2. E
3. A
4. H
5. L
6. F
7. C
8. K
9. D
10. N
11. I
12. B
13. G
14. J

Exercise 3

1. foregut
2. esophageal atresia
3. foregut
4. lesser sac
5. epiploic foramen
6. foregut, midgut
7. distal
8. stenosis, atresia
9. umbilical, two
10. hemopoiesis
11. midgut
12. Meckel's diverticulum

Exercise 4

1. fluid-filled
2. 20 to 30
3. portal, umbilical
4. color
5. swallowing
6. meconium
7. hyperechoic
8. peristalsis
9. haustral folds
10. colon
11. hypoechoic
12. left, right
13. 20

Exercise 5

1. situs inversus
2. partial situs inversus
3. pseudoascites
4. proximal
5. diameter
6. esophageal atresia
7. absent, hydramnios
8. proximal
9. meconium ileus
10. anorectal atresia
11. subjective
12. abnormal

Exercise 6

1. In Figure 58-3, the *P* is the portal sinus, the *PV* is the umbilical portion of the left portal vein, the *S* is the stomach, and the *sp* is the spine.

2. Based on Figure 58-16, bowel obstruction is demonstrated.

3. Meconium peritonitis secondary to bowel obstruction is shown with an irregular appearance of the bowel in Figure 58-19. In image *A,* there are distended loops of bowel with bowel clumping (arrows). The amniotic fluid was slightly increased. In image *B,* the bowel is slightly more echogenic when compared with the liver, which is normal.

4. Fetal ascites are present in Figure 58-20.

CHAPTER 59

Exercise 1

1. D
2. F
3. B
4. G
5. C
6. A
7. E

Exercise 2

1. J
2. C
3. G
4. A
5. I
6. E
7. L
8. F
9. B
10. K
11. D
12. H

Exercise 3

1. C
2. F
3. H
4. A
5. E
6. B
7. D
8. G

Exercise 4

1. kidneys, bladder, amniotic fluid
2. mesoderm
3. nephrogenic
4. genital
5. metanephros
6. 11th to 12th
7. major
8. placenta
9. pelvis
10. echogenic, right

Exercise 5

1. agenesis
2. divided
3. horseshoe
4. urogenital
5. exstrophy
6. allantois
7. urachus
8. fistula
9. urachal cyst

Exercise 6

1. 13
2. hyperechoic
3. 25
4. 4, 7
5. 45 to 60
6. hypertrophied
7. urethra
8. large
9. multicystic
10. polycystic renal
11. hydronephrosis, reflux
12. pelvis, vesicoureteric
13. bilateral

Exercise 7

1. amniotic fluid
2. 11, 14 to 16
3. 30
4. incompatible
5. adrenal
6. ectopic
7. Potter's
8. kidneys, liver
9. oligohydramnios, absent
10. cystic
11. noncommunicating
12. large, echogenic
13. obstruction
14. ureteropelvic, ureterovesical, megacystis
15. early
16. late

Exercise 8

1. 4, 10, 7, 10
2. pyelectasis, calyectasis
3. ureteropelvic junction
4. ureterovesical
5. ureterocele
6. bladder, keyhole
7. oligohydramnios, ascites

Exercise 9

1. turtle
2. hamburger
3. uterus didelphys
4. bicornuate
5. unicornuate
6. hydrocele
7. cryptorchidism
8. hermaphroditism
9. hydrometrocolpos

Exercise 10

1. In Figure 59-7, image *A* shows a small separation in the renal pelvis measuring less than 1 to 2 mm. Images *B* and *C* show severe hydronephrosis with loss of renal parenchyma.

2. This coronal image of the fetal pelvis shows a large distended fetal bladder with extension into the ureters in Figure 59-8. The fetus has a bladder outlet obstruction. Note the thickened bladder wall.

3. Based on Figure 59-9, "keyhole bladder" found in bladder outlet obstruction is the term for this image.

4. Bilateral renal enlargement with the kidneys occupying more than half of the abdomen is visible in Figure 59-12.

5. Unilateral dysplastic multicystic kidney is present in Figure 59-15.

6. In Figure 59-18, image *A* shows a unilateral ureteropelvic junction obstruction with dilatation of the renal pelvis communicating with the renal calyces (hydronephrosis). Image *B* shows a normal contralateral kidney.

7. Bilateral posterior urethral valve syndrome with severe hydronephrosis is present in Figure 59-29.

CHAPTER 60

Exercise 1

1. E
2. C
3. A
4. H
5. F
6. B
7. I
8. D
9. G

Exercise 2

1. mesoderm
2. somites, mesoderm
3. ectoderm
4. 8th
5. 9th
6. dysplasia

7.

   a. Assess limb shortening. All long bones should be measured. A skeletal dysplasia is suspected when limb lengths fall more than 2 standard deviations below the mean (Tables 60-2 and 60-3).

   b. Assess bone contour. Thickness, abnormal bowing or curvature, fractures, and a ribbonlike appearance should be noted.

c. Estimate degree of ossification. Decreased attenuation of the bones with decreased shadowing suggests hypomineralization. Special attention should be focused toward this assessment of the cranium, spine, ribs, and long bones.

d. Evaluate the thoracic circumference and shape. A long, narrow chest or a bell-shaped chest may be indicative of specific dysplasias.

e. Survey for coexistent hand and foot anomalies, such as talipes and polydactyly.

f. Evaluate the face and profile for facial clefts, frontal bossing, micrognathia, hypertelorism, and other facial anomalies that may be associated with skeletal dysplasias.

g. Survey for other associated anomalies, such as hydrocephaly, heart defects, and nonimmune hydrops.

Exercise 3

1. thanatophoric dysplasia
2. short, cloverleaf
3. achondroplasia
4. rhizomelia, macrocephaly, trident hands (short proximal and middle phalanges), a depressed nasal bridge, frontal bossing, and mild ventriculomegaly may be identified
5. bone, hypomineralization
6. brittle, sclera
7. osteogenesis imperfecta
8. hypophosphatasia
9. bowing
10. limbs
11. narrow, atrial septal defect
12. sirenomelia
13. 3, single
14. amniotic band
15. talipes
16. rocker-bottom

Exercise 4

1. In Figure 60-3, thanatophoric dysplasia is visible. Images *A* and *B* show right arm micromelia. Images *C* and *D* demonstrate a narrow thorax with shortened ribs and protuberant abdomen in image *E* and *F*.

2. In Figure 60-4, image *A* shows decreased ossification in the fetal head, which is compressible. There is severe micromelia in the femur (image *B*) and humerus (image *C*).

3. In Figure 60-6, image *A* shows the small thoracic cavity as compared with the fetal abdomen. Image *B* shows the hypomineralization of the fetal skull.

4. Image *A* shows a normal femur compared with image *B* in which a femoral fracture is shown in Figure 60-7. Osteogenesis imperfecta Type I or IV is suspected.

5. Image *A* shows rigid legs with hyperextended knees in Figure 60-18. Image *B* shows the fetal arms contracted and crossed over the chest with clenched fists.

6. Bilateral talipes is shown in Figure 60-27.

IMAGE ANALYSIS EXERCISES

CASE 1

ANS: coarse, nodular liver compatible with cirrhosis; ascites, look for reversal of flow in the portal system

CASE 2

ANS: appendicitis—the appendix is inflamed and does not reduce in size with transducer-initiated graded compression

CASE 3

ANS: thrombus within the bilateral internal jugular veins, occlusive without significant flow

CASE 4

ANS: Twin gestation—the two sacs are identified in the late first trimester. The crown rump is seen in the anterior sac.

CASE 5

ANS: renal carcinoma

CASE 6

ANS: Pyloric stenosis was found. The wall of the pylorus is thickened, which causes obstruction whenever the neonate consumes liquids, therefore causing the projectile vomiting.

CASE 7

ANS: Chronic pancreatitis—look for calcification within the pancreatic tissue. The pancreas may be small and hyperechoic. The pancreatic duct may be dilated with tiny calcifications within.

CASE 8

ANS: Thyroid adenoma—note the fine halo of sonolucent echo band surrounding the mass.

CASE 9

ANS: right epididymoorchitis with accompanying simple hydrocele

CASE 10

ANS: pancreatic pseudocyst

CASE 11

ANS: cholelithiasis

CASE 12

ANS: hydrocephalus with interventricular bleed

CASE 13

ANS: Hydronephrosis of the renal transplant. The presence of a ureteral stent is noted. The renal artery and veins are patent.

CASE 14

ANS: Amebic abscess or biliary disease. The diagnosis is acute cholecystitis.

CASE 15

ANS: Dilated pancreatic duct with atrophic pancreatic parenchyma and multiple calcifications. Findings are compatible with chronic pancreatitis. There is sludge within the gallbladder without evidence of cholelithiasis or cholecystitis.

CASE 16

ANS: Large mass within the testes represents a scrotal tumor.

CASE 17

ANS: hepatoma

CASE 18

ANS: multiple lymph nodes in the porta hepatis; hepatosplenomegaly, normal directional flow and waveform patterns of the hepatic artery and veins and portal vein

CASE 19

ANS: hepatocellular carcinoma

CASE 20

ANS: uterine myoma with intrauterine pregnancy

CASE 21

ANS: Two regions of large nonocclusive thrombus within the middle hepatic vein. The left hepatic vein, portal vein, and hepatic arteries demonstrate normal flow.

CASE 22

ANS: Subhepatic or subphrenic abscess or intraabdominal abscess. He developed a splenic abscess when a piece of the spleen was nicked during the exploratory surgery.

CASE 23

ANS: anencephalic fetus with polyhydramnios

CASE 24

ANS: epididymitis

CASE 25

ANS: choledocholithiasis

CASE 26

ANS: endometrioma

CASE 27

ANS: pancreatitis (not shown) and cholecystitis

CASE 28

ANS: omphalocele

CASE 29

ANS: abdominal aortic aneurysm

CASE 30

ANS: staghorn calculus—may cause obstruction with subsequent infection

CASE 31

ANS: left atrium

CASE 32

ANS: breast cyst: anechoic, well-defined borders, good through transmission

CASE 33

ANS: two hyperechoic areas in the liver near the right hepatic vein, likely hemangiomas versus focal fatty infiltration

CASE 34

1. liver function tests and serum amylase and lipase
2. fatty infiltration
   chronic hepatitis
   cirrhosis (mild to severe)
3. ANS: ascites

CASE 35

ANS: hepatocellular carcinoma, ascites, and thrombus invasion of the hepatic venous structures

CASE 36

ANS: fibroadenoma

SELF TESTS

General Ultrasound Review

1. d	36. c	71. a	106. a
2. b	37. b	72. d	107. d
3. c	38. c	73. d	108. d
4. c	39. a	74. c	109. d
5. a	40. c	75. b	110. a
6. c	41. d	76. c	111. a
7. a	42. d	77. a	112. b
8. b	43. b	78. d	113. a
9. c	44. d	79. b	114. b
10. a	45. b	80. c	115. c
11. d	46. a	81. d	116. a
12. b	47. c	82. c	117. a
13. b	48. a	83. d	118. c
14. b	49. d	84. c	119. b
15. b	50. d	85. c	120. b
16. b	51. b	86. c	121. b
17. c	52. d	87. d	122. c
18. b	53. d	88. a	123. d
19. b	54. d	89. b	124. c
20. a	55. c	90. b	125. d
21. d	56. b	91. d	126. a
22. b	57. c	92. c	127. c
23. b	58. b	93. c	128. a
24. b	59. b	94. d	129. d
25. a	60. c	95. d	130. c
26. c	61. d	96. b	131. a
27. b	62. b	97. c	132. c
28. c	63. a	98. c	133. a
29. a	64. c	99. a	134. c
30. c	65. d	100. b	135. d
31. a	66. a	101. c	136. b
32. b	67. c	102. d	137. d
33. c	68. a	103. a	138. b
34. c	69. a	104. c	139. d
35. d	70. c	105. d	140. b

141. a	156. b	171. d	186. b
142. d	157. a	172. d	187. c
143. b	158. d	173. a	188. d
144. c	159. d	174. d	189. b
145. a	160. c	175. b	190. c
146. a	161. b	176. d	191. b
147. c	162. a	177. a	192. c
148. b	163. c	178. b	193. b
149. c	164. b	179. d	194. d
150. b	165. b	180. b	195. b
151. b	166. b	181. b	196. b
152. a	167. a	182. d	197. b
153. d	168. a	183. a	198. b
154. d	169. b	184. c	199. c
155. d	170. a	185. c	200. d

Pediatric Review

1. a	14. b	27. d	39. b
2. b	15. c	28. c	40. c
3. a	16. b	29. a	41. b
4. b	17. c	30. c	42. b
5. b	18. a	31. d	43. a
6. c	19. a	32. b	44. c
7. c	20. a	33. d	45. d
8. c	21. b	34. a	46. c
9. d	22. d	35. b	47. a
10. a	23. a	36. b	48. c
11. b	24. d	37. d	49. d
12. b	25. a	38. a, d	50. b
13. a, c	26. b		

Cardiovascular Anatomy Review

1. a	10. d	19. b	28. c
2. a	11. b	20. b	29. b
3. d	12. b	21. b	30. b
4. b	13. b	22. b	31. a
5. b	14. d	23. a	32. c
6. c	15. a	24. d	33. a
7. d	16. d	25. c	34. b
8. b	17. d	26. d	
9. c	18. d	27. d	

Obstetrics and Gynecology Review

1. c	6. a	11. c	16. a
2. b	7. d	12. a	17. d
3. b	8. c	13. c	18. c
4. c	9. a	14. b	19. b
5. b	10. b	15. a	20. d

21. b	63. a	105. c	147. b
22. a	64. c	106. c	148. c
23. c	65. d	107. b	149. b
24. b	66. c	108. c	150. b
25. b	67. c	109. a	151. c
26. c	68. d	110. b	152. c
27. a	69. b	111. c	153. a
28. a	70. c	112. b	154. b
29. b	71. b	113. c	155. b
30. b	72. c	114. c	156. d
31. b	73. a	115. c	157. c
32. c	74. a	116. a	158. a
33. b	75. d	117. b	159. a
34. c	76. a	118. b	160. b
35. a	77. d	119. c	161. d
36. c	78. a	120. b	162. c
37. d	79. d	121. a	163. d
38. c	80. a	122. b	164. a
39. b	81. c	123. b	165. c
40. a	82. c	124. a	166. a
41. a	83. a	125. b	167. c
42. c	84. b	126. d	168. b
43. a	85. d	127. a	169. d
44. a	86. c	128. b	170. a
45. d	87. b	129. a	171. a
46. c	88. c	130. a	172. d
47. c	89. d	131. c	173. c
48. b	90. b	132. b	174. b
49. b	91. c	133. c	175. c
50. d	92. b	134. d	176. a
51. d	93. c	135. b	177. b
52. d	94. c	136. a	178. a
53. b	95. c	137. c	179. c
54. a	96. a	138. d	180. d
55. a	97. a	139. a	181. b
56. d	98. c	140. b	182. d
57. a	99. b	141. b	183. c
58. b	100. a	142. c	184. a
59. b	101. a	143. d	185. c
60. c	102. d	144. b	
61. d	103. d	145. b	
62. d	104. c	146. a	